HIV/AIDS
ISSUES AND CHALLENGES

INTERNATIONAL ENCYCLOPAEDIA OF AIDS-2

HIV/AIDS

ISSUES AND CHALLENGES

Part-I

Editor

Dr. Digumarti Bhaskara Rao

M.Sc. , M.A., M.A., M.Ed., Ph.D.

R. V. R. College of Education

Guntur–522 006

Andhra Pradesh. (INDIA)

2000

DISCOVERY PUBLISHING HOUSE

NEW DELHI 110 002

First Published-2000

ISBN 81-7141-524-5 (Set)

Published by:
DISCOVERY PUBLISHING HOUSE
4831/24, Ansari Road, Prahlad Street,
Darya Ganj, New Delhi-110 002 (*INDIA)*
Phone: 3279245
Fax: 91-11-3253475

Printed at:
Arora Offset Press
Laxmi Nagar, Delhi 110 092.

Preface

The HIV/AIDS is a new phenomenon in the human society. HIV destroys the immune system of human individuals, producing a defenselessness fatal state known as AIDS. The World Health Organisation has estimated that already one in every two hundred and fifty adults in the world is infected with Human Immunodeficiency Virus and according to WHO's projections a total of forty million men women and children worldwide will have been infected with HIV by the turn of this twentieth century. Visualising the devastating effects of the HIV/AIDS epidemic within our life times and beyond is difficult. Probably, no other disease in recent times has had the impact on human society generated by HIV/AIDS.

The HIV/AIDS epidemic has brought into focus many health related ethical, legal and human rights issues. This epidemic requires immediate and effective responses in new programming areas: attitudinal and behavioural changes, community-based care and support initiatives, and the maintenance of human development in the face of increasing rates of illness and deaths. At this point, education enters the scene as it can alter the HIV/AIDS situation since it brings change in the behaviour of the people.

This *International Encyclopaedia of AIDS* presents the worldwide information about HIV/AIDS, issues and challenges, reports and reviews, ethics laws and human rights, and educational activities and programmes to keep the policy makers, planners, professionals, activists, researchers, educationists, teachers and students well informed of the epidemic.

Dr. Digumarti Bhaskara Rao
26 January 1999
The Republic Day of India

Acknowledgements

I am thankful to the World Health Organisation and its associated offices for using their material namely School Health Education to prevent AIDS and STD: A Resource Package for Curriculum Planners-Handbook for Curriculum Planners. Student's Activities, Teachers' Guide, Global Programme on AIDS-HIV Prevention and Care: Teaching Modules for Nurses and Midwives, Global Programme on AIDS. Community HIV Prevention Handbook; STD care Management-workbooks 1-7, Facing the Challenge of HIV/AIDS STDs: A Gender-based Response; HIV/AIDS and STD surveillance Data Management and Use-Report, Bangkok, 1995; Carrying out HIV Sentinal Surveillance-A Guide for Programme Managers, AIDS Prevention and Care in the workplace: Enhancing the Role of Private Sector; HIV Testing Policies and Gidelines; Carrying out HIV Sentinel surveillance; AIDS Prevention; Understanding and Living with AIDS; AIDS: A Modern Epidemic; HIV/AIDS in South-East Asia: IXth meeting of the National Programme Managers, New Delhi, 1993; Information, Education and Communication: A Guide for AIDS Programme Managers, Handbook on AIDS Home Care; HIV/AIDS in South-East Asia: A Pictorial summary; etc.

I am thankful to the United Nations Development Programme, UNDP's HIV and Development Programme, and UNDP's Regional Projects on HIV and Development for using their material namely Economic Implications of AIDS in Asia; Socio Economic Implications of the Epidemic; NGOs Working with Sex workers; NGO Responses to HIV/AIDS in Asia-Case Studies; HIV in the Workplace: Dealing with the Issues-Role Plays, Development and the HIV Epidemic, Law Ethics and HIV; HIV Law and Law Reform; Issue Papers; Study Papers; Working Papers; etc.

I am thankful to the Health and Nutrition Centre, Republic of Philippines for using its material namely sourcebook on HIV/AIDS Prevention Education for Tertiary Educational Institutions.

I am thankful to the Curriculum Development Programme, Ministry of Education, Government of Thailand for using its material namely Institutional Modules for AIDS Education.

I am thankful to US Department of Health and Human Services: Whitman-Walker Clinic, Inc., USA; East-West Centre, USA; National AIDS Control Organisation, Government of India; Academy of Culture Communication Education Science and Service, Guntur, United Nations and its agencies for using their material.

I am grateful to Bhaskar Bhattacharji; V. Alexeev, Geeta Sethi, Elizabeth Reid, Mina Mauerstein-Bail, A. A. Trinidad, Palomi Cuchi, D. Pushpa Latha for their kind co-operation.

Dr. Digumarti Bhaskara Rao,
Secretary
ACCESS
D-43, S.V. N. Colony,
Guntur-522 006

Contents

1

The Global Epidemiology of HIV/AIDS

Geoff Manthey
Technical Officer WHO's
Global Programme on AIDS, Manila, Philippines.

Today, by WHO's conservative estimates, more than 12 million men, women and children are infected with HIV — the virus which causes AIDS. By the end of 1992, over 600,000 cases of AIDS had been reported to WHO; however, our estimates are that figure is closer to 2.5 million. The gap between reported and estimated cases can be explained via under reporting, misdiagnosis and reporting delays.

In the Asia/Pacific region, WHO estimates that close to 40,000 adults have developed AIDS since the start of the pandemic. But it must be remembered that AIDS takes 10 years on average to develop from the time an adult first becomes infected with the human immunodeficiency virus (HIV). So these cases reflect infections that probably occurred a decade ago.

WHO estimates that of the 12 million HIV infections, more than one and a half million people have been infected with HIV in the Asian and Pacific regions. Although 1.5 million is an enormous figure, it may not sound frighteningly large when compared with other parts of the world. After all, sub-Saharan Africa has more than 7 million cumulative infections. Unlike Africa, Asia is at the early stage of the pandemic. Here, the virus is spreading at an alarming rate. In the first six months of 1992, WHO estimates that one million new infections occurred globally. Of these infections, over 30 per cent occurred in Asia.

The problem in the Asia/Pacific region may be illustrated with some examples. HIV infection has been explosive among injecting drug users. In India's north-east states, prevalence rose from less that 1 per cent to 50 per cent in just one year. Drug injectors in China's Yunnan Province had infection rates ranging from 10 per cent to over 50 per cent in 1990, and those in Myanmar had a rate of 72 per cent in 1991.

HIV transmission due to injecting drug use has become an alarming problem in Malaysia, where prevalence in one sample of 9,000 injecting drug users in a rehabilitation centre was found to be 11 per cent in 1991 and up to 26 per cent in smaller samples. In the first 3 months of 1993, 9 per cent of injecting drug users in Ho Chi Minh City, Vietnam were found to be HIV-infected. Surveys in the Philippines, Singapore and Japan, however, have not discovered HIV infection among injecting drug users tested.

Among men attending sexually transmitted disease (STD) clinics, national rates in Thailand have grown from zero in mid-1989 to 6 per cent in mid 1992, and in Myanmar from 2 per cent to 9 per cent between 1990 and 1991. Where results are available in other countries in the Asia/Pacific region, HIV infection among STD clients remains at low levels, less than 1 per cent, except Cambodia where a recent survey found that 4.2 per cent of 72 persons were infected.

Seroprevalence rates as high as 50 per cent or 60 per cent are now being seen among female commercial sex workers (CSWs) in parts of Asia. HIV infection was first documented among female CSWs in Thailand in 1989, when the first national serosurvey detected a prevalence rate of 44 per cent among "lower class" brothel sex workers in Chiang Mai. HIV prevalence in female CSWs in India has also risen rapidly. In Bombay, prevalence has been estimated at between 30-50 per cent while in Delhi it has been found to be over 30 per cent among female CSWs.

In other parts of Asia, information suggests that spread has not yet occurred to the same degree as Thailand and India. The highest prevalence among female CSWs to date has been found in Cambodia. Some surveys have seen infection rates of 10-15 per cent. There has been a gradual increase in prevalence among female CSWs in Malaysia from zero in 1988 to 1.3 per cent in 1991.

In the mid-1980s the prevalence among female CSWs tested in the Philippines was between 1 per cent and 2.5 per cent. Surprisingly, recent surveys in parts of the country, including Cebu City, have found no infection among the 800 CSWs tested, although testing bias cannot be excluded. In Vietnam and Korea, very low levels of infection have been found. No infection has been documented recently among female CSWs in Singapore, Hong Kong, Australia and Japan.

Surveys among men who have sex with men have found relatively high levels of infection —up to 30 per cent in Sydney and 11 per cent among foreign homosexual/bisexual men in Japan.

However, studies in Singapore, Philippines and Taiwan revealed a low prevalence of HIV.

It must be remembered that by the time HIV infection is perceptible in these vulnerable groups, it has spread far and wide in the population.

Seroprevalence in the general population has reached 4 per cent in northern Thailand and 7 per cent in southern Myanmar. Cumulative infections in India totalled half a million at the end of 1991 and may have reached one million by the end of 1992—a doubling time of one year.

Statistics such as these tell us several important things. Firstly, Asia and the Pacific have the same mix of transmission routes as we have seen in other parts of the world. The same risk behaviours exist here as elsewhere in the world. In Asia and the Pacific, the number of HIV infections has tripled in the last two years. And, by the end of the century, WHO predicts that in Asia and the Pacific, over one million adults will become infected with HIV each year.

An epidemic of AIDS will follow this great epidemic of HIV infection. By the year 2000, close to 2 million adults in this region will have died of AIDS. During that year alone some half a million HIV-infected people will develop AIDS and require care.

Globally, by the end of the century, WHO projects that there will be a cumulative total of 30-40 million HIV infections in men, women and children, of which 90 per cent will be in developing countries. The projected cumulative total of adult AIDS cases will be close to 10 million, of which 90 per cent will be in developing countries. And there will be 10 million or more children less than 10 years of age orphaned as a result of AIDS, primarily in the developing countries.

But there are still facts and fiction about HIV that seem not to be fully understood by the public. Until they are, the epidemic will continue to spiral out of control. Getting these facts known and accepted, and the fiction identified and removed, are challenges facing Asian and Pacific countries.

HIV is not casually contagious. Fortunately for us, HIV is not one of the viruses that spreads through air or water, through saliva or through urine or faeces. It is spread via blood, semen, vaginal fluids and breast milk. People need to understand that they cannot catch HIV by eating food prepared by an HIV-infected person, or by sharing toilet or bathing facilities or through sneezing, shaking hands, hugging or even kissing.

Health care workers need to understand that they must carefully handle the body fluids, particularly blood, of all patients as it is always a potential source of HIV, hepatitis virus and other pathogens. And just as there is no reason to isolate HIV-infected

Cumulative AIDS cases in Men, Women and Children, Late 1992

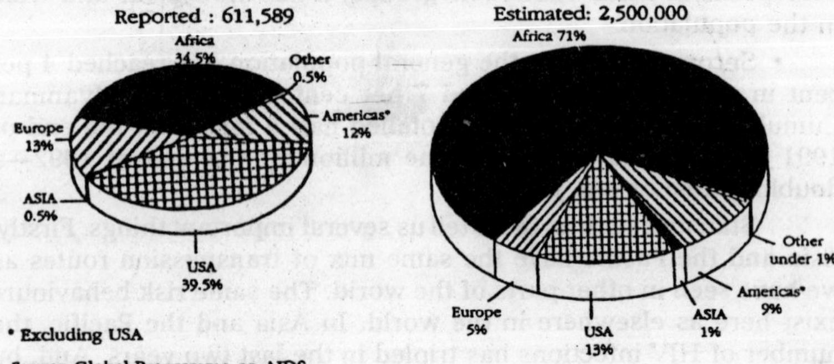

* Excluding USA

Source: Global Programme on AIDS January 1993

ESTIMATED GLOBAL NEW HIV INFECTIONS From early to mid 1992

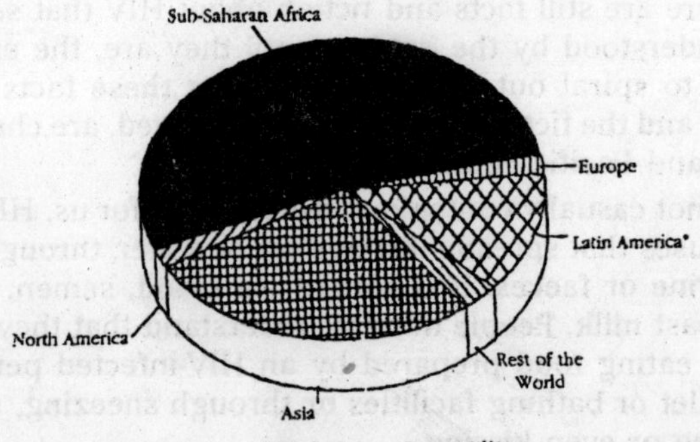

Total about One Million

* Including the Caribbean

Source: Global Programme on AIDS, July 1992

Fig. 1.1 Estimated Distribution of Cumulative HIV Infections in Adults, by Continent or Region Late 1992

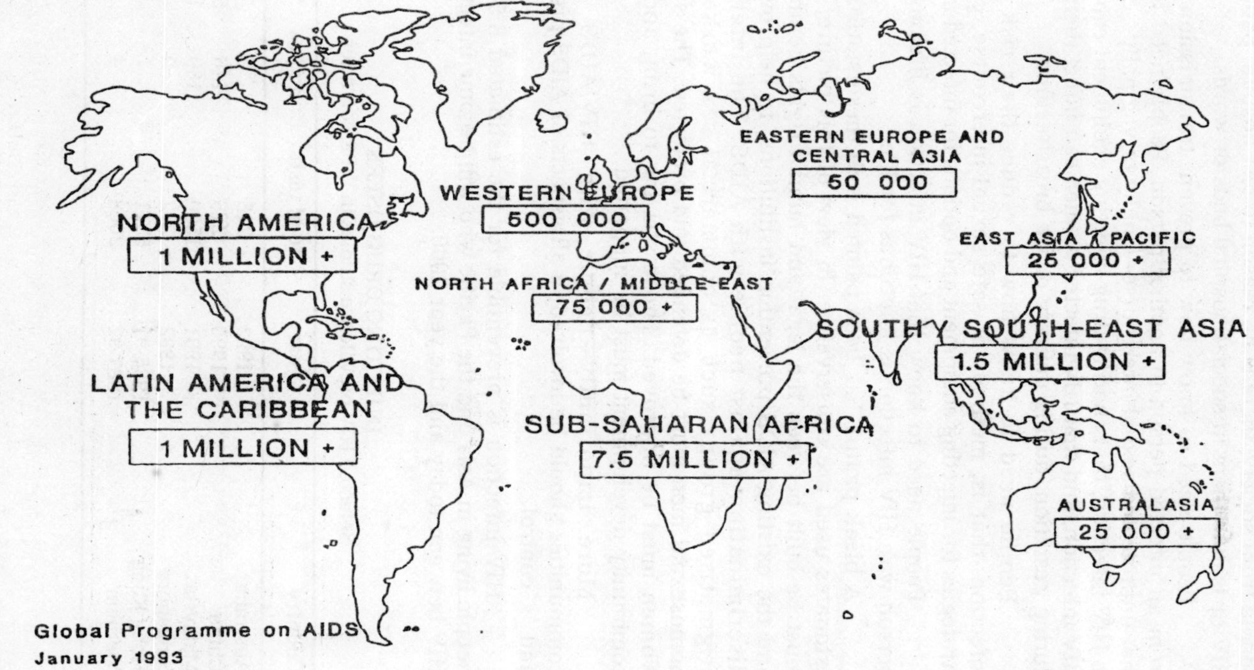

people from society, there is no reason to test hospital patients for HIV or isolate them in special hospital beds or wards.

People need to know how to prevent transmission of HIV from an infected person to another person. People need to know that unprotected sexual intercourse—anally or vaginally—can lead to HIV infection, that sharing drug injecting equipment can lead to HIV infection, and that HIV-infected women can infect their babies during gestation, during delivery or via breastfeeding.

People need to know how to reduce their risk of HIV infection, that is, methods of safe sexual intercourse, cleaning strategies for injecting equipment and options for infected mothers.

People need to know that HIV infection is lifelong and a person with HIV infection is infectious for life.

A bleak picture has been painted with these statistics. The estimates used are conservative. In view of this picture, bridges must be built between the legal and human rights communities and the existing AIDS prevention institutions, to help overcome discrimination against people with AIDS. The interests of stigmatised groups such as commercial sex workers and homosexual men must be defended and protected. The status of women must be improved. Those striving to bring about true community development must be supported.

More importantly—people with HIV/AIDS in our communities should be involved in all aspects of AIDS prevention and control.

HIV infection is preventible for the estimated 8.5 million people living in Asia and the Pacific who will become infected with HIV between today and the year 2000.

INJECTING DRUG USERS
Selected HIV prevalence studies in WPR countries

Country	year	no of tests	no pos	% pos
Australia	1992	218	5	2.30
China	1990	276	146	52.90
Malaysia	1991	1500	169	11.30
Singapore	1992	212	0	0.00
Hong Kong	1985-91	5371	1	0.02
Vietnam	1987-92	2008	4	0.20

STD CLINIC ATTENDERS

Selected HIV prevalence studies in WPR countries

Country	year	no of tests	no pos	% pos
Australia	1992	5100	17	0.33
Cambodia	1992	72	3	4.20
Hong Kong	1992	2146	2	0.09
Vietnam	1987-92	8572	5	0.06
Papua New Guinea	1992	6035	5	0.08

Source: Global Programme on AIDS, as of 6 April 1993.

FEMALE SEX-WORKERS

Selected HIV prevalence studies in WPR countries

Country	year	no of tests	no pos	%pos
Cambodia	1992	207	19	9.18
Hong Kong	1985-91	12950	0	0.00
Philippines	1992	227	0	0.00
Rep of Korea	1992	411425	11	0.003
Singapore	1992	2740	0	0.00
Vietnam	1987-92	11745	3	0.03

HOMO/BISFXUAL MEN

Selected HIV prevalence studies in WPR countries

Country	year	no of tests	nopos	% pos
Cambodia	1992	499	9	1.8
Japan	1985-89	786	24	3.1
Singapore	1992	111	4	3.6
Philippines	1992	300	0	0
FR Polynesia	1990	156	6	3.8

Source: Global Programme on AIDS, as of 6 April 1993.

2

Approaching the HIV Epidemic

Ms. Elizabeth Reid
UNDP, New York

The HIV Epidemic comes to people 's attention through the language of its texts and its spokespersons. The way it is brought to people's attention will be critical determinant of how they will respond to it. Currently, the discourse is based on metaphors of epicentres of spread identified as core transmitter groups. These are metaphors of distancing which encourage blame and denial. There are, however within affected communities, new discourses emerging of inclusion, empowerment and processes and of the complexity of the reality of the epidemic. These discourses are associated with a new way of responding to the epidemic described here as one of community mobilization.

"We are not prostitutes. It has nothing to do with us."

(Women in Latin America)

INTRODUCTION

Determining how best to approach this epidemic is neither an idle nor an academic exercise. At stake are people' s lives and well-being and the capacity of communities, businesses and economies to continue to function.

Some people are more likely to come to unsafe contact with an infected person. If they alone are targeted as transmitters or as epicentres of spread, others fail to understand that everyone must change in the face of the epidemic.

The epidemic must and can be slowed down, quickly and effectively. The first decade of the epidemic has shown us what approaches are effective and under what conditions. These lessons have been learned from the response in affected communities, be they in Sydney, Kampala or Madras. The community mobilization approach is an attempt to apply these lessons more broadly and to implement them more effectively.

For too many people, the HIV epidemic is still a distant spectre. As exemplified in the quote above, the way the epidemic is brought to people' s attention will be the critical determinant of how they will respond to it and thus whether they, personally, protect themselves from infection and whether effective and sustainable programmes are established in response to its presence in their midst.

An epidemic comes to people's attention through the language of its texts, its presentation and its programming (Watney, 1989; Patton, 1990; Siedel, 1993, for example). There are four dominant and overlapping discourses which have been constructed:

the public health discourse
the epidemiological discourse
the biomedical discourse
the educational discourse.

These discourses derive from the beliefs and assumptions about the nature and causes of the epidemic. They reflect the moral, social and institutional values of those who have constructed them and constitute the analytical framework of national responses. It is timely to cast a critical glance over the assumptions and logic of these discourses.

The Dominant Discourses: Metaphors and Misapprehensions

All four of these dominant and overlapping discourses are dominated by metaphors of small, physically locatable epicentres of spread of the HIV virus which if contained by condoms or bleach or segregation will ensure that the epidemic is held in check. Those who are assumed to fill this description are referred to as 'core transmitters'. Prostitutes, injecting drug users, STD patients and, more recently, truck drivers are the accepted target groups for intervention. In these discourses, there are no metaphors of spread which include whole populations or which include the speaker as well as the others. They are metaphors of distancing: epicentres are located elsewhere, not in groups of doctors. IEC experts or public servants. Such metaphors encourage blame and become their own justification for restrictive or punitive measures.

The metaphors of the dominant discourse have reinforced the ancient view of women as spreaders of disease, as vessels of infection for men and vectors of transmission to their infants. Women who work as prostitutes have been scapegoated by this approach and the very dangerous myth born that only such women are at risk of infection. This myth is widespread. The women whose voices began this paper are many. Patterns of HIV infection in women in general should seriously call into question the very concept of epidemic spread by a limited group of sexually active people. The HIV epidemic is propagated by accepted norms of sexual behaviour, particularly of men.

The Distortion of the Metaphors

The dominant discourse and its associated programme interventions, particularly the focus on mass education, condom distribution and STD treatment, create an illusion that nations are responding to the HIV epidemic in an effective and sustainable manner. However, there is no evidence that these approaches have been effective in slowing down the epidemic, and there is much evidence to the contrary. For example, there are studies in the US which show that HIV infection rates in female prostitutes are comparable with other women in the same geographical areas (Corea, 1992).

It is not that frequency of unprotected sexual intercourse with different partners or the existence of sexually transmitted infections are irrelevant to the analysis. Rather they have their origins in social, psychological, economic and gender relationships and it is these that determine to whom and how rapidly the virus spreads (Reid, 1992b). Furthermore, the disproportionately high infection rates in girls and young women in all populations should force us to add to this list of determining factors the biological immaturity and vulnerability of the female genital tract (Reid & Bailey, 1992).

The language of core transmitters and targeted programme approaches is drawn from STD epidemiology and control programmes. Computer models have been used to justify the claim that even a small number of highly sexually active individuals can maintain an STD epidemic in an otherwise low-risk population (May & Anderson, 1987, for example). The public health discourse has centred around the assumption that this analysis provides a basis for programme development, justifying the targeting of resources to groups assumed to be most critical for transmissions, the 'core transmitters'. It has led to the simple imperative: trace them and treat them. This orthodoxy has been transferred to HIV programming (WHO, 1992; Over & Piot, 1991, for example). This is an excellent sample of a programme fitting a model. The pressing question is whether the model fits the world.

Programming approaches targeted to 'core transmitters' are based on the following assumptions:

that identifiable groups of people, rather than dispersed individuals, fill this specification;
that all or most members of such a group are locatable and are accessible to targeted programmes;
that the groups of 'core transmitters' targeted in the programmes are the most active of such groups.

Core Transmitters?

It is either assumed that these models fit the world or reality is forced to fit the model like the feet of the Ugly Sisters into Cynderella's glass shoe. Thus women who work in prostitution, rather than the men who infect them, are singled out as core transmitters. Even among these women, only the more easily accessible are targeted: the bar 'girls', street workers or workers in brothels. All other women who have multiple sexual partners are unrecognized and untargeted.

Furthermore, research data have long indicated that it is not only those who have multiple sexual partners who are most prone to sexually transmitted infections (STIs) but also girls and young women. STI infection rates globally are extremely high in adolescents and young adults. Within this group, it is the young men who tend to have frequent sexual intercourse with multiple partners while the young women, who are less sexually active, are more likely to be infected with STIs (Bell & Hein, 1984), for example. These data have long been ignored (Reid 1992a). Nor is it the case that an STI programme approach targeted at core transmitters has reduced these epidemics. Indeed, the global prevalence and incidence rates of STIs are rising both among and beyond so-called core transmitters groups (Mann et al., 1992). These facts alone should cause us to pause before applying either the STD-based core-transmitter analysis or its associated programming to the HIV epidemic.

HIV programmes targeted at core groups are justified by the claim that most people are not at risk of HIV infection and that it is not possible and not cost-effective to target whole communities or populations yet the concept of being at risk relates to a person's likelihood of becoming infected. It is clear that those at risk of infection are the spouses and other sexual partners of those who are infected, when unsafe sexual intercourse takes place. Many of these people at risk are not even sexual transmitters; that is, they have no sexual partners others than those who place them at risk. They are identifiable neither as individuals nor as groups, nor are they reachable by targeted programmes.

The metaphors of core transmitters and of onwards

transmission are embedded within an over-arching metaphor of health as a battle ground and its language of surveillance, targets, control and campaigns. They distort our vision and our language. A paradigm shift is required from those who are assumed to be transmitting the virus, to those who are becoming infected and to those who are not protecting themselves from infection or who cannot do so. This shift could radically change surveillance systems, research agendas, national HIV/AIDS programme approaches and resource allocations. A simple example would be to shift to the recording of HIV infected people by age, gender and occupation as well as classification by risk situation. Such a shift would force a broadening of focus from pathogenic transmission from one individual to another, to the complex socio—economic and other conditions which lead each person to unsafe behaviour. Such a simple paradigm shift would immediately enrich the discourses and their analytical basis.

Emerging Discourses

The dominant discourses are being increasingly challenged by new discourses. A language of optimism is being developed within affected communities as they learn to live with the presence of the virus. This new discourse is about:

face-to-face discussion leading to changes in community norms and values relating to gender and sexuality;

stories of living with HIV breaking down false divisions into Us/Them and relocating the epidemic within each of us;

how knowing someone infected lessens fear and denial and opens up the possibility of respect for self and others;

ownership of knowledge, decision making and programme development leading to appropriate and sustainable responses.

This emerging discourse of optimism and empowerment is constructing a new programming discourse: a language of processes rather than interventions, of people as responsible actors rather than as manipulable objects of interventions. The approach that emerges is based on community mobilization for change. It respects and acknowledges the expertise of those directly affected, and its sources of leadership and counselling come from within the community. This new programming approach contrasts sharply with the current programming focus on impersonal technologies, condoms, STI services, blood safety kits, for example, and on directive educational interventions.

This is not to deny that the correct use of good quality condoms or the treatment of sexually transmissible infections (and other infections of the genital area) are protective against HIV infection. But these goods and services must be desired by people. People must want to protect themselves from infections, know what their protection options are and must be able to practice them. This will require radical changes in community norms and values relating to sexuality and to gender. Only when these processes are in place can the current interventions be embedded within them and only when this occurs will these interventions contribute to programme effectiveness.

The third emerging discourse links the epidemic to development (Museveni, 1991; Kaunda, 1989) and argues that the epidemic has the potential to touch every facet of human, social and economic life. It locates the reasons for the spread of the virus and the nature of its consequences in the psychological, social and economic determinants of people's daily lives. It identifies the factors which predispose individuals and populations to unsafe behaviour as including inequalities of wealth, power and autonomy, sexual norms and social values, attitudes to women, mobility patterns and the legal, ethical and human rights environment.

A country's development choices influence the speed and pattern of spread of the virus. In turn, the spread of the virus determines how the epidemic will affect national development and weaken the national capacity to respond. Those countries that are developing participative, community-based institutions, strong social cohesion and adequate redistributive policies will find the epidemic much easier to overcome.

There remain discourses yet to be articulated. HIV and AIDS evoke complex and powerful emotions and psychological states. In those as yet untouched by the epidemic, these may include hatred, anger, fear, righteousness, disgust, guilt, shame, humiliation or denial. There has been a reluctance to acknowledge the existence of this side of the epidemic and to address it. There is a deep, culturally-instilled unease which inhibits families and nations from using a language of emotions, vulnerability, sexuality and mortality.

There is silence about the dark side of the epidemic, the reality of living with the knowledge that one is infected or that someone one loves dearly is infected: the haunting presence of death, the hesitancy of desire, the longing for love, the uncertainty, the sadness. Even the emotional states, which are central to the belief that the epidemic can be overcome, are unacknowledged in its discourse. There seems to be a reluctance to use words such as 'respect', 'caring', 'compassion', 'love,', 'happiness', 'spirituality', or 'concern' in this context. These emerging and yet to be spoken discourses recognize a basic truth: to understand and respond to this epidemic, one must understand daily life and human nature in all its complexity.

Placing People and their Communities at the Centre of the Response

The language of empowerment leads to a programming approach that places people and their communities at the centre of the response to the epidemic and which builds upon the complex nature of people's daily lives. It recognizes that poverty, wealth, power, subordination and debt, to mention just a few, are essentially interlinked with the HIV epidemic.

It should be made clear what is not involved in this paradigm shift. This approach, which could be called community mobilization, is not an argument in favour of existing IEC approaches to the general population. Nor is it an argument for the geographical targeting of prevention messages or indeed any targeting. These approaches have the wrong direction of fit. The role of the outsider must be supportive, not directive. One of the starkest lessons to be learned from the first decade of the response to the epidemic is that whilst information or education may change knowledge, alone they rarely change attitudes or sexual or drug-using behaviour. It is not that information and education have no place; they must be there to be drawn upon by individuals, couples and communities. This is the correct direction of fit and is intrinsic to a community mobilization approach. Nor is this approach an argument against programmes for and within particular communities and groups, including gay men and injecting drug users. At present these programmes are amongst our richest sources of lessons relevant to a community mobilization approach. However, these group-specific programmes must be embedded in broader mobilization networks. It is not only members of particular groups who participate in unsafe behaviour but is also the case that an exclusive group-specific focus will not create conditions of sustainability. The wider community is an important source of volunteers, of workers and of financial, moral and other forms of support. However, it can also be a source of discrimination, indifference, rejection or antagonism, all of which negatively affect programmed. Hence the whole community must understand the need for and be involved in processes of attitudinal and behavioural change.

These processes are stimulated by stories of the need for support, of changing attitudes and behaviour, of concern. They consist primarily of face-to-face discussion. They require local leadership and sources of information, advice and counselling within the community. They create agents of change, people who wish to ensure that we respond effectively and compassionately.

These are the processes that are already taking place in affected communities (Carr, 1991; UNDP, 1993). However, as yet there are few such communities globally and we cannot wait for them to emerge for by then too many people will be infected. Experience in Africa and elsewhere shows that these processes can be stimulated by local organizations (Williams, 1991), by political, religious and other leaders (Hampton, 1991) and by certain research initiatives (ICRW, 1993).

A community mobilization approach will have radical implications for social research design. The research agenda must be influenced or determined by communities and reflect their needs. Social research methodologies will need to be participative and interactive and lead to a process of group and individual introspection, including reflection on socio-cultural norms and values, and on individual and collective behaviour. the process itself of carrying out HIV-related research in such cases become critical and its findings only a part of the stimulation of change.

Setting Priorities

An approach which is centred around community mobilization does not pre-empt the possibility of setting priorities. Firstly, assistance should be given to communities with higher rates of infection. More sophistication will be needed in surveillance systems in order to be able to identify such communities, occupations or locations.

Secondly, enough is now known about the physiological, social and economic causes of spread of the virus to be able to identify communities or countries where the virus is most likely to spread rapidly irrespective of present rates of infection. Their identifying characteristics include:

economically vital areas and areas with mobile populations;
communities and cultures which do not value women and which tolerate or encourage certain patterns of sexual behaviour, particularly in men;
communities which are stratified by wealth, income and/or power;
communities without strong traditions of respect and concern for others;
communities with little capacity for reflection or change.

Thirdly, assistance should be given to all groups or communities who actively seek it. These foci of assistance need to be complemented by a more general mobilization and sustained by appropriate forms of assistance, by the availability, accessibility and affordability of the required goods and services and by appropriate legal, ethical and human rights policies and practices.

The appropriate entry points for community points for community mobilization are still being explored. Approaches based on the creation of fear and revulsion have been shown to be counter-productive. We know that those who are living this epidemic in their daily lives are powerful catalysts for change. A discussion within a group about how they would react if one of their sons or husbands returned infected can initiate the concern for self and others. Mass media can also be used effectively for attitudinal change. The primary role of outside technical assistance may lie in the transfer of the concepts that are the essence of a sustainable response (Campbell, 1992):

the justifiability of faith and hope;
the interrelatedness of care and behaviour change;
the possibility of peaceful co-existence with the virus;
the language of emotions, vulnerability, sexuality and mortality;
the resources of time, compassion, labour, food and money within communities;
the reality that we are all affected.

To the transfer of these concepts will need to be added assistance in the management, monitoring and evaluation of the process and skills in drawing down the required services and technologies.

There are no methodologies yet developed for determining the cost-effectiveness of processes as distinct from discrete interventions. However, it is likely that the cost of such an approach compares reasonably with the cost of the current components of national HIV/AIDS programmes, including extended surveillance systems, KAP and similar studies, extensive mass media IEC campaigns and securing blood supplies. Furthermore this approach, based on local resources and capacities, creates the conditions for its own sustainability and for the effectiveness of other interventions.

REFERENCES

Bell, T.A. & HEIN, K. (1984). Adolescents and sexually transmitted diseases, in K. HOLMES (Ed.), *Sexually Transmitted Diseases, pp. 72-84 (New York, McGraw-Hill).*

Campbell, I. (1992), *An Integrated Response to HIV/AIDS, An Opportunity for Community Development and Change,* (London, Salvation Army).

Carr, A. (1991) *Behaviour Change in Response to HIV/AIDS. Some Analogies and Lessons from the Experience of the Gay Communities (New* York, UNDP).

Corea, G. (1992) *The Invisible Epidemic* (New York, Harper Collins).

Hampton, J. (1991) Meeting AIDS with Compassion: AIDS Care and Prevention in Agomanya, Ghana, *Strategies for Hope. No. 4* (London, Actionaid).

International Center for Research on Women, ICRW (1993) Preliminary report on the Women and AIDS Research Programme: evolving a model for AIDS prevention education among underprivileged adolescent girls in urban India (Personal communication).

Kaunda, K. (1989), Address to the 6th International AIDS Conference (Montreal).

Mann, J., Tarantola, D. & Netter, T. (Eds.), (1992), *AIDS in the World,* (Cambridge, Harvard).

May, R.M. & Anderson, R.M. (1987), Transmission dynamics of HIV infections, *Nature,* 326, p.137

Museveni, Y. (1991), New Vision, Address to the 7th International AIDS Conference, (Florence).

Over, M. & Piot, P. (1991), *HIV infection and sexually transmitted diseases* (Washington, D.C., World Bank).

Patton, C. (1990), *Inventing AIDS* (New York, Routledge).

Reid, E. (1992a), Gender, knowledge and responsibility, in J. MANN *et al* (Eds.), *AIDS in the World 1992* (Cambridge, Harvard).

Reid, E. (1992b), *The HIV Epidemic and Development. the Unfolding of the Epidemic,* (New York, UNDP).

Reid, E. & Bailey, M. (1992). *Young Women: Silence, Susceptibility and the HIV epidemic,* AIDS in Society Infold (October/November, 1992).

Seidel, G. (1993). Competing discourse of HIV/AIDS in Sub-Saharan African, *Social Science and Medicine,* 36, pp. 174-194.

United Nations Development Programme (1994). *Report on the Asian and Pacific Informal Consultation on Attitudinal and Behavioural Change,* (New York, UNDP).

Watney, S. (1989), Taking Liberties: an Introduction, in: E. Carter & S. Watney (Eds.) *Taking Liberties,* pp 11-57 (London, Serpent's Tail).

Williams, G. (1991). From Fear to Hope: AIDS Care and Prevention at Chikankata Hospital, Zambia, *Strategies for Hope. No. I (London,* Actionaid).

World Health Organization, (1992). *The Global Strategy for the Prevention and Control of AIDS,* (Geneva, WHO).

3

The HIV Epidemic as a Development Issue

Ms. Elizabeth Reid
Director
HIV and Development Programme
UNDP, New York. USA

INTRODUCTION

The immense impact of the psychological, social and economic consequences of the epidemic is already being experienced in communities throughout the world. Families have been scattered, villages abandoned, food production diminished, enterprises forced to close and public and private health care systems overwhelmed.

In sub-Saharan Africa, it is estimated that one adult in 40, men and women, are already infected with HIV and in some areas it is as many as one in four or higher. Data on communities in Asia, the Caribbean and South America show or predict similar levels of infection. Moreover, every indication is that the number of new infections will increase exponentially over the next decade. Many of these countries face the loss of whole generations of people within their communities and the decimation of their productive workforce.

Without effective responses at the community, national and international level, the efforts of the last 25 years to strengthen the human and capital resources required for national development may have been to little avail.

The Setting of the Epidemic

The impact of the HIV epidemic in developing countries must be understood in the context of the critical social and economic problems already experienced by these countries: poverty, famine and food shortage, inadequate sanitation and health care, the subordination of women and adjustment policies that allocate insufficient resources to the social sectors.

These factors create a particular vulnerability to the devastating consequences of the epidemic. Economic need and dependency lead to activities that magnify the risk of HIV transmission and mean that many people, particularly women, are powerless to protect themselves against infection. Inadequate standards of health and sanitation further exacerbate the spread of HIV and accelerate the progression from HIV infection to AIDS.

The setting of the HIV epidemic in developing countries creates a downward spiral whereby existing social and economic deprivation produces an environment in which the spread of HIV can occur and, in turn, the HIV epidemic compounds and intensifies the deprivation already experienced by those countries. Not only must the epidemic itself be directly addressed in programmes of assistance but its consequences will impact upon all existing development initiatives which themselves will need to be reformulated in order to encompass these new situations.

The Consequences of the Epidemic

The consequences of the epidemic will continue to unfold for many decades after the spread of the virus within a community. This is because those infected are productively engaged, have established households and support dependants. The cost to society, and to individuals, includes not only illness and death but also the effects of this loss on those who survive, on their communities and on nations.

Just as a stone thrown into a pond will create ripples that reach to the farthest edges of the pond, so too will the effects of HIV infection be experienced at all social, cultural and economic levels. Figure 3.1 describes the chain of consequences associated with the spread of the virus and the wide range of policy needs and concerns created by these consequences. An understanding of the full dimensions of the epidemic requires a recognition of the way in which the epidemic, while appearing first in the form of infection and illness in individuals, moves rapidly and inevitably towards a far-reaching and catastrophic impact upon communities and nations.

The invisibility of infection during its early stages and the subsequent failure to recognise its threat has allowed reluctant parliaments and bureaucracies to delay in acting to protect their populations. However, the failure to implement effective policy interventions at the earliest possible stage will result in many more serious and far-reaching consequences in the future.

Figure -3. 1 The HIV Epidemic and its Consequences

Spread of the Virus	Illness and Death	Survivors	Social and Economic Impact	Long-term Potential Impact
Description Initial spread hidden but increasing numbers of people becoming infected.	Spread of virus continues and infected people become increasingly ill and die.	Children, spouses, elderly and others left without support, grief and bereavement.	Depletion of the labour force, adverse impact on productive and social sectors, loss of military strength	Possibility of social and political unrest, destitution, social and economic disintegration
Policy-Context Behaviour change Education Prevention Legislation Other preventive measures Surveillance Human rights	Living positively Coping with fear and powerlessness Social and psychological support Employment Income maintenance Confidentiality Care and treatment Legal rights	Integration within community Emergency assistance Counselling and social support Education and health services Income generation Legal protection	Monitoring impacts Strengthening and financing health and social sectors Public sector allocations Labour market Policies Revenue generation Economic production	Minimising adverse impact on individuals, communities and nations.

Individuals and Communities

The immediate impact upon those people infected with HIV and their families is devastating. In addition to the psychological and emotional distress caused by illness and death, the HIV epidemic creates a critical need to care for those infected and to find ways of replacing their contribution to the household and the community.

Because the majority of infected people in developing countries are men and women in the age group 15 to 45 years, most will have families and dependants. There will be a decrease in family income and, at the same time, an increased need for expenditure on health care. The death or disability caused by AIDS may lead to increasing numbers of families without parents or providers, of single parent families, and of orphans, some of whom are themselves infected with HIV.

Steps will need to be taken to reorganise the division of labour within households in order to reallocate productive tasks to uninfected household members. Children may need to be withdrawn from school to assist in food production and in caring for the sick. The resulting adverse impact on children and on long-term national development may be serious.

With growing numbers of women falling ill and dying and with surviving women becoming increasingly occupied with the care of the ill, women will have less time for caring for their own children and for productive work in the fields, in self-employment, or in the paid workforce. Much of the work performed by women is not measured in cash value and therefore does not appear in economic indicators such as gross national product. Thus, it is difficult to monitor the macro-economic impact of these losses, despite their serious consequences for the survival of families and communities and the role of women within these communities.

In coping with the threat to household units, community-based programmes will be essential in order to establish support networks between households at both the emotional and economic levels. Collective action of this kind represents an indigenous, affordable response to the HIV epidemic. Community-based organizations can play multiple roles within HIV strategies, ranging from home care, counselling and emergency support for families, to training and employment programmes, income generation and co-ordination of external assistance. They permit local resources to be utilised most effectively and can assess and respond to the full spectrum of needs of their particular community.

National Level

The increasing illness and death among people formerly

productively engaged will have a serious impact upon national economies. At the national level, deaths from AIDS will lead to a loss of economic output and, hence, of national income. Many sectors of the economy may be threatened by the sudden depletion of the workforce: mining, agriculture, transport, and construction, for example. The sectors most vulnerable are those which depend on highly trained personnel or upon occupational groups which may have high rates of HIV infection, such as truck drivers, construction workers, teachers, etc.,

Because of the way that infection is clustered in families, occupations and geographical areas, the impact of multiple illness and death is much greater than the accumulated individual losses. Households and communities can quickly cease to be viable social or economic units. The trauma of grieving death after death can induce a feeling of powerlessness and an inability to act. Support systems falter with the seemingly endless demands made upon them. The lost labour becomes more and more difficult to replace and the concomitant loss of output, skills, experience and aspirations can discourage investment, force the closure of enterprises and lessen national income. Population growth rates and economic growth will be reduced.

The direct costs of the epidemic will escalate as the demands for health and social services increase creating the possibility of the withdrawal of investments in the productive sectors. At the same time, the tax base will be increasingly depleted. Foreign exchange earnings will be affected by drops in production of export commodities or crops.

In the longer term, there is the possibility of the disintegration of communities, abandoned children turning to banditry and other socially disruptive survival strategies, widespread destitution, strategic imbalances caused by the depletion of military forces, and changes in the economic bases of societies.

These long-term consequences are not inevitable. If effective steps can be taken at an early stage to minimise the spread of HIV, to provide appropriate support for the individuals and communities affected, and to implement economic and social policies that redress the harm caused by the HIV epidemic and the factors that make communities vulnerable to HIV, the potential long-term consequences may be contained. However, this requires that any denial of the magnitude of the problem cease in order to permit immediate and decisive action. The extent and seriousness of the consequences will depend directly on the timeliness and effectiveness of prevention programmes and of policies adopted to respond to the needs of the infected, the ill and the survivors.

Critical Choices

The severity of the consequences just described will depend upon how early effective policy interventions are implemented. If this is not understood, competing demands on limited national resources could mean that programmes in response to the epidemic, prevention programmes in particular, are not allocated sufficient resources.

Each different kind of consequence of the epidemic has its own set of policy and programme requirements, and these are cumulative rather than sequential. That is, as different phases of the epidemic emerge, a new set of policies and programmes will have to be developed while those already in place will need to be continued and strengthened. Further, as can be seen in Figure. 3.1, responsibility for most of these policies and programmes will lie with sectors and ministries other than health. The earlier the epidemic ceases being solely the responsibility of the Departments and Ministries of Health and begins to be a multi-sectoral concern, the greater the possibility of minimising the severity of the impact.

Along the spectrum depicted in Figure. 3.1, there are a number of critical points at which choices must be made by governments, choices which will either minimise or aggravate the subsequent impact of the epidemic. These include:

The type of policies and the extent of resources directed to the epidemic in its early stages. Policy decisions must be made which anticipate future needs that may not yet be visible.

The extent to which effective prevention programmes are implemented to minimise the adverse impact of the epidemic. These may require political courage to adopt. Programmes and information directed towards minimising sexual transmission may need to be gender specific. Different information, skills and support may be required by women and men.

The extent to which the community response is integrated into and complemented by the government response. The most effective national strategies will be based on the diversity of responses arising within the community.

The extent to which governments assist all people affected by the epidemic, that is, those infected, their families, and those that survive them, to remain an integral part of their communities.

At what stage communities, the government, the private sector and others begin to address the adverse social and economic impacts of the epidemic.

Human Development Challenged

This epidemic will force a rethinking of approaches to development. A focus on human development highlights the need to ensure that the benefits of growth be used to address critical needs and to improve the human condition. The modalities currently used to achieve this include credit and social investment schemes, labour market flows, employment creation and investments in education and training. These very modalities are being challenged by the epidemic.

Credit is usually seen as an instrument to achieve positive developmental objectives, for example, through public lending for low cost housing or for financing the supply of agricultural inputs. The need for low cost housing will rise as the epidemic leads to a worsening of living standards. However, the capacity to repay will be affected by illness and death and where this is widespread, the viability of such schemes will be in question. Repossession, whilst it may preserve the viability of such schemes, will worsen social stability and increase destitution. Thus, a rethinking of the use of credit for achieveing social and economic objectives will be required or a new way found of responding to these needs.

Mobility of labour too has been a positive factor in development but it is now instrumental in the spread of the virus. High rates of infection occur in most mobile or relocated populations, especially unaccompanied males. Mobility destroys both its mechanisms through the collapse of transport networks and its purpose, the redistribution of labour. Epidemiological studies have shown that truck drivers, seafarers, pilots and other transport sector personnel have relatively high rates of infection. Yet the transport sector is essential to knitting together markets, both for outputs and inputs. Lahour mobility occurs in response to labour market demands and, on a local basis, these will increase as a result of the epidemic.

Education and training play an important role throughout the spectrum of social, technical and economic development. High incidence countries will need to ensure that those infected can continue to contribute productively to the economy so that this investment is not necessarily lost.

New approaches to training may have to be devised because of increased mortality rate. one Ugandan study found an annual mortality rate of 2.5 per cent among staff of government institutions who had studied abroad between 1986 and 1988. The epidemic will also further erode the capacity to plan, manage and implement in those countries where there is little depth in trained personnel.

There will be immense costs to communities and nations. The early illness and death of the active labour force will generate a need for replacement of social investment at a time of shrinking public and national resources. The anguish of the illness and deaths of so many young adults will be difficult to bear. However, an understanding of the extent of the personal, social and economic costs will strengthen the demand for effective prevention programmes, the most effective way of minimising the adverse impact of the epidemic.

4

The HIV Epidemic and Development:

The unfolding of the Epidemic

Ms. Elizabeth Reid
Director
HIV and Development Programme,
UNDP, New York

THE DEVELOPMENT IMPLICATIONS OF THE HIV EPIDEMIC

The HIV epidemic will pose an unprecedented challenge to communities, nations and to the international community: a challenge to human survival, human rights and human, development. It is difficult to visualize the devastating effect of the HIV epidemic within our lifetimes and beyond.

The consequences of the spread of the virus will be inexorable and awesome. The challenge facing national and international communities is to act speedily and effectively to limit the further spread of the epidemic and to minimize its impact.

The impact of the HIV epidemic in developing countries must be understood in the context of the critical social and economic problems already experienced by these. countries: poverty, famine and food shortage, inadequate sanitation and health care, the subordination of women and adjustment policies that allocate insufficient resources to the social sectors.

These factors create a particular vulnerability to the devastating consequences of the epidemic. Economic need and dependency lead to activities that magnify the risk of HIV transmission and mean that many people, particularly women, are powerless to protect themselves against infection. Inequitable power structures, a lack of legal protection and inadequate standards of health and nutrition all further exacerbate the spread of the virus, accelerate progression from HIV infection to AIDS, and aggravate the plight of those affected by the epidemic.

The setting of the HIV epidemic in developing countries creates a downward spiral whereby existing social, economic and human deprivation produces a particularly fertile environment for the spread of HIV and, in turn, the HIV epidemic compounds and intensifies the deprivation already experienced by people in those countries. Not only must the epidemic itself be directly addressed in programmes of assistance but its consequences will impact upon all existing development initiatives which themselves will need to be reformulated in order to encompass these new situations.

The important lessons learned from the first ten years of responding to the epidemic are that behaviour change to stop the transmission of HIV can and does occur but that it needs the support of community and an enabling and supportive legal environment. Behaviour change is a process which must essentially involve changes in community and sexual norms and values, the availability of voluntary and confidential counselling and testing services and the creation of an environment which creates the possibility of open and honest discussion of sexuality and dying.

We have also learned that for sustainable behaviour change to occur, there has to be a belief in the future, or at least a reason for hope. This, we have found, comes about when communities and individuals become involved in the care of those living with HIV. We know this care leads to compassion and caring, rich and valuable human attributes which are at the centre not only of the response to the epidemic but of human development itself. The coping strategies of communities must be central to national responses.

For there to be a future in the face of this terrifying epidemic, the infrastructure required by communities must continue to function. As we respond to the immediate needs of behaviour change and the care and support of those infected and affected, the need to maintain the physical, social and economic infrastructure of communities and nations must not be overlooked. The impact of the epidemic begins to affect this infrastructure when increasing numbers of people sicken and die.

The challenges posed by the epidemic to human well-being and development are so immense that collaborative and complementary action is essential for our assistance to be timely and effective. Our efforts must also be sustainable. Effective responses to the epidemic will be needed for many years to come and we must recognize this in the care with which we develop and co-ordinate our efforts.

Co-ordination occurs when there is mutual respect, a common vision, the exchange of experience and a shared sense that the policies and programmes established are effective and sustainable.

THE EPICENTRE : THE SPREAD OF THE VIRUS

The analysis presented here places people and their communities at the centre of the exploration of the repercussions of the spread of the virus. At the epicentre (Figure. 4.1) of the inexorable chain of consequences is the transmission of the virus from person to person, from adult to child. We are still struggling to understand the factors which determine to where and how fast the virus spreads and who gets infected. An improved understanding of these factors will enable us to better understand how the virus moves from place to place, person to person, day to day so that we can more effectively limit its spread and anticipate its repercussions.

Inequalities of Wealth, Power and Autonomy

The first factor is inequalities of wealth, power and autonomy. The greater the disparity, the more stratified a society, the faster and further the virus spreads. Both the rich and the poor are likely to have higher infection rates.

The rich, like the powerful, are more mobile, less constrained by community norms and can afford the lifestyles they choose, which often place them at risk of infection. The poor and the powerless alike are less able to make choices about their life circumstances, more often forced into work away from home and family, or commercial sex work. Their health and nutritional levels are low and they cannot afford to use health services.

Attitudes to Women

These inequalities and stratifications are linked to the second determining factor, namely that of attitudes towards women which are demeaning or which deny women value and. dignity. The indicators of these attitudes will include levels of domestic violence, physical and sexual abuse, abortion laws and practices, and whether women are listened to when they speak. For example, one study of couples who describe themselves as true equals shows that, whereas 97 per cent of conversations initiated by the husband succeeded, only 30 per cent of those begun by the women were continued.

Cultural prescriptions, myths and jokes all embody these attitudes to women, along with the popular and serious literature of communities and nadons. Where women are denied dignity and respect, the virus spreads.

FIGURE 4.1
The Waves of Impact of the HIV Epidemic

EPICENTRE	WAVE I	WAVE II	WAVE III	WAVE IV
Spread of the Virus	*Trauma, Illness and Death*	*Survivors*	*Social and Economic Impact*	*Long term Potential Impact*
Description Spread hidden, but Increasing numbers of people becoming infected.	Psychological trauma; HIV opportunistic diseases appear; Increasing illness and death.	Grieving and bereavement, children, elderly and others left without support.	Depletion of the labour force, adverse impact on productive and social sectors, shrinking revenues, loss of military strength.	Possibility of social and political unrest, destitution, social and economic disintegration.
Determining Factors Inequalities of #wealth #power #autonomy Sexual norms and community values Condition of genital area Attitudes to women Mobility Ethical/legal env.	Extent of spread Attitudes to affected Ethical and legal environment	Clustering of infection in households and communities Dependency ratios Attitudes to survivors Ethical and legal environment	Morbidity in productive adults Clustering in occupations and geographically Gender role differentiation Structure of labour market and economy	Effectiveness and type of earlier policies and programmes Clustering in occupations and geographically Dependency ratios

The type of attitudes that lead to the spread of the virus may co-exist with a quite high status for women in terms of access to education, training and employment.

Community Norms and Values

The third determining factor is community norms and values. Communities where the social construction of gender leads to quite different paradigms of masculinity and femininity have higher infection levels. Similarly, communities and families which tolerate or encourage male sexual behaviour patterns that separate sexual satisfaction from responsibility to others and which value passivity and self-effacement in women will be disproportionately highly infected.

Pathology and Immaturity of the Genital Area

The fourth determining factor of the speed and extent of spread is the pathology and immaturity of the genital area. When unprotected, penetrative intercourse takes place, the virus is much more likely to be transmitted if there are lesions, secretions, inflammation or scarification of the genital area. The existence of these conditions is related to hygiene practices, nutritional status, access to sensitive health services, cultural practices and reproductive practices. In women, transmission may also occur more easily at different stages in the hormonal cycle or if the genital area has not reached maturity, which does not usually occur until young women are in their twenties.

This factor is clearly implicated in the high infection rates in young women and probably in infection rates in uncircumcised men, and contributes significantly to the different rates of infections between developed and developing countries.

Mobility

The fifth determining factor is mobility. The patterns of spread of the virus follow the movement patterns of people: the criss-crossing of armies across countries, the transport routes, the commercially vigorous trading centres, job markets, seasonal flows for agriculture or for ceremony.

Mobile groups of people—senior civil servants, parliamentarians, teachers, students, migrant workers, pilots, truck drivers, the military and so on—have higher infection rates than others.

People Telling Their Stories

The final factor which determines the speed and extent of the spread of the virus and who gets infected is whether conditions exist for people to tell their stories, stories of being infected and stories of changing their behaviour to prevent themselves from becoming infected.

For this to happen, there must be a strong legal and ethical framework which will lessen the almost inevitable discrimination and stigma surrounding HIV infection. There must be community and family support systems. There must be supportive government policies relating to continuation in employment, in school, etc., Finally, there must be the courageous people to tell their stories, for the cost to the individuals and their families of speaking out is usually very high.

If we bear in mind these determining characteristics, we can now put some faces to the estimated 12 million adults already infected in the world today. We now know that soon there will be as many, or more, women infected as men. Many, perhaps most, will be couples, husbands and wives. Many, of not most, will be poor. Although there will be a not insignificant number of the infected among the rich and powerful, many will be in situations that take them away from their families and communities and most will come from communities which accept and even value the behaviour which puts men, women and their families at risk of sexual transmission. We can now begin to see our own faces amongst those 12 million.

THE WAVES OF CONSEQUENCES

The consequences of this spread radiate out over time and will continue to spread. Over time, various types of repercussions are becoming apparent. Their extent and nature are determined by many factors but there is a small number of dominant ones. The first wave of consequences follows directly from the spread of the virus: Those who are infected will, in time, start falling ill and dying.

The second wave of consequences arises from two dominant characteristics of the epidemic:

those who are infected are overwhelmingly at a stage in their lives when they have the maximum number of dependents: children, parents, others living with them, others that they are supporting; and

the virus is clustered in households and so their dependents will be left with few or no means of support.

The third wave of consequences arises from those other

dominant characteristics of the epidemic:

those who are infected are at their most economically productive and active period in their lives;
the virus is clustered occupationally and geographically; and
the rigidity of the gender division of labour, skills and responsibilities.

The extent and nature of the fourth wave of consequences is determined by two dominant characteristics:

the response of communities and nations to those infected, those caring for them and those who survive after their deaths, in particular by whether or not they remain an integral part of their communities, supported and cared for by them; and
the clustering in certain occupations and geographically.

The personal, psychological, social and economic consequences of the spread of the virus will unfold for decades after the virus has taken hold in a community and will continue to unfold for as long as the virus continues to spread.

Let us look at the overlapping waves of consequences more closely.

The first wave of impact to emerge is centered on the infected person and her or his family, partners and carers. It includes the trauma of diagnosis, community reactions (acceptance or stigma and discrimination), economic and emotional impact on their households, reaction of health care workers, illness and death. As indicated in Figure 3.2, those primarily affected are individuals and families, and the ways in which they are affected and the resources that they and others can bring to bear on their problems determine the policy and programme requirements.

In developing countries, most women and men are faced with the probability of their being infected when a baby or young child is clinically diagnosed with HIV. The lack of confidentiality, which is too frequent in these settings, often leads to the mother being singled out for blame. Fear and denial on the part of the father can lead to the woman's rejection and repudiation. The family may be torn apart and the women and her children left destitute and homeless. Strict confidentiality and the disclosure of the child's HIV status with counselling to both parents, not just the mother, can often protect the women and enable the family to continue as a basic nurturing and socializing unit for the children.

The immediate concern of infected women, and often men, is the future well-being of their children. Who will look after them after their deaths? Where the receiving family cannot be the extended family, many women would like to participate in the choice of an alternative form of care and help prepare their children for the future. Already at this stage, long before the children are left without parents, attention needs to be given to identifying or establishing forms of care for these children.

The second area of immediate concern is that the parents continue to be able to provide for and nurture their children for as long as possible. In one Kigali community, the women identified one nutritious meal a day and the treatment of any opportunistic infection, oral thrush, for example, which might impair their ability to look after their children.

As more and more children and adults fall ill, the demand for the treatment of opportunistic infection and for anti-virals will increase as will the demand on hospital beds. Whilst neglect of these demands may cause political unrest, addressing these demands may not be possible because of a lack of a basic health infrastructure and because of resource constraints. There is thus the need to achieve an informed and widespread consensus in the community, as well as in the health sector and among bureaucrats and politicians, on a treatment strategy.

The formal health care system will have to rationalise its role as it ceases to be able to provide institution-based care for all those with HIV-related illnesses. New modes of care management and collaborative and complimentary home and institutional-based care regimes will need to be designed. The increasing burden of care will be to a great extent borne by family and friends, but probably disproportionately by women and girls.

In this latter case, women's other roles and responsibilities, including child rearing and their productive roles, will be seriously affected if the burden of care is added to women's illness and death. Young girls may be withdrawn from schools to help care for the sick and for siblings and to keep the family together as long as possible.

As the burden of illness increases, household incomes and provisioning will be directly affected. Those unable to pay rent or repay mortgages may lose their homes. School fees and food requirements may become unaffordable. Furthermore, the use of household savings and assets in the futile search for a cure can seriously impoverish the family. There will need to be programmes of assistance to meet the basic needs for food, shelter, counselling and school fees in affected households.

The effectiveness of programmes for affected individuals, families and communities will ultimately depend on the legal, ethical and human rights milieu pre-existing or established to respond to the epidemic. Respect for the rights and dignity of those affected,

FIGURE 4.2
Programming the Epidemic and its Impact

EPICENTRE	WAVE I	WAVE II	WAVE III	WAVE IV
Spread of the Virus	*Trauma, Illness and Death*	*Survivors*	*Social and Economic Impact*	*Long term Potential Impact*
Level of Primary Intervention				
Individual Community	Family Community	Family Community	Workplace Nation	Nation Community
Primary Programme/Policy Focus				
Change in norms and behaviour Voluntary testing and counselling sites Legal, ethical and human rights Prevention technology Socio-economic causes	Social/sexual development Social inclusion Psychological support Legal, ethical and human rights issues Welfare maintenance Care and treatment Future planning	Legal, ethical and human rights Assistance programme social/sexual development Social inclusion Psychological support legal ethical and human rights issues	Labour market and social services planning Productivity maintenance Governance	Governance Decentralization Community survival strategies External Aid flows

guarantees of confidentiality, anti-discrimination provisions and a policy context of support and commitment that all affected people remain an integral part of their communities are sine qua non conditions for an effective response. Furthermore, without this legal framework, the affected will not speak out and tell their stories so that others may learn and change their behaviour. Such stories are amongst the most effective motivaters for behaviour change.

Often it is not until large numbers of the population are infected and many have progressed to AIDS or associated diseases such as tuberculosis that there is the possibility of a national consensus on the urgency of the matter. It is usually only at this stage that the voices of public health officials, health workers and the infected and their families finally begin to be heard.

As more adults die, the second wave of impact begins to emerge: increasing numbers of children and the elderly left without support and of single-headed households (Figure 4.1). For every adult dead, there could be on average two to three dependents. Thus the amplitude of this phase could be two to three times greater than the mortality rates in the previous phase. Poverty will also be spreading: households disintegrating; children scattered.

The most striking feature of this wave is the psychological impact on individuals and communities of so many lives lost, so many parents, siblings, friends, children, colleagues, neighbours dead. In young children this often induces an almost catatonic state, a withdrawal from the world of pain and despair. One story from the Kagera region in Tanzania is of a young girl sitting day after day at the edge of the yard, rocking on her heels and staring into space. Both her parents are dead, brothers and sisters, aunts and uncles. There is little food but she is not hungry. She rocks, grieving.

The grandmother takes time away from her overwhelming burden of care of all her other grandchildren to come and sit quietly beside the young girl. she knows she must gently draw her back into the land of the living or she will slowly die. The little girl has no will to eat, to go to school, to help out in the house. Unless programmes find a means of reaching out to such children, and similarly affected communities, other assistance programmes will be less than effective.

Grandmothers and grandfathers are bearing a crippling burden of care although, as the epidemic deepens, they too are increasingly numbered among the infected. The extent of homeless, destitute and traumatised children and elderly will be largely determined by the extent of caring environments that can be found or created for them.

Extended family and neighbourhood forms of care will soon become overwhelmed unless they, themselves, are supported. A recent study in Kigali, where the impact of the epidemic in creating dependent survivors has already become visible, shows that already one in every two households is caring for one or more children other than their own.

There are various different ways to provide assistance to the survivors and their communities (Figure 4.2): direct transfer programmes, subsidies, entitlements, credit and social services including housing, feeding and child care programmes. These must complement and support the initiatives which arise within the communities themselves. The striking feature of this epidemic is that wherever the virus spreads, individuals and communities respond. Leaders emerge, caring and coping strategies spring up and programmes are developed.

For the survivors as well as the infected, a supportive legal, ethical and human rights environment is essential if they are to be supported by their communities and if they are to be able to retain their property, inheritance and custody rights. This is particularly true for women and for orphaned children.

The third wave of impact centres around the loss of so many members of the workforce and the impact of the epidemic on household and domestic savings and on foreign exchange earnings (Figure 4.2). The epidemic will cause a reduction in the quantity and quality of labour available to produce output in both the formal and informal sectors and both measured and unmeasured activities. Women's labour, both productive and domestic, is disproportionately unmeasured. The loss of women's labour will threaten the living standards of households and communities as well as national productivity. Patterns of labour supply and demand will change, the determining factor being the clustering of the virus occupationally and geographically (Figure 4.1).

There will also be a reduction in and changing patterns of use of savings. The quantity of savings available and how this is employed influences the rate of growth of Gross National Product (GNP). Decreasing levels of savings will occur at the same time as the direct and indirect costs associated with the epidemic escalate.

Economies most vulnerable will be those that depend on a single or a limited number of sectors, agriculture alone or mining and agriculture, for example. The sectors most vulnerable will be those which require a critical number of trained personnel for whom replacements are difficult to find, pilots and mining engineers among many others, or occupations with high infection rates, transport sector workers, construction workers, senior public servants, students, for example.

The transport sector knits together producers and markets, raw materials and finished products, matches migrant labour supply to labour demand, links urban and rural economies, holds families together, enables centralised military and police control. A slow down in this sector will have extensive economic, social and political repercussions.

In the agricultural sector, farming systems which are labour intensive throughout the agricultural cycle or where labour demand peaks at certain times, as well as those with which is associated a strict gender division of labour, are most vulnerable to shortages in the labour supply. In subsistence farming systems, crop mixes are already changing, swinging away from cash crops and certain food crops to less demanding crops such as manioc. Farming systems based on the availability of wage labour, for example, plantation crops, are also vulnerable. Significant changes in patterns of production will adversely affect household nutrition and income levels as well as urban food supplies and foreign exchange earnings.

With growing numbers of women falling ill and dying, and with women being increasingly occupied with the care of the ill, women will have less time for caring for and socialising with their own children and for productive work in the fields, in self-employment or in the paid workforce.

This work is often unrecognised and undervalued. Too much of it does not appear in systems of national accounts nor is much of it included in economic measures such as GNP. It will be difficult to monitor the impact at the macro level of the loosening of these social and economic networks or parenting, providing, coping and caring. However, their absence will be widely felt. This work of women is essential for the economic and social well-being of families, communities and societies.

Increasing morbidity will eventually affect all sectors of the economy: financial institutions, education and health sectors, water and electricity supplies, industry and governance (Figure 4.2).

The fourth wave of impact is directly linked to the failure of previous interventions. If the spread of the virus is not slowed down as early as possible in the epidemic, and if those affected by it are not adequately supported, then the very survival of communities and nations will be in jeopardy. The survival tactics of the bands of destitute children could lead to the terrorization of populations. Strategic vulnerability will increase with the morbidity rates in the military. Basic services, water, electricity, road maintenance, financial services, will be impaired. Price increases and service decreases will lead to discontent and unrest. National governance could come to a halt. Households, communities and countries will disintegrate.

At this stage, even international interventions to prevent the total disintegration of the nation state may be too late. Such interventions will need to occur much earlier and in an intensive and systemative way.

These longer-term consequences are not inevitable. The extent and seriousness of the consequences will depend directly on the timeliness and effectiveness of behaviour and attitudinal change programmes and of policies adopted to respond to the needs of the infected, the ill and the survivors.

The phases identified in Figure 4.1 are not discrete; they overlap. However, there is often a time lag before the problems associated with each stage becomes visible and the phase recognised. The severity of subsequent phases will depend upon the efficiency of earlier interventions. If this is not understood, competing demands on limited national resources could mean that programmes for earlier phases, behaviour change programmes in particular, are not allocated sufficient resources. Furthermore, in each phase there are policy options which are best decided in advance, so that people can be educated to understand and accept them and planning for them commenced.

The proportional costs of delaying the start of an effective HIV programme. This displays, on the right hand side, the proportional costs at year thirty of the epidemic in a particular country. The difference in levels of cost depend on the stage that the epidemic has reached before an effective programme is implemented. The cost of starting an effective programme rises with the stage of the epidemic. This is because there will be more sectors and programme components and a greater demand for services. The different levels of cost at thirty years probably differ from each other by factors of ten or more. Thus there is a disproportionate advantage in starting effective HIV programmes early.

Each phase has its own set of policy and programme requirements and these are cumulative rather than sequential. That is, as different phases of the epidemic emerge, a new set of policies and programmes will have to be developed while those for previous phases will need to be continued. Thus the demand on human and financial resources will expand rather than change over time.

Furthermore, as can be seen from Figure 4.2, responsibility for most of these policies and programmes will lie with sectors and ministries other than health. An early understanding of this can create a broader consensus on the need for timely expenditure on effective prevention programmes. The epidemic then ceases being the responsibility solely of Departments or Ministries of Health and begins to be a multisectoral concern. The earlier this happens, the greater the possibility of minimising the severity of subsequent phases. The most powerful intervention to minimise the impact of the epidemic is an effective programme to reduce the further spread of the virus.

Thus, an effective strategic response to the epidemic would

be a phased response consisting initially in support to communities responding to the epidemic and the establishment of an appropriate ethical, legal and human rights framework. Next, the underlying socio-economic causes which determine the pattern and speed of spread need to be identified and programmes to address them established.

As communities mobilize and respond, the demand for technology and services, for voluntary testing sites, condoms, health services, sterile needles, etc., will increase and, at this stage, these should be accessible and affordable. Finally, the socio-economic consequences of the spread of the virus will need to be identified, monitored and minimised.

The spread of the virus initiates an inevitable chain of consequences which will continue for decades, for generations. The nature of these repercussions is so devastating that despair and fatalism would seem to be the only rational responses. However, this bleakness is held at bay by the extraordinary response that the epidemic evokes. Wherever the virus spreads, individuals and communities respond.

THE CHALLENGES OF THE HIV EPIDEMIC

There are a number of challenges for communities and governments (Figure 4.2), choices which will either minimise or aggravate later waves of impact. **The first challenge will be the type of behaviour change and prevention policies adopted and the extent of resources directed to the epidemic in its early stages.**

Choices made will affect the number of people infected and hence the numbers who die and the numbers of survivors. They will determine the extent of the impact. For as long as the virus continues to spread in the community, high priority will need to be given to behaviour change and attitudinal change programmes. In the economic situation of most countries, initiating new programmes requires commitment, courage and effective arguments. Cabinet members will need to be convinced of the need for adequate financing and be active participants in policy development and planning processes.

However, even if all future cases of HIV infection could be prevented from today, every year for the next twenty years approximately five per cent of those already infected will develop AIDS and die. Thus, if in a city or country half a million people are already infected, around 25,000 people will die each year for the next two decades. In countries with an already high rate of infection, the impact would be long felt.

The second challenge will be the extent to which the

community response is integrated into and is complemented by the governmental response. Affected communities have already begun initiatives that respond to their own needs, build on their resources and use their networks and forms of social organization. They must be given the political and social space and resources to continue. Other players in the community response include community leaders, health professionals, traditional non-governmental organizations, employers, trade unions, religious and political bodies, youth groups, women's organizations and many more.

The most effective national strategies will be based on and give coherence to the diversity of responses arising within the community and will, in balancing, supporting and shaping these initiatives, command widespread support.

Another challenge will be whether and the extent to which governments assist the affected, that is, those infected, their families and carers and those that survive them, to remain an integral part of their communities. For this to occur, there need to be guarantees of confidentiality, protection against discrimination and repudiation, assistance to the infected to live positively and productively, respite and child care, access to health and education services, income and housing maintenance, assistance to families to stay together as long as a parent is still alive and programmes to keep survivors within the community.

Without such policies, increasing numbers of children and the elderly will be without the, care and support of their families or communities. The consequent lack of socialization of these children and their isolation could lead, as numbers increase, to a dissolution of social relations and the possibility of civil unrest and lawlessness. Thus the seriousness of the long-term impact is dependent upon responses to the previous challenge.

If the choice is made to assist the infected and their survivors to remain living and cared for within their communities, it will be essential for governments to create a climate of acceptance and support for this policy. People's fears and misconceptions will need to be addressed in education programmes and every means found to lessen rejection, blame and stigma and to oppose discrimination. A further challenge is whether and at what stage governments, the private sector and others should begin to plan to minimise the adverse social and economic impacts.

The epidemic has come to be in a world already shaped by a multitude of factors and these in their turn influence and determine its dimensions. Poor nations burdened with debt are unable to honour the basic rights of women and men to health care, education, shelter and employment. This has created a backlog of deprivation which both facilitates the spread of the virus and aggravates its consequences. The poverty of individuals, and of women and children in particular, has led to their increasing vulnerability to infection. Poverty caused by HIV-related illness and death deepens existing poverty, creates new poverty and increases indebtedness. This interrelatedness between the epidemic and the setting within which it is occurring will make government attempts to plan to minimise the adverse impact of the epidemic more difficult.

The challenges identified so far all occur at the level of households, communities and nations.

There is a further critical challenge which will occur at the global level: whether the world community will provide the direct foreign investment in human capital and technological development and in social safety nets to allow poor nations and nations rendered poor by this epidemic to survive.

The free working of the global market tends to increase the disparities between rich and poor nations. National governments try to offset such tendencies, nationally, by redistributing income through systems of progressive income tax. They also supplement this with social safety nets to prevent people from falling into absolute destitution.

No such systems operate at present at the global level. The closest the world comes to a global safety net is the current system of development assistance. But this system is fatally flawed, not only in the inadequacy of its extent but because its allocation at present is unrelated to the level of poverty.

Some examples. South Asia receives $5 per person while aid-receiving countries in the Middle East, with more than three times South Asia's per capita income, receive $55 per person. India has 34 per cent of the world 's absolute poor, yet receive only 3.5 per cent of total aid flows . Indeed, the 10 countries that together have more than 70 per cent of the world's poorest people receive only 25 per cent of global aid.

If overseas aid is to be able to serve as a social safety net for the world's poor, it will have to be based on principles requiring that aid should be directed to priority concerns for human development.

The final challenge rests with us. Ultimately, our hope lies in understanding the centrality of the will to live, to stay together, to cope and survive at all levels— individuals, families, communities, nations and internationally.

If we keep quiet, if we think that this is not our problem, HIV will change the world despite us. We can make a difference. We can overcome the epidemic by speaking out, by using our influence within our families and communities. By changing our lives and our behaviour, we can create a world in which we can peacefully coexist with the virus.

5

AIDS and Asia: A Development Crisis

Ever since cases of AIDS began to appear in Asia during the mid 1980s, chose involved in efforts to contain the global epidemic have warned that the spread of HIV, the virus responsible for AIDS, could inflict social devastation in the world's most populous region.

This up coming toll as yet remains in the future: there is so far no Asian city or rural area where the impact of HIV infection has reached close to that experienced in some pockets of Africa. However, AIDS is no longer a stranger in the Asian environment. Although the caseload of actual AIDS is still very low, over one million HIV infections are already thought to have occurred in Asia and the Pacific. If the rate of spread continues at its current pace, Asia can expect around one million new infections a year by the year 2000, by which time many of those now infected will have become sick with AIDS-related illnesses and died.

The relatively late arrival of HIV in Asian and Pacific countries confers on their governments an advantage not enjoyed in much of Africa, where the caseload of HIV-induced sickness and AIDS was already high by the time the presence of the virus was recognized. Governments in the region are in a position to draw from the body of knowledge and experience already accumulated about the epidemic both to prepare at the earliest opportunity to meet its many consequences, and to take urgent action to contain—so far as possible—its spread. In the absence of both a vaccine against HIV and affordable, widely applicable therapies for AIDS, at present the only means of blocking HIV transmission is to encourage people to adopt self-protective and other-protective behaviours.

Most governments have established national bodies to address issues associated with HIV and AIDS and develop strategies for prevention. Their existence can be seen as an encouraging sign that the vision of the damage HIV could wreak in the region is being taken seriously at the highest levels. However, these national AIDS bodies are not immune to the tendency which has occurred elsewhere: postponement of significant action until there is a significant AIDS caseload, by which time HIV infection levels are high and may be spiralling beyond control.

One of the key lessons from experience is that the presence of AIDS in a population has far wider implications than those exclusively concerned with health. There are a number of social and economic attributes in a given population—such as the degree of occupational mobility, the role and status of women, and taboos on the discussion of sexual behaviour and sexually-transmitted disease—which contribute to the spread of HIV. These, in turn, affect the ethical and legal environment informing responses to the HIV-affected.

Since AIDS is both incurable and fatal, the presence of the HIV virus tends to arouse fear, denial, and victimization of those infected. These emotions, operating within the family, community, and society at large, are an important characteristic of the epidemic, negatively influencing personal and official responses to it. However, there have also been positive social reactions to AIDS, within affected communities or from health or social service Non-Governmental Organizations (NGOs), which have helped prolong life and reduce social distress. There is much to be learned from these experiences.

In addition to the many social and economic factors which are part of the context of the epidemic, there are also a number of socio-economic impacts stemming from it. The most important of these is the loss to sickness, and ultimately death, of a large number of adults in the prime of their economic life: most cases of HIV infection occur in men and women between the ages of 20 and 45. This has major implications for family dependents of those with AIDS, particularly the elderly and the very young, as well as for the workforce, and ultimately for a country's productivity. The cost to social services budgets of care for AIDS patients and HIV related sickness, including paediatric cases and of the care of destitute dependents, are charges which the community and state will somehow have to bear.

In July 1991, the United Nations Development Programme (UNDP) established a Regional Project based in India to stimulate awareness of the upcoming social and economic consequences of the spread of HIV infection in Asia and the Pacifie, and to catalyze early action in response to the epidemic . The Project's authority stems from the "Alliance to Combat AIDS" entered into by WHO and UNDP in 1987, which brings to the global effort to contain HIV the strengths of both organizations, recognizing WHO's primacy in health and biomedical affairs and UNDP's international leadership in social and economic development. The Regional Project co-operates closely with UNDP's. HIV and Development

Programme, based in its New York headquarters, and with its Interregional Programme to strengthen UNDP's capacity to respond to the HIV epidemic. The Project also provides assistance to existing HIV- and AIDS-related initiatives in which UNDP is involved at country level in the region.

HIV AND AIDS

What is AIDS? Acquired Immunodeficiency Syndrome (AIDS) is caused by HIV, human immunodeficiency virus. The means of HIV transmission are few and very specific. They include the use of HIV-infected blood and blood products during transfusions; injection with HIV-contaminated hypodermic needles; and transmission from mother to child in the womb or at delivery. But by far the most important route of HIV transmission is via unprotected sexual intercourse.

HIV erodes the body's defense system, exposing the infected person over time to lung diseases, cancers, fungal infections, wasting, rashes, and sores. These eventually overpower the body's ability to fight back, causing physical—and sometimes mental—ruin and death.

There is as yet no cure for AIDS, although treatment can relieve distress from opportunistic infections. One or two new drugs slow down the rate of progress from HIV infection to serious illness, but they are very expensive and have toxic side-effects.

AIDS, a threat to humankind: AIDS is one of the most serious threats to human health and life ever faced because:

The major mode of HIV transmission is sexual, and the urge for physical intimacy is fundamental in all human beings.

An important means of transmission is from mother to unborn child, in the womb. AIDS therefore presents a major threat to bearing healthy children.

The period between HIV infection and onset of illness can last several years. A person with no knowledge of being infected can infect others unwittingly.

There is no cure. Prevention is dependent on following a self-protective behavioural code, and one which protects others.

Human capacity for denial is so great that the adoption of self-protective behaviour tends to become widespread only when deaths from AIDS are close to home; by which time many people have already been infected.

Responses to the HIV epidemic: The fight against HIV and AIDS at international, national, and local level requires engagement by all groups within society, not only medical scientists and health workers. These include community-based organizations and those in the business sector. Responses to the epidemic take many forms:

Research into all aspects of HIV, to understand its epidemiology and develop curative and preventive therapies against its invasion and onslaught.
Spreading information about HIV and AIDS through all possible channels to dispel stigma, ignorance, and false conceptions, and guide people to self-protective behaviour.
Providing care and counsel for those with AIDS, and for family members affected by their illness and death.
Ensuring that hospital practices, blood and blood products, and hypodermic needles are consistently HIV-free.
Challenging the immense human capacity for denial about the threat of HIV and AIDS, and lifting taboos surrounding the discussion of sexually-transmitted disease.

With the collaboration of UNDP and WHO country offices, as well as that of other local, national, and regional partners, the Project has been exceptionally active. Drawing on lessons from other parts of the world, initiatives have aimed to strengthen understanding of the full dimensions of the HIV epidemic among decision-makers in all fields, not only that of health; establish, by research and analysis, the soeial, economic, cultural, and political factors influencing the epidemic, and their implications for policy-making and the application of the law; build capacity to meet HIV infection and AIDS in a variety of sectors, within government and outside it; and harness from a number of sources the energy and creativity needed to develop preventive strategies which will work. A number of other donors have lent support, including SIDA (Sweden), USAID, ODA (UK), the UN Drug Control Programme (UNDCP), and the Ford Foundation.

All initiatives fall within UNDP's own policy framework for HIV and AIDS, articulated by the HIV and Development Programme of UNDP in New York. They are also designed to dovetail with existing country plans for the control of AIDS, developed throughout the region with assistance from WHO's Global Programme on AIDS, within which socio-economic factors are increasingly becoming a feature. The Project has also played an educational role within the international donor community, familiarizing its members with the development implications of the epidemic and embedding within tJNDP's own regional consciousness the need to review constantly efforts in other sectors in the light of HIV and AIDS.

The vely special nature of the HIV epidemic, whose life-damaging potential is almost certainly unprecedented in the history of public health, demands an unusual degree of programmatic innovation and experimentation. To help create a supportive limate towards HIV containment, the Project has enlisted many partners inside and outside governmental networks. These include NGOs, especially community-based organizations, as is consistent with UNDP's contemporary programming philosophy; and partners in the private business sector, Chambers of Commerce, and the legal and media worlds. The urgency of the HIV and AIDS situation has prompted a variety of effort. Some results may be disappointing; others may cut corners in identifying effective strategies for behavioural change—corners which must be cut if what has been described as a 'smouldering volcano' threatening Asia is to be prevented from erupting.

Already, there are signs that leading politicians, government officials, and economic analysts are taking on board the social and economic implications of HIV and AIDS. In November 1992, the 2nd International Congress on AIDS in Asia and the Pacific will be held in New Delhi. The Conference, of which UNDP WHO, the AIDS Society for Asia and the Pacific, and the Government of India are co-sponsors, indudes on its agenda a prominent concern fòr the economic, social, and cultural aspects of HIV, and exploration of lessons from the educational and behavioural sciences to help develop preventive strategies. This indicates a broadening of the perspective in which the epidemic and responses to it are now being addressed.

Plans are in progress for a four-year Second phase of the UNDP Regional Project. In response to the increased level of awareness in the region, a number of new project and programme initiatives are coming forward. New Strategies for communlicating the key messages about AIDS need to be thoroughly piloted and tested. New approaches for responding to the HIV-affected through community based approaches and human rights networks need support. The special challenges of protecting women from HIV need to be given extra attention.

With Project expansion in view, this publication has been prepared in the hope that the sharing of information and ideas will help to build the necessary alliances throughout the region to control the social and economic damage that HIV and AIDS will otherwise surely bring.

6

The Impact of HIV on People and Society

Up to now, the protential impact of HIV infection on people and society in Asia has largely been analyzed in terms of medical issues: the costs of testing for HIV infection, of clinical care for AIDS patients, of protecting the blood supply, of sterilization practices, and of publicizing health information about AIDS. Little attention has been given to analyzing the impact on the families of patients, or on patients' and their dependents' needs for counselling and other kinds of support.

These are elements of the much broader human and economic development perspctive conerning the HIV epidemic in Asia and the Pacific which the UNDP Regional Project is setting out to illuminate. The development of capacity to analyze upcoming impacts is pre-emptive, drawing on experience from elsewhere to identify in advance the contexts in which those impacts will occur.

AT THE PERSONAL AND FAMILY LEVEL

At presents there is little other than anecdotal evidence about the impact of HIV and AIDS at the personal level in Asia and the Pacific. However, a recent paper prepared for UNDP underlines that the dominant share of the costs of the epidemic will be borne by the affected individuals and their families; and that the onset of HIV-related illness will tend to strain the resources of those affected to a point, where they and their families become seriously disadvantaged. The costs faced at the personal and family level include the direct costs of medical are and the loss of livelihood from the death of a breadwilnner. This situation contrasts with that in most western economies where many such cost are met by state or private insurance provision and where —accordingly- there is more incentive for the institutionalized public and private sectors to invest in HIV prevention.

There is another cost, not easy it to quantify, represented by the trauma of victimization for the person with HIV. This too often follows the discovery of a person's HIV-positive status. In 1988, when a blood bank in Goa, India found HIV in the blood of a donor, he was forcibly held in isolation for 64 days under the Goa Public Health Act although he had no knowledge of his infection, was not sick, and presented no risk to society.

This case illustrates the negative impact of a legal and ethical climate which is unprepared to deal with HIV; which is governed by unjustified fear of contagion; and which inappropriately applies public health legislation designed in another era for the containment of infections with a totally different pathology, such as cholera or smallpox. In the Goa case, relatives acted on the individual behalf and the Public Health Act was eventually adjusted so that isolation for HIV-positive individuals became optional, and he was allowed home.

Another case of victimization was recently reported from a village in Kochi. A young man returned from a spell of employment in Bombay and the Gulf fell sick as an outcome of HIV infection. When the source of his illness became known, his elderly parents were made socially out cast and destitute and the young man was hounded from the village. Not only does this case illustrate the need for confidentiality in HIV diagnosis, but many other social and economic impacts and interactions: the vulnerability of migrant workers; loss of livelihood for the patient and dependents; loss of shelter and community support.

Among low-income groups, the impact of HIV related disease, or of social stigma engendered by it, is far more devastating than among those with economic reserves and social out. Poorer families have no margin to absorb the cost of health care, the loss of earnings vital to meet food bills and other basis needs. The costs of the HIV epidemic will fall most heavily on the poor in Asia, and will further entrenh their poverty thereby augmenting existing soeio-economic inequity. Thus, there is an urgent need for research into impacts at the personal and family level within all ineome groups but especially among the least well-off.

Experience from Africa, USA, and elsewhere has shown that the person with HIV needs support and confirmation of his or her intrinsic value as a human being. This is demanded not only by considerations of humanity, hut as a strategy to maximize the development of individual and family resources to offset the impact of infection. The person who is able to "live positively with HIV" can prolong his or her healthy and active life, and make provision for the future of dependents. A person reconciled to HIV infection is also motivated to protect a spouse or sexual partner from exposure, by abstinence or the use of condoms.

UNDP initiated research into the economic impacts of HIV/AIDS in Asia and the Pacific

Who is Bearing the Cost of the HIV/AIDS Epidemic in Asia? David Bloom and Sherry Glied, April 1992.

The Economic Impacts of AIDS in the Republic of Korea, Bong-minYang, July 1992.

Economic Implications of AIDS in Southeast Asia: Equity Considerations, Myo Thant, April 1992.

Economic Impact of HIV and AIDS on the Transport Sector: Developing an Assessment Methodology, Patrick Giraud, May 1992.

The implications of AIDS for the agricultural sector in Lao PDR, Anthony M. Zola, September 1992.

Overseas Contract Workers and the Economic Consequences of HIV/AIDS in the Philippines, Orville Solon and Angelica Barrozo, 1992.

The Impact of AIDS on Malaysian Industrialization, David Lim, April 1992.

The Economic Impact of AIDS, Desmond Cohen, 1992.

When family members fall sick, womenfolk provide nursing care and absorb other parts of the household maintenance burden, such as income or food provision. This is another component of the special impact of the epidemic on women, and on their daughters, some of whom may have to minister to parental sickness and death at a vely young age. When death occurs, grandparents and other relatives often have to take in bereaved offspring. Again, the additional domestic onus falls most heavily on women household members. In Africa, children in HIV-affected families are often forced to give up schooling and shoulder adult responsibilities, proscribing their life prospects one of the key impacts of HIV on atfected individuals has been the lead they have taken in providing support services. AIDS patients and their relatives have often been the courageous initiators of responses at community level which help to replace stigma with sympathy, fear and denial with correct information about HIV, despair with life-enhancement, and risky with protective behaviours. Community based action provides the best comfort for the HIV affected, and the best hope for HIV containment.

AT THE COMMUNITY LEVEL

In certain Asian communities, HIV has already made an

impact even though its full effects in tellls of sickness and socio-economic fall-out have yet to be felt. Slum communities, typified by low standards of living, significant public health hazards, a fluid populations and common resort. to illegal or semilegal methods of Subsistence, are regarded by public health experts as likely 'distribution eentres' for HIV. In Northeastern India, community leaders are already aware of the need to respond to the rising level of infection among drug-users, and the UNDP Regional Project held a workshop to help them do so. This is but one example of the Project strategy to promote and assist community-based initiatives throughout the region.

Foremost among the impacts on communities of a growing toll of HIV-related sickness will be the implications of many households' inability to bear the economic loss of key productive members. Inevitably, there will be a transfer of responsibilities and e osts onto Community Coping mechanisms. In many families where men fall sick, women will not be able to manage financially on their own, or with relatives' help, and the community will be forced to provide additional child-care facilities, scholarships, and other types of support. Existing strains on available resources for community and social services, in both urban and rural areas, will deepen. Family fragmentation and the juvenile crime rate may also rise. The UNDP Consultation on the Economic Implications of HIV and AIDS in May 1992 pointed to the need for more interdisciplinary study at the community level, particularly regarding the dynamics influencing information flows and their impact on behaviour and attitudes.

At present, to place any figure on such future impacts is bound to be speculative. But certain social behavioural determinants which predispose people to HIV—such as recreational behaviours and patterns of sexual contact—are well-established, and hypothesis is practicable. The UNDP Regional Project is active in this area. Even speculative research is valuable in providing ammunition to impress upon policy-makers in all sectors the need to inject more resources into strategies for AIDS prevention. However difficult it is to promote behavioural change, there are ways to encourage it: for example, the insistence by brothel owners (with police support) on condom use by all clients, as in northern Thailand. And it is vital that, at the moment when people are prompted to change their sexual or drug-injecting behaviour, they have the means of doing so, and a clear sense of social, cultural, legal, and political endorsement.

AT THE LEVEL OF THE WIDER SOCIETY

Certain industries and sectors, notably those employing migrant, mobile or seasonal workers, have workforces particularly vulnerable to HIV infection. Industries involved in transport, tourism, entertainment, mining, fishing, and the armed forces, can anticipate economic costs as a result of HIV infection among workers. Productivity in these sectors, and in agriculture, is also likely to be affected, as has already been shown in Africa. The UNDP

UNDP support to community-based initiatives

The UNDP Regional Project places a high priority on the need to foster community-based activity for care and counselling of the HIV-affected, and containment of HIV spread. The Project acts as a facilitator, to help organizations plan, resource, implement, and monitor, their interventions; and enables them to share experiences.

Workshops

Development implications of HIV/AIDS in the NE States of India, Manipur, January 1991; a sub-regional workshop for government policy-makers and representatives of NGOs to increase awareness of strategies for limiting HIV/AIDS.

NGO writing and communications skills, Delhi, January 1992; a workshop for Indian NGO representatives, designed to help them write up their experience and "lessons learned", for use in workshops and seminars.

Promoting NGO/Business Sector Partnerships for AIDS Prevention, Thailand, June 1992; a regional consultation attended by representatives of 24 NGOs and members of the Asian business community.

Publications

NGO HIV/AIDS Project Development Manual: A manual for use by NGOs and CBOs (Community-Based Organizations) embarking on HIV/AIDS related activity; the project planning and implementation process is broken down into nine steps, from needs assessment through planning, funding and implementation, to evaluation, and is designed to help NGOs accomplish the process smoothly.

Community Responses to HIV/AIDS in Asia: Experiences from India and Thailand: Case studies of pioneering examples of community-based NGO HIV/AIDS action in

India and Thailand, for advocacy among other NGOs and CBOs.

NGO responses to HIV/AIDS in Asia: Exploring Programmatic and Organizational Issues. Six discussion cases of NGOs designed to explore the programmatic and organizational issues they face in implementing HIV/AIDS prevention and service delivery interventions. Intended for training and teaching purposes, for use in seminars, workshops or with project or programme practitioners. NGOs examined include: Southern India AIDS Action Programme, Madras; Planned Parenthood Association of Thailand; Community AIDS Service, Penang; Duang Prateep Foundation, Bangkok.

Regional Project has set out to develop a framework of research into the up coming economic impacts of HIV/ AIDS in Asia and the Pacific.

Since up to now the epidemic has mainly been seen as a health problem, its economic impact on the wider society has only been calculated— where it has been calculated at all — in terms of its burden on health care systems. Thailand is the only country in the region to estimate the up coming costs of HIV and AIDS in terms of public and private expenditures, and has found that health care costs could grow from $1.7 million in 1991 to $65 million by 2000. However, although many non-health care costs to families are noted, including the care of up to two million parentless Thai children, no attempt has yet been made to calculate the extra burden to society or the social services imposed by increased dependency ratios and the breakdown in family life.

HIV and AIDS will soon begin to have a major impact on the workplace, particularly in Thailand and India, with companies and industries experiencing losses in workdays, in trained manpower in recruitment costs, and burdens on benefits schemes UNDP-which has established its own personnel in relation to HIV - is doing its best to ensure that managers concern is directed away from responses such as exclusion or expulsion of workers whom testing reveals as HIV-positive.

Since the average period between infection and the onset of HIV-related sickness is several years, those living with the virus enjoy a long period of fitness in which they are as capable of productive work as the non-infected. Existing research indicates, moreover, that the costs of such testing, combined with the inaccuracies and short shelf-life of results obtained, disqualify workplace surveillance as an effective strategy for AIDS control. UNDP has 'begun the task of communicating this to the Asian business sector so as to avoid wastage of resources on methods of

HIV containment that not only offend human rights, but will not work.

The upcoming economic impact of HIV/AIDS in Asia and the Pacific: Towards a Framework of Research

The UNDP Regional Project hosted a Consultation on the Economic Implications of HIV/AIDS in Bangalore, India, in May 1992. A number of researchers subsequently developed proposals for action in their own environments. All focussed on HIV prevention, on expanding resources for HIV and AIDS, and on the need for epidemiological data; other priorities varied:

The cost-effectiveness of re-orienting information campaigns towards migrants and the workplace *(Bangladesh, Malaysia, Thailand)*

Market analysis of the commercial sex industry; socio-economic profiles of workers and clientele *(India, Nepal)*

Vulnerability of tourists travelling overseas; promotion of AIDS-free tourism *(Korea, Thailand)*

Cost estimates for prevention, treatment, and rehabilitation of HIV/AIDS cases *(Malaysia, Indonesia)*

Socio-economic causes of cross-border trafficking in girls and programmes for alternative opportunities *(Nepal)*

The need to factor into economic analyses considerations other than those purely related to cost-effectiveness; for example, the right of hospital patients to be transfused with HIV-free blood (India)

Impact of HIV/AIDS productivity, consumption, and labour supply within the household; costs of interventions *(Philippines, Indonesia)*

Understanding of social, economic and cultural factors to do with condom use *(Thailand)*

Integration of existing STD programmes with HIV prevention *(Bangladesh, Vietnam)*

With the Population and Development Association of Thailand and ILO, UNDP sponsored a workshop on issues related to HIV/AIDS in the Workplace, held in Bangkok in March, 1992. Presentations focussed on familiarizing managers with the relevant personnel issues, and the creation of a supportive climate towards HIV in the workplace by personal example, by training and education of staff, by providing counselling services and at access to condoms, and by promoting open debate. The workshop

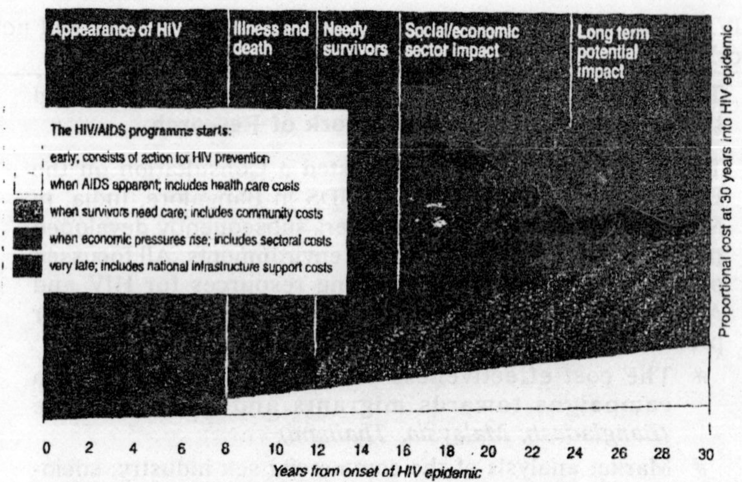

Escalating costs due to delaying the start of an effective HIV programme

conclusions placed a strong emphasis on the duty of employers to provide information services; on their obligation to desist from mandatory HIV testing of job candidates and employees; and to respect their rights to confidentiality, and to equal rights with others affected by serious illness in thus event of developing AIDS.

Certain members of the travel industry, notably hotel companies in Thailand concerned about erosion of tourist confidence, have begun to develop a workplace response. Attention is needed by other industries, such as construction companies, which similarly employ large numbers of seasonal or migrant labourers. Outflows and inflows of labour within countries and between them, are becoming a common feature of Asian economies. Between 1969-89, nearly 12 million Asians -worked as contract labour in the Middle East and in labour-short countries such as Singapore and Malaysia. In 1991, the receipts in Thailand alone from workers abroad were as high as $1 billion.

There are implications both for sending countries, and for receiving countries. Analysts in the Philippines and Thailand have already noted the possibility that their workers might be excluded from certain countries on the grounds of possible HIV infection, with implications for foreign earnings. Receiving countries will be concerned to reduce the prospect of transmission within the migrant labour community, and from it to the local population. Since migrant workers are often of low socio-economic status, their vulnerability to HIV infection is enhanced. Thus, AIDS also has the potential to reduce the labour supply, leading to higher wage levels and lowering investment from overseas.

One certain calculation about the upcoming costs of the HIV epidemic in Asia is that investment in prevention now, to reduce both the rate of HIV spread and its costs to society, is a major economy by comparison with the costs of AIDS damage control at a later stage. These costs will grow exponentially unless action is taken pre-emptively. (see chart).

Again, only Thailand has made cost calculations based on various scenarios. If Thailand were to meet its HIV behavioural change targets (reducing sexual partners, doubling condom use, timely STD treatment) the savings by the year 2000 would amount to $5.1 billion. Even if the national AIDS control and prevention budget were to trilple in the immediate future, the cost of prevention would yield a 17 times return on investment. UNDP hopes that Thailand's example in promoting the economic advantages of HIV/ AIDS prevention will have an impact throughout the region.

7

Development Practice and the HIV Epidemic

Ms. Elizabeth Reid
UNDP, New York

Development practice with respect to HIV is paradigmatically the practice of human development. This is so for two central reasons. Firstly, the focus of HIV is people's sexual, psychological and social relations and behaviour. No roads, fertilizers, procurement systems or stock exchanges are available to distract attention from or mask the fact that people are the focus of its practice. Secondly, all the classical components of development—transportation systems, labour markets, economic growth, governance, poverty and more —are within the causal framework which determines patterns and speed of spread of the virus and will also themselves be affected by the impact of its spread, its associated mortality and morbidity and the burden of dependency and social disruption it will create. No longer are failures to alleviate poverty or success in employment creation just that; they each and each of the others affect what happens with the HIV epidemic.

Thus, there is now for UNDP a double imperative: improve our development performance whilst at the same time addressing the epidemic. The tools, approaches and practices for each may well be the same. The focus must be on development practice: learning the lessons of what approaches and initiatives are most effective and of how one can catalyze and support them.

Team and Constituency Building within the Organization

Exploring new approaches to development practice involves changing accepted ways of thinking about issues and accepted procedures and practices. The inertial tendency is always towards the status quo. The HIV and Development programme has the responsibility to ensure that there is a common understanding of the epidemic and a consensus on effective ways of using development assistance to respond to it throughout the organization. As more staff are recruited to HIV specific positions, especially in the two regional projects and as HIV and Development NPOs in country offices, more resources have had to be directed to collegial team building activities amongst the HIV dedicated staff. The priorities and approaches adopted and advocated by UNDP are drawn from an ongoing exploration of and quest for effective and timely responses. It is important that all parts of the organization understand and have the human and other resources required to integrate the lessons learned about effective approaches into their work.

These team building activities have involved dialogue, guidance and skill building and the development of adequate managerial and supportive capacities in the regional bureaux. It also involves building an informal constituency throughout the organization, informed not only about HIV but also about the causal interrelationships between development and the epidemic and knowledgeable about how they take this into account in their own work: the "But what should I be doing about it?" questions. Although increased time and resources were directed to this, there was only limited success achieved and significantly more effort will need to be directed at this in 1995.

Designing Development Assistance

Many, perhaps most, country offices who have fielded HIV project design missions, whether small or large, single or multi agency, have been disappointed with the resulting proposals and documentation. As have most of their government counterparts. This should not be surprising. The issues involved are complex, and often contentious. UNAIDS and most national HIV/AIDS programmes admit that what they are doing is not having a sufficient impact on the problem.

A technological resource base has been developed—condoms, information, drugs, test kits, etc.,—but even if the problems associated with accessibility and affordability of these technologies were able to be overcome, much more is needed to protect people from HIV infection. The missing factors include areas into which development has not yet ventured: male sexuality, discourse taboos, the abuse of women, the forces of traditional patriarchy, individualism, moral corruption and others. There is no tradition to guide the development practitioner in such areas, yet this is where HIV is leading development .

However, little change will occur until those involved themselves, as individuals, as communities, as economic actors, want to change: wherever people want beer, it can be found, whatever the state of disintegration of roads or markets or the formal economy. Thus, one of the basic programming challenges is to determine/how the collective will to change can be created and strengthened. Telling people to change or to behave differently or to do things differently does not work, as the history of development has taught us.

In response to the repeatedly expressed frustration of country offices, HDP has developed two alternative approaches to the traditional project design missions: the process consultancy approach developed by the MDG group in BPPS and the use of preparatory assistance to build local capacities for programme design. The former defines a different role for the outsider, the consultant who enters into a context. It is neither that of expert, source of knowledge and authority, a disempowering and ineffective role, nor one which denies to the outsider the exercise of the skills, knowledge and experience which she or he brings into the context. The process consultant is a facilitator of and contributor to processes which draw out from those involved their primary concerns and resources and strengthen their capacity to determine how themselves to achieve their self determined ends. Perhaps the most telling performance criterion for the process consultant is who writes the mission report or project document: those involved or the outsider?

In the latter approach, the whole concept of a project design mission is laid aside and ways are explored of building a national consensus on what should be done by whom with what resources. Two different approaches have been tried: a process, facilitated by external institutions or individuals, of a critical mass of key concerned nationals

reflecting on need and identifying areas where learning is needed,
learning from others and other countries (facilitated study tours),
applying the lessons to the particulars of the national situation,
programme and policy development, implementation and redesign (Djibouti)

and a process initiated by a facilitator/consultant within a country, stimulating discourse, bringing into the process all those involved and building a local consensus on what should be done (Cambodia, Bangladesh).

These approaches involve increased management and oversight responsibilities in the country office, a more profound knowledge of development practice and a capacity to work with processes rather than inputs and outcomes. Backstopping support to country offices, the role of the regional bureaux, is also more resource demanding and involves substantive as well as managerial guidance.

Identifying and Redefining the Expert

Robert Chambers, in Poverty and Livelihoods, poses the question: whose reality counts? He answers that, for an understanding of poverty, it is that of the poor and that this imperative must redefine the role of the professional. Chambers argues that the basic challenge for the professional is to learn to see things from the perspective of the poor, to allow the poor to analyze and express what they know, experience, need and want.

In the case of the HIV epidemic, this is particularly pertinent. The epidemic is new, unexperienced in the lives, personal or professional, of those normally considered as experts and development specialists. It has and will have no parallel in living or even recorded history.

Those with the subtlest and most extensive knowledge of it are those living with it as a part of their daily lives. Amongst these, those infected with the virus and those that love and care for them, there are very few leaders, public figures, elites or elders who have disclosed that they are infected. The educated, the rich and the leaders are absent by choice. Those who speak out and commit themselves to respond to the epidemic, to work for change, are mainly drawn from the ranks of the less asset or access endowed. They are the people. In donor countries, those with expertise in sexuality and HIV, in community development, are mainly, at this time in history, drawn from the ranks of the socially marginalized, from the gay men's movement and the movements of women.

These agents of change often do not have the profiles or professions that organizations like UN/OPS or UNDP are accustomed to classify, renumerate or even regard as experts. Yet experts they are because they know intimately the nature of what we are facing. And so they are becoming the trainers, consultants, speakers, partners and advocates of the response. In this way, the response becomes grounded in the reality of the epidemic. It is they who must reskill development professionals and organizations.

It has been a challenge to the programme to find ways, for example, of working with people from oral rather than written traditions, to assist those affected to develop the self-confidence and the skills necessary to use their expertise, to legitimize their presence in fora where people are unaccustomed to and uncomfortable with their being present, to work in situations of recurrent illness and dying, to deal with the loss of respected colleagues and to forge partnerships of equals within differences.

UNDP as a Development Partner

One of the emerging concepts of development practice is that of partnership. This has been formulated in reaction to felt imbalances in worth or agency between donors and recipients. This imbalance has existed in the discourse of development as well as its practices: note the acceptability of words such as "recipient".

But redressing these imbalances has not been easy. Here are the words of the Co-ordinator of the Women and AIDS Support Network in Zimbabwe:

One of the principles of partnership is equality. Can we be equal when our resources are mainly human resources and we rely on our partners for material resources? Whatever we call ourselves, partners, or donors and recipients, this inequality in money can translate into inequality in power.

... I see the dialogue that is emerging as a positive one. Increasingly, the relevance of our experience and skills is being grasped by our partners To the extent that we can exchange experiences, we build ties not only based on the flow of funds but on a recognition that we have something to offer each other.

In the response to the HIV epidemic, UNDP' s contribution has been knowledge and skill based rather than grant based. We have functioned with minimal financial resources. This has assisted the programme to develop new ways of achieving its developmental ends for, like technology, knowledge and skills cannot be transferred or shared, or even given away, unless someone wants them. Thus, we have entered into partnerships with a number of networks, consortia and institutions (LACCASO, AFRICASO, APCASO, GIPA, NAP+, GNP+, FAO, PAHO, etc.,).

The defining characteristics of these partnerships have been that the purpose of the partnership has been determined through extended discussions of each partner's priorities, capacities and ways of operating, from which a work programme was developed (or not). This has created relationships of mutual respect, based on a proper understanding of each partner's interests, roles and responsibilities, has created the possibility of partnerships of equals, equal in self esteem and self confidence, and has enabled development assistance to be an empowering rather than a disempowering set of international relations. This approach is time consuming and requires skills of dialogue and conflict resolution, but it changes the pattern of relationships from the binary and unbalanced centre-periphery or directive-receptive relations to decentralized and equitable network patterns.

Governance Capacity Building

Development practitioners have come to realize that the causes of development failure may not only reside in inadequate project design or implementation but may also exist in the actual setting of the development intervention: bureaucratic ineptitude, corruption, vested interests, lack of legal redress or safeguards, people's indifference, the suppression of dissent and such like. There is, thus, a growing awareness that development must also encompass the many elements of governance, including electoral support, strengthening of legal systems, support to legal activism, participatory politics, accountability of the armed forces, the strengthening of the institutions of civil society, decentralization and other political, legal, governmental and strategic initiatives.

There is also a growing awareness that the strengthening of the institutions of governance alone may not be sufficient to address these problems. Such institutions function best in societies where there is trust, respect and concern for others as well as self, family and kin, and where there are ways for people to come together in shared pursuits. This is referred to as the social capital of a society.

The aspects of governance critical to an effective response to the HIV epidemic include not only stable government (Rwanda, Cambodia, Zaire as illustrative) and bi-or multi-partisan support but also

a supportive legal, ethical and human rights framework,

the inclusion of those directly affected, including their non-marginalisation and non-discrimination,

the existence of concerned civil society organizations and groups, and

mechanisms and formal processes for the participation and co-ordination of all involved.

One important means of governance capacity building is the establishment and support of activist and professional networks: Ethics, law and HIV, People Living with HIV and AIDS the Global Civil-Military Alliance, AIDS support organizations and HIV researchers.

The human rights, ethics, law and HIV networks, which have been established in Africa, Asia and the Pacific, Latin America and the Caribbean, and are now beginning in Eastern Europe, draw their members from legal, governmental and academic institutions and from the organizations of civil society. They only indirectly contribute to institutional capacity building or to human resource development. Their main function is social capacity building around a common purpose, in this case,/the establishment of an agreed upon legal and ethical framework for the response to the epidemic and the provision of appropriate services to those affected.

These networks contribute to social capacity building through drawing together a diverse group of those interested or implicated to enable the addressing of issues of common interest. They broaden the base of discussion and contribute consensus building within the community sector and amongst civil society, the public and the private sectors. They contribute to governance capacity building in this way and also through advocating for law reform, changes in legal practices, the provision of appropriate services, policy and programme development and through a guardianship rule in determining the legal and ethical appropriateness of the response.

Networks of people living with HIV and AIDS are forms of social organization which assist in both building capacity for representation and participation in policy and programme development and in ensuring that their expertise and commitment contribute to the strengthening of local and national responses. Such networks are important vehicles for protecting the rights of those affected and of providing protection and sanctuary. They enable those affected to enter into partnerships collectively rather than individually and provide the possibility of a continuing organizational form and presence despite the illness and death of their founders and activists.

Social Capacity Building

Social capacity building is the facilitation of collective decision making, collective commitment to a purpose, people' s participation and the building of inclusion within communities and nations. It is a means of building the social capital identified as the neglected component of sustainable human development in the 1994 UNDP/BPPS publication *Sustainable Human Development: From Concept to Operation: A Guide for the Practitioner.*

Social capacity building provides an accountability framework for institutional capacity building and a social framework within which human resource development can contribute to the collective as well as the individual good. It provides a participatory alternative to existing sources of power within communities and nations and a more equitable mechanism for redistribution of access and benefits and for programme and policy development.

The publication *Sustainable Human Development: From Concept to operation: A Guide for the Practitioner* describes development as impossible unless people making up collectivities have a chance of engaging in activities that are meaningful to them, that build on their strength and resources and that increase their well-being, however they define that. This captures an important truth about development but leaves one grappling still with the How questions: how can a development institution like UNDP assist in bringing this about?

This question has been an important focus of HDP's work. For example, to date, virtually all HIV related socio-economic research has been "turn-key' research, the antithesis of local capacity building. HDP has been exploring ways of assisting the strengthening of national capacity to undertake socio-economic research and to use the results in programme and policy research (Senegal, Central African Republic, Kenya, Zambia, Myanmar, Nicaragua and Econet—the Asian and Pacific network of economists).

This initiative is based on the recognition that sources of learning must be local, that for ideas and programmes to take root within communities, they must spring from within, be based on the realities of the lived experiences and must be disseminated and defended from there. Participatory research initiatives support and create local processes of social learning which are an essential pre-condition for social change. These local processes of social learning must, in their turn, be complemented by strengthened national capacities for reflection and analysis so that social learning can be transformed into policy and programmes.

In addition to building local capacities for social learning, the programme aims to create new approaches to the provision of supportive technical assistance. National teams and local communities take direct responsibility for the establishment of research priorities and methodologies and the development of the ethical principles to govern the research. They set the conditions under which technical assistance is provided and determine the areas where their own research competence is in need of supplementation or strengthening. Outside expertise is fitted into local processes of social learning. The programme facilitates the drawing down of assistance from external academic and development sources, national, regional and international. The provision of technical assistance becomes more complicated but more relevant and more sustainable. The processes of learning and skills building occur within, facilitated from without.

Another challenging example of local capacity building and social learning is post-war Rwanda. HIV infection rates before the genocide were amongst the highest in the world, probably around 40 per cent or higher in the urban areas. Both the nature of the slaughter and its social and political aftermath will have significantly increased the rate of infection and spread the virus into rural populations. Now, in the post-war period, no one wants to think or talk about the epidemic. They are haunted and pre-occupied by other things. As is UNDP, in country and at headquarters. No one is listening.

How can a nation address this issue in such circumstances? The approach developed and discussed intensively with the government and civil society was based on creating mechanisms within communities to enable them to begin to talk about betrayal, pain, hatred and fear, in all their causes, supported at the national level by the development of proper governance arrangements, including the re-establishment of the legal system and the creation of national consensus on an appropriate ethical and human rights framework. It also included the provision of the required services and technology—voluntary testing and counselling services, protective technologies, etc., The government of Rwanda has presented the programme to the donors and it has generated interest. This is an important example of a development practice which creates and contributes to social capacity building: the capacity of collectivities to reflect on needs, take collective decisions, resolve conflict and plan for, indeed create the possibility of, a future.

Community and National Mobilization

The fear, the pain and the denial around HIV and AIDS are so great that they are impeding the creation of the processes of social change necessary for communities to be able to support each other and survive the epidemic.

There is a need to better understand how these processes could be stimulated. An analytical framework has been developed and broadly discussed. The right for people to be able to find out whether or not they were infected was identified as a basic but neglected right. Most Africans, and many others in the developing world, cannot find out whether or not they are infected. There are few or no voluntary testing and counselling services available. The existence of such services is essential if the silence which wraps this epidemic and its paralyzing pain and fear is to be broken and a mass movement for social change created.

The quality of people's lives is affected and often determined by how they are perceived and treated by their communities. A UNV programme in Zambia stumbled across an important way of initiating a process of community mobilization. In Livingstone, the UNV team has trained women volunteers from the compounds in basic techniques of home care. These women have few, if any, resources, often not even soap to wash bodily fluids off themselves. They are concerned about the extent of the illness and dying that is happening in their compounds. They can offer little but comfort to those they visit.

Yet the social importance of their care lies in their entering the house of someone suspected or rumoured to be dying of AIDS. Through this gesture of concern and solidarity, fear and rejection are wordlessly challenged and soon the attitudes to those infected begin changing. This gesture is an essential first step in the transition from passivity and fatalism to the mobilization of the communities own resources to care for and comfort their own. This work needs to be followed up and documented as a means whereby other communities can hear and understand the story of these courageous women. HDP has been exploring how processes of community and national mobilization can be initiated in other communities (civil-military alliance, legal and ethical networks, NGO networks, political leaders, etc.,).

Collaboration and UN System Reform

The focus on UN system reform through the establishment of the joint and cosponsored prograrnme on HIV and AIDS has created the conditions for increased collaboration between and amongst the participating agencies. Non-token collaboration presupposes an extensive knowledge of the culture, mission and modus operandi of all collaborators. It requires a great deal of staff resources, good will and mutual respect and a shared understanding of what needs to be done and how to do it. Social capital building is as essential in this collectivity of organizations as it is elsewhere.

The central elements of the HDP's contribution to the process of HIV related institutional reform have focussed on the strengthening of this social capital. It has tried to contribute to creating a common vision and understanding of the nature of the epidemic and of effective responses through discussion and analysis of the overlapping and complementary conceptual frameworks and approaches of the cosponsoring agencies. In this way, it was hoped to build trust and create the necessary preconditions for collaboration. There is a need for a similar drawing together in the wider global community.

The programme was also inward turning in its efforts to strengthen UNDP's ability to contribute to the mission of the new programme through the mainstreaming or integrating of HIV into all aspects of the work of the organization and through the mobilizing of the resident co-ordinator system. UNDP has particular responsibility within the UN system for the management of the resident co-ordinator system and for the training and capacity building of the system.

For country level activities of the new programme to be able to be effective, the UN resident co-ordinator and the country office must have the capacity to undertake those tasks critical to the operation of the country Thematic Working Groups. Strengthening UNDP's capacities in both of these areas will place new demands on HDP specifically and UNDP in general.

The issues raised by the epidemic require an understanding of the structural origins of transmission of the virus and of the epidemic's consequences for societies. As an organization whose purpose is to strengthen the operational activities of the UN system through the instilling of good development practice, UNDP's contributions will be critical to the success of the new programme.

8

Gender, Knowledge and Responsibility

Ms. Elizabeth Reid
UNDP, New York

One of the most striking features of the response to the HIV epidemic to date is how few of the policies and programmes we have developed relate to women's life situations. The daily lives of women and the complex network of relationships and structures which shape them are well known to women and well documented. Despite this, our theories, research agendas, policies and programmes have not been grounded in and informed by these experiences.

This failure to take into account existing knowledge or sources of knowledge, to seek to understand and explore relevant facts and strategies, I wish to call a failure of epistemic responsibility.

Epistemic responsibility is marked by an openness to the acquisition of knowledge and a certain kind of orientation to the world and to one's knowledge-seeking self within it.[1] Certain kinds of knowledge are contingent on experience which itself is mediated by the gender, ethnicity, class, academic discipline and geographic location of the experienced. The value of what is known is dependent upon the alternatives or perspectives considered. If assumptions have not been questioned and alternative sources of knowledge sought, then the knowledge can be faulted. Claims to knowledge can not only be verified. The claimant can be faulted for not having looked enough, for the way he or she comes to knowledge.

The concept of epistemic responsibility has already been used in the context of the HIV epidemic. It has been accepted that those in charge of blood and blood-product services in a number of countries can be held accountable for not exercising their responsibility to know, to take existing knowledge and techniques into account which could have significantly lessened the contamination of the blood supply before HIV test kits were available. Individuals, not only the systems within which they operate, can and should be held responsible for their lack of interest, commitment or sense of urgency.

Responsible knowledge of human experience in general and women's experiences in particular is essential to effective HIV-related research, policy and programme development. Since the cost of ineffectiveness in these areas is an increasing toll of human despair, destitution, illness and death, epistemic responsibility is also a moral imperative.

This article will focus on the urgent need to ensure that women's knowledge and their varying life situations are systematically taken into consideration in the formulation of responses to the epidemic. Clearly, HIV-related research, policies and programmes must be grounded in human experiences, that is, those of men and boys as well as of women and girls. However, to a great extent, the life situations of men and boys have been more accessible to those responsible for developing HIV programmes. The reason for this differential access needs exploring and provides a justification for the specific focus on women's experiences.

The strategies developed in response to this epidemic have been marked by the absence of a grounding in women' s various life situations. The cost has been high. Over 4 million women are infected, ill or dead. The majority of these women are in the age group 10 to 30, with the highest prevalence in the age group 15 to 25. In men, high prevalence occurs ten years later in the age group 25 to 35. In developing country regions, Africa, Asia, Latin America and the Caribbean, the proportion of women to men is almost equal or rapidly becoming so (China 1991). Elsewhere, the proportion is also approaching one to one, although more slowly.

Most women are at risk of infection by sexual transmission. Yet the prevention strategies advocated to prevent sexual transmission have offered women little or no protection from infection.[2] Prevention strategies in general and education (IEC) messages in particular have focused on the reduction of the numbers of sexual partners, fidelity within relationships, safer sexual practices, in particular the use of condoms, and more recently, the treatment of sexually transmitted diseases (STDs). However, these measures are grounded in men's physique, lifestyles and experiences, rather than women's, and should be directed at men. As means by which women can protect themselves from HIV infection, they are inadequate.

Advocating the reduction of sexual partners as a prevention strategy is irrelevant to the lives of the many women who have no sexual partner other than their husband or regular partner. Where women do have multiple sexual partners, this is often a choice forced on them by economic necessity. For as long as this situation and the socio-economic system that gives women few choices for economic independence remain, women will not be able to adopt this strategy.

Neither is the second strategy, faithfulness within relationships, enforceable bv women. It is estimated that between 50 and 80 per cent of all infected women in Africa have had no sexual partners other than their husbands. Having no sexual partners other than their husbands may be under women's control but their husbands' behaviour is not.

Condom usage could be an important prevention strategy for women who cannot negotiate the nature of their relationships. However, condoms are used by men not women, who can only ask for their use, and so the same structural determinant of women's lives as sketched above means that they may have no power to control the use of condoms or to negotiate abstinence.

Advocating the treatment of STDs as a prevention strategy can be faulted in a similar way: it does not adequately reflect the reality of women's lives and is, therefore, based on incomplete knowledge. Rarely are these services provided in culturally acceptable circumstances or by women. They need to be paid for by cash and are usually not easily accessible.

The probability of infection by the virus during unprotected intercourse with an infected partner may be significantly increased when there are lesions, secretions, inflammation or scarification of the genital area. In men's lives, such conditions are usually caused by the presence of sexually transmitted infections and, again, this has determined the research and intervention agendas. But even in men, it is possible that factors such as a lack of circumcision may cause conditions which increase the likelihood of infection or increase infectiousness. This needs to be better understood.

In women, the situation is more complex. Lesions, secretions, inflammations or scarifications may be caused not only by sexually transferred pathogens but as much or more by sexual practices, by cultural practices in particular female infibulation and severe forms of circumcision, by non-infectious inflammatory genital conditions or other common conditions, fistulas, for example, arising from women's reproductive role.

Few data exist indicating the incidence of these latter conditions but they are pervasive. An estimated 84 million women and girls have been infibulated or circumcised worldwide causing conditions of the genital area which could place them at high risk of infection when intercourse takes place with an infected man. More than one million women will suffer disabling illnesses and conditions from reproductive causes this year alone (Jacobsen 1991). These chronic disabilities are higher among poor women everywhere and 99 per cent occur in developing countries. The most common reproductive-related disabilities, particularly in young women, occur during illicit abortions or during childbirth and could certainly increase the efficacy of HIV transmission.

Many of these conditions, including most sexually transmitted infections in women, are treatable conditions.[3] Some will require changes in cultural practices, including child brides, pregnancies in pre-puberty girls or reproductively immature young women, assaultive sexuality, including rape and incest, and other sexual practices causing lesions or inflammation as well as in infibulation and circumcision practices.

The social, sexual and economic subordination of women places them at risk of HIV infection in different ways from men. Strategies must differ when addressed to those put at risk of infection through behaviour or circumstances over which they themselves do or could exercise control and those at risk of infection through behaviour or circumstances over which they cannot exercise control. Prevention strategies have particularly not worked for those young women who become infected immediately they commenced sexual activities. For these young women, too often the circumstances in which they became sexually active allowed them little opportunity for choice or control. The behaviours that are unsafe are determined and controlled by others.

Whilst the social construction of masculinity, reinforced by peer norms and community acceptance, may include a disdain for condoms, along with multiple sexual partners, including during marriage, these are behaviour within men's ability to change. Similarly, there may be behaviours which place women at risk of infection which are within women's ability to change.

For prevention or behaviour change strategies to be able to protect women, they must fit their lives in two directions. They must be based on the contexts in which women's sexuality is expressed and, at the level of the individual, they must be strategies that women can exercise, that are under their control.

There are few possible strategies which fulfil these conditions. The diaphragm plus spermicide may protect both women and men from HIV infection and, when necessary, can be used clandestinely by women. There is clear evidence that it protects men and women from sexually transmitted infections other than HIV (Stein 1990, Alexander 1990, Lancet 1990). However, little or no research has been done in this area. Indeed, little is known about how the virus enters women's genital tract, whether infection occurs at the level of the vagina, the cervix or the uterus or about how infected women infect men. If the virus ascends through the cervix then a diaphragm could give considerable protection but if the virus crosses the vaginal wall, it will be less effective.

The female condom effectively protects both women and men, although it cannot be used without the man's knowledge since it is visible or palpable to the man when in use. However, it has not been aggressively advocated nor means explored to make it more affordable and reusable.

All genital conditions which may facilitate HIV transmission should become a focus of attention. Those conditions which are treatable should be treated. However, the reality of women' s lives forces another question: where? Many women have genital conditions which could be treated but an insignificant number of these women attend STD services. In fact, very few women are ever internally examined throughout their life, despite repeated pregnancies (McNamara, 1990).

The protective strategy most widely adopted by women is that of talking to men and attempting to help them see the importance of protecting themselves from infection and the consequences of not so doing for their families (Mongola, 1991). This is a strategy that may best be undertaken by women collectively. Women individually may feel and be powerless but women together can both change community norms for male behaviour and change that behaviour itself (Reid, 1991).

If these strategies are not available or effective, the only other strategy that may be possible is leaving her partner. This is happening with increasing frequency in seriously affected areas. However, it is only an effective protective strategy if the woman is then able to support herself and her children, where she is able to take them with her, by means other than prostitution.

If there are no strategies which adequately fulfil the two conditions identified above, then this must be clearly acknowledged and the focus of behaviour change strategies be found elsewhere: in men's sexuality and life situations or in communities. Changing men's behaviour and changing community standards to support the required behaviour changes are the most effective way of protecting women and their children from infection.

In summary, then, we have seen that those prevention strategies advocated to date have not emerged from or responded to women's experiences; they were not even based on a responsible knowledge of human experience, of men's as well as women's. Yet all of the facts about women's and men's lives upon which this analysis is based are well documented. The failure to seek them out and use them can be measured in terms of lives lost through this irresponsibility.

Both experience and knowledge are shaped by the gender of the experienced It is, therefore, necessary to find appropriate ways of knowing women' s experiences and the structures that shape them and to develop research priorities, policies and programmes which retain contiguity with these experiences.

What men and women know differs because their experiences are different.[4] A paradigm of this would be experiences relating to biological differences between men and women. Only women can experience pregnancy, childbirth, conditions resulting from childbirth or because of her reproductive capacity. Men cannot be the knowing subject of these experiences. They can be accessible to men only through the stories women tell.

Other areas where difference in gender may preclude the possibilities of common knowledge would include sexuality, parenting, strictly gender specific tasks and, in certain circumstances, some psychological and emotional states. This is not to argue that such knowledge is necessarily or intrinsically gendered but that, where experiences are not available to one gender, the knowledge arising from these experiences is not directly available either. In many of these latter cases, the difference is a matter of cultural, social or historical contingency. Men could be knowledgeable about growing manioc, tending the sick, nurturing children, expressing grief through crying, etc., Where they are not, this can be made a matter of choice not necessity.

The need to draw upon women' s knowledge and to remain in touch with the reality of women's lives will become more critical as the epidemic deepens and increasingly people begin to fall ill and children and the elderly are left without support. As the limits of the capacity of institutionally-based services to cope become clear, community- and family-based services are being advocated (Baldwin and Twigg, 1991). The terms "community-based" or "family-based" systematically obscure the reality that these services are provided by women: caring for the sick, feeding and caring for the elderly and the young, healing the traumatised, easing grief. All the work women do in holding together families, communities and their societies. Furthermore, to the extent that caring for the sick and the dependent means women's exclusion from the labour market, this will reinforce their economic and emotional dependence on men and so their inability to protect themselves from infection.

Policies which build upon and reinforce the assumption or stereotypes of women as carers presume the availability of women to undertake these tasks, and to the extent required, as demand for the services increases with the epidemic. But at the same time that demand will increase for women's labour as nurturers, networkers, copers and carers, the economic and demographic changes induced by high adult mortality rates will increase the demand and the need for women' s participation in productive labour. The complex network of responsibilities and relationships that women exercise in families and communities may be resistant to its collapse into the single function of caring.

These considerations must be taken into account as strategies are sought to satisfy the increasing demand for care and support services and the expressed desire of the infected and the survivors to remain within their communities. We will need to recognize that care must be a collective responsibility of all involved: governments and communities, men and women, families and communities. Each has a role to play in the provision of support services to carers or in direct care provision. These strategies may vary from place to place as the details of women's lives, and men' s, vary but the responsibility for them must be collectively held and exercised for us to survive the epidemic.

It follows from this analysis that women experience and know things that men do not experience or know. The same is true for men. It also follows that it is impossible to understand the epidemic without drawing or women's knowledge and experience. We must free ourselves from the limited and limiting perspective of a particular gender, class or race.

Unfortunately, such a limited and limiting perspective has dominated the HIV research and programme agendas, irrespective of discipline: epidemiology, clinical research and trials, intervention design, biological research, behavioural research, economics and so on (WHO/GPA/91.2, Stein 1990, for example)[5]. Women have been missing from clinical trials; they have been tested without consent and denied access to the results; they have not been informed that their husbands are infected; their clinical conditions have not been included in case definitions or research priorities; stereotypes of prostitutes or wives have closed off possibilities of understanding. The primary focus of attention was elsewhere. The lack of awareness or acceptance that experience is gendered has left too many women without the possibility of knowledge of their infection status, without the capacity to plan for their children's future, with increased responsibilities and with a greatly increased chance of dying.

Because most HIV research touches experiences that are gender specific —sexuality, oppression, reproduction, labour, domestic responsibilities, etc., — it must remain continually in touch with women's lives, experiences and knowledge as well as with men's. This will require that a critical intelligence be brought to bear on it. A serious constraint to this is that women are more aware than men that experience and knowledge are gendered,[6] that social, political, moral research, policy, programme and other agendas relating to all facets of their life are drawn up on the basis of men's experiences. Daily reminders of this are rare for men, for many quite absent. As a result, the relevance of women's perspectives may not be realised by those developing responses to the epidemic and gender specificity not seen as critical to the value of the outcome. There is not a felt need to know.

This lack of a felt need to know can lead to a failure to seek further in the face of dissonant facts, to set aside stereotypes and to search to know. Let us turn to a well and long known fact, already mentioned, which should be deeply disturbing. It has been noted above that the prevalence of HIV infection is highest in young women aged 15 to 25 but peaks in men ten years later in the 25 to 35 age group. This is a consistently different pattern between women and men. It was known as early as 1986 in the earliest data sets from the epidemic, the first 500 diagnosed AIDS cases in Kinshasa. The pattern is the same in recent data sets from Uganda where the epidemic has significantly deepened and from Thailand where the epidemic is still recent.'.

However, only rarely in the literature have the possible causes of this disturbing difference been explored. Decosas and Pedneault (1991) argue that this difference is due to the fact that sexual partnerships are usually formed between older men and younger women. This is doubtlessly a contributing factor but cannot be the complete explanation, if only because it is true for women in almost all age groups and so cannot explain the striking difference in infection rates in young women compared to older pre-menopausal women.

Let us rephrase the question in order to highlight it: Why do young women (15-25) have such significantly higher rates of HIV infection than, for example, young men in the same age group? Both groups are sexually active; but young men more so than young women (United Nations, 1989). Both groups have sexually transmitted infections; but young men more than young women. Young women often have different sexually transmitted infections from young men. Both older men and young men form sexual partnerships with the women who are sexually active in this young age group. These facts are not adequate to explain why the rate of infection in young women is so steep at the onset of sexual activity and so high. The question can again be rephrased: why are more young women infected than older pre-menopausal women [8]. In one South African study, 50 per cent of all infected women were aged 15-19 years, were young women with limited sexual experience, and had significantly higher rates of infection than young men of the same age and women in all other age groups (O'Farrell and Windsor, 1991). Similar patterns are found in a study of Rakai district in rural Uganda (Wawer *et al.* 1991; Cohen, 1992).

In this case, the principle of epistemic responsibility would require urgent and high priority be given to the identification of possible determining causes of this high infection rate in young women. But this has not happened to date. Frequency of sexual intercourse with infected men is insufficient to explain the data.

Thus, it is highly probable that the condition of the genital tract in young women significantly increases the likelihood of transmission whenever unprotected sexual contact occurs. A number of possible hypotheses come to mind. The efficacy of HIV transmission to young women may be increased by.

(a) the sexually transmitted infections found in young women and/or other infections of their genital area;
(b) cervical ectopy in young sexually active women;
(c) hormonal changes at the onset of menstruation and during the menstrual cycle;
(d) the changes in the anatomy of the genital tract as young women reach puberty; and
(e) the immaturity of the genital tract in post-puberty young women.

The biology of the female genital tract remains poorly understood. We know more about the cellular structure of lungs, for example, or about the increased protection from HIV infection offered by an intact genital mucosa in monkeys (Miller and Gardner, 1991, for example). In young women, the explanation for their shocking rates of infection may be a combination of some or all of these or other factors. The research agenda is in urgent need of realignment.

Since in so many facets of the HIV epidemic experiences are gender specific, it must become part of responsible epistemic and programme practice to move on from the constraints of single gender knowledge — for both men and women — to an approach that is grounded in human experience. This is only possible if gender specific experience and knowledge can be made accessible to others and if how to let experience shape and reshape theory and practice can be learnt.

Women's gender specific experiences and knowledge can be accessible in a number of ways: by ensuring that women as well as men shape and determine the agendas, through first person narratives or through the devolution of responsibility for interventions to women and their communities.

First person narratives provide access which can be subtle and various. Some stories from the epidemic are now being told, a few by women (Rieder and Ruppelt, 1988; Willmore and Roy, 1989; Reid, 1990; UNDP, 1992). Noerine Kaleeba's moving story (1991) presents the experienced in the complex, interrelated way life usually asserts itself. First person narratives can bring to light different perspectives, different points of view and so make them accessible across gender.

Since, as discussed above, women are more aware of the dynamics of gender, the way these effect the epidemic emerge more clearly in their narratives. It is clear to them that one can understand life situations—being infected, caring for someone infected, for example—only if gender roles and relationships are taken into account. These narratives both present and interpret the relationship between the individual and society and the dynamics of power between women and men. They provide glimpses into men's lives as well as their own and relate individual agency to social and economic structures.

First person narratives increase understanding. Their truth or falsity or the justification of their knowledge claims will be determined in the same way as first person narratives in general: in their closeness of fit to reality and the extent of agreement with other stories. However, listening to and interpreting such narratives, whether as stories, on film or in consultations, is an acquired capacity. The interpreter must be sensitive to the narrator's purposes in telling her story. Interpretation demands a profound respect for the narrator, for what she says and for the lives from which the stories are drawn.

Narratives can identify new research and programme needs. A simple example: stories told by women of the discrimination and rejection that happened to them when a newborn child was diagnosed with HIV has led to the proposal that parents be counselled, informed and tested together (Willmore and Ray, 1990).

Patterns and structural factors will emerge as more women's voices are heard. The less these voices are muted or silenced, the more they will speak with authority and relevance, even when the knowledge and experiences recounted cut across the grain of received knowledge. Women know the nature and causes of their lives.

A critical strategy of this epidemic will be to ensure that women's perceptions, experiences and capacities are able to be expressed, valued, understood and acted upon. In so doing, the discontinuity between HIV—related experiences and HIV-related research and programmes will be lessened.

Narratives, however, do not capture systems of relationships which affect individuals but whose locus is beyond the individual and her realm of vision. The relationships between poverty and her infection status may form a critical part of her narrative but the relationships between structural adjustment programmes, poverty and the tragedy of being infected may not. Narratives need to be complemented by system level analyses. A full understanding of the nature and impact of the epidemic requires both kinds of analysis.

The second way in which women's gender specific knowledge can be accessible is through devolving responsibility for programme development and delivery to women. If solutions are to be found for men' s refusal to protect themselves and others, for women' s powerlessness to prevent themselves from becoming infected, bring women together to seek them (Willmore and Ray, 1990; Mongola, 1991). The strategies so decided upon may or may not integrally involve men. We may believe that this is essential but it is not ours to decide. If there is a collective responsibility for the care of people unable to survive independently, bring communities, women and men, together with governments to work out how it can be exercised. Women's knowledge and experiences are essential to the development of effective solutions.

Once it is recognised that responsible knowledge of human experiences in general and women' s experiences in particular is essential to developing effective responses to the epidemic and once people are more at ease and more skilled at acquiring or expressing that knowledge, we will be in a position to face the coming decades with some hope. We will then be able to develop programmes grounded in human experience to address the three central programming areas of the epidemic: changing attitudes and behaviour, caring for the affected and maintaining the social and economic infrastructure of seriously affected communities and countries.

NOTES

1. I am indebted to Professor Lorraine Code (1988) for an elaboration of the concept of epistemic responsibility and its relevance as a means of measuring the adequacy of theories.
2. This critique is more fully elaborated in Reid 1991 and Hamblin and Reid 1991. See also Worth 1989, Stein 1990 and Carovano 1991.
3. For many sexually transmitted infections in women, the problem is one of diagnosis rather than treatment.
4. This is not to argue that all women or all men know these aspects of their lives in the same way. It is a point about the lack of such experience and direct knowledge across gender.
5. There are three contributing factors. Firstly, that the early research populations were infected men, secondly, that male researchers have predominated in all disciplines and, thirdly, because of the severe inequalities of wealth between the developed and developing worlds, all early research populations were drawn from developed countries. It should be remembered that there were more infected women than gay men or men with haemophilia in the world at every stage of the epidemic.
6. Professor Anne Jacobson, University of Houston, Texas, drew to my attention that men may have to be reminded to worry about their daughters. It seems harder for men to believe that there is a perspective on the world different from theirs. I am indebted to Professor Jacobson for assisting in clarifying the conceptual issues in this paper.
7. A fuller discussion of these data sets can be found in the Reading the Data module of the UNDP training material on HIV and Development.

See also, on Uganda, Cohen 1992.

8. There is some evidence that the efficacy of transmission is also high in post-menopausal women, that is, that when post-menopausal women have unprotected intercourse with infected men, the likelihood of their becoming infected is quite high.

REFERENCES

Alexander, Nancy J. "Sexual transmission of human immunodeficiency virus: virus entry into the male and female genital tract." *Fertility and Sterility,* Vol. 54, No. 1: 1-18, 1990.

Baldwin, Sally and Julia Twigg. "Women and Community Care - reflections on a debate." In Mavis Maclean and Dulie Groves (eds.) *Women's Issues in Social Policy,* Routledge, London, 1991.

Bassett, Mary and Marvellous Mhloyi. "Women and AIDS in Zimbabwe: The Making of an Epidemic." *International Journal of Health Services,* 21,1, 127-130, 1991.

Carovano, Kathryn. "More Than Mothers and Whores: Redefining the AIDS Prevention Needs of Women." *International Journal of Health Services,* 21:1, pp. 131-142, 1991.

Chin, James L. "The Increasing Impact of the HIV/AIDS Pandemic on Women and Children." Paper presented at the APHA meeting, Atlanta, November, 1991.

Code, Lorraine. "Experience, Knowledge and Responsibility." In Griffiths, Morwenna and Margaret Whitford (eds.) *Feminist Perspectives in Philosophy.* Indiana University Press, 1988.

Cohen, Desmond. "AIDS in Uganda." Report on a Programming Mission for UNDP Fifth Cycle Support to Uganda, 1992.

Decosas, Josef and Violette Pedneault. "The Demographic AIDS Trap for Women in Africa." Paper presented at the VII International Conference on AIDS, Florence, 1991.

Hamblin, Julie and Elizabeth Reid. "Women, the HIV Epidemic and Human Rights." Paper prepared for International Workshop on AIDS: A Question of Rights and Humanity, The Hague, May 1991.

Jacobson, Jodi. *Women's Reproductive Health: The Silent Emergency.* Worldwatch Paper 102, June 1991.

Kaleeba, Noerine with Sunanda Ray and Brigid Willmore. *We Miss You All.* Women and AIDS Support Network. Harare, 1991.

Lancet Editorial. "Barriers and Boundaries". Lancet 335: 1497-8, 1990.

McNamara, Regina. "Female Genital Health and the Risk of HIV Transmission." Literature review commissioned by UNDP, 1991.

Miller, Christopher and Murray Gardner. "AIDS and Mucosal Immunity: Usefulness of the SIV Macaque Model of Genital Mucosal Transmission." *Journal of Acquired Immune Deficiency Syndromes;* 4:1169-1192, 1991.

Mongola, Margaret. Interview for *Reflections on the Impact of the HIV Epidemic,* 1991. Forthcoming UNDP publication.

O'Farrell, Nigel and Isobel Windsor. "Sexual Behaviour in HIV-1 Seropositive

Zulu Men and Women in Durban, South Africa." Letter to the Editor, *Journal of Acquired Immune DeficiencY Syndromes,* 4:1258-59, 1991.

Reid, Elizabeth. "Placing Women at the Centre of the Analysis" in *Women and AIDS: Strategies for the Future.* Canadian International Development Agency, 1991.

Reid, Elizabeth. "Two Voices". *World Health,* WHO Geneva 1990.

Rieder, Ines and Patricia Ruppelt. *AIDS: The Women.* CLEIS Press. San Francisco, 1988.

Sabatier, Renee. "Women and AIDS," in *Women and AIDS: Strategies for the Future.* Canadian International Development Agency, 1991.

Stein, Zena. "HIV Prevention: The Need for Methods Women Can Use." *American Journal of Public Health;* 80:460-462, 1990.

United Nations. *Adolescent Reproductive Behaviour.* New York, 1989.

United Nations Development Programme (UNDP). Report of the Informal Consultation on Behaviour Change. Dakar, 1991. Forthcoming.

Willmore, Brigid and Sunanda Ray. *AIDS: An Issue for Every Woman.* Proceedings of the Women and AIDS Support Network Conference. Harare, 1989.

World Health Organization. Global Programme on AIDS. *Report of the Meeting on Research Priorities Relating to Women and HIV/AIDS.* GPA/DIR/91.2. Geneva, 1991.

Wawer, Maria J., David Serwadda, Stanley D. Musgrave et al. "Dynamics of the spread of HIV-1 infection in a rural district of Uganda." *British Medical Journal,* 303: 1303-6, 1991.

Worth, Dooley. "Sexual Decision-Making and AIDS: Why Condom Promotion Among Vulnerable Women is Likely to Fail". *Studies in Family Planning,* 20:6 November/December 1989.

9

HIV and the Challenges Facing by Men

Ms. Kathryn Carovano
The University of Michigan

INTRODUCTION

Since the beginning of the HIV epidemic, scores of men have been directly and indirectly affected by HIV. As of 1 January 1996, the Global AIDS Policy Coalition estimates that men represented 59 per cent of the projected 20.5 million HIV infected adults around the world, and their numbers continue to grow. The large majority of all people living with HIV (21.4 million; 92 per cent) are from the developing world, and men are no exception. Of the approximately 2.5 million men infected with the virus between January and December 1995, some 95 per cent were from the developing world.[1]

The Global AIDS Policy Coalition projects that by the year 2000, there will be a minimum of 38 million adults living with HIV, and possibly as many as 110 million.[2] New infections among men during 1993 were estimated at 139.73 per 100,000, compared to 99.15 new infections for every 100,000 women.[3] Sexual transmission is currently held to be responsible for 86 per cent of all HIV infections, and while men with HIV tend to be older than the women infected, they are still primarily young adults at the prime of their lives. Finally, while many men are coping with being infected with HIV, there are even more who are experiencing losses due to HIV-related illness and death among their family, friends and colleagues.

Against this backdrop, it is reasonable to wonder why, more than a decade into the epidemic, we feel it important to focus this Issues Paper on the challenges that HIV poses to men. In its simplest form, the answer is that we must examine HIV from every angle, ignoring none in order to improve our capacity to respond to the epidemic. Every day, more and more people are becoming infected with HIV, caring for family and friends who are suffering, and grieving the passing of those they have loved. While substantial efforts to respond are being made around the world, the epidemic continues to grow and to have a devastating impact on the lives of far too many of us. The need for more effective strategies to respond to HIV demands that we rethink old issues, re-examine previous assumptions, and leave no questions unasked. Michael Helquist, an expert in HIV communication based in San Francisco points out, "[h]ow we think about men—and women—affects how we try to fight AIDS."[4]

Men have always been a part of the HIV "problem", and they have played vital roles in the search for an effective response. Examples of their involvement includes speaking out as individuals livine with HIV, providing care to familv and friends, working as professional researchers, educators and care providers, and assisting in the development of local, national and global programmes and policies to respond to the growing epidemic. However, there has been no systematic examination of men's multiple roles in the epidemic, the many factors that influence them, as well as the obstacles that prevent more men from becoming involved. While many men have responded to HIV with a sense of urgency, responsibility, and compassion, they often appear to be the exceptions rather than the norm in their communities or professions.

At an individual level, there are many men who continue to engage in behaviours that place them and others at increased risk for HIV. Their actions may reflect a lack of awareness or understanding, or simply human frailty in the face of the immensely difficult task of maintaining safer sexual behaviours over time. Yet there are many others whose actions — or lack of action—can only be considered irresponsible, selfish and even cruel. These men do not heeds the warnings, do not see themselves as responsible, or seem to simply care more about their own pleasure than the risk their actions pose to themselves and others. In the extreme, they are the men who lie to their partners about their sexual history and even their HiV status, sexually exploit those with less power, and use sex as a form of violence against women, children and other men.

In many communities, the broader response to HIV has divided the infected from the uninfected, perpetuated stigmas, and aggravated the suffering of people living with the virus. Throughout the world, people have been tested for HIV against their will, dismissed from jobs, kept out of schools, incarcerated, abandoned by their families, denied medical care, beaten and killed in reaction to HIV. Because men hold most positions of power in families and communities, they must also bear the greater part of the responsibility for these misguided responses.

And finally, in nearly every region of the world, national and international governmental bodies have failed to act in a timely and effective manners. Governrnents—male dominated in nearly every country in the world—continue to bar admission to those with HIV infection, test suspect populations without consent, and simply refuse to acknowledge that those affected "matter"[5] and that something needs to be done. Many international agencies also continue to let the politics of power define their agenda and their actions, impeding the development of effective and sustainable local responses to HIV.

With this bleak scenario in mind, it is imperative to ask why this is so and what men—together with women—can do to make it different. The following discussion will focus on three primary areas of concern: HIV-related behaviour and behaviour change, illness and care, and death and its impact on survivors. The discussion in each area will attempt to illuminate ways in which men in different circumstances and different parts of the world are responding to these challenges. It will also focus on obstacles to an improved response and ways to assist men in the effort to face the challenges of HIV. The goal of the paper is to serve as a starting point for further discussion and understanding of the challenges that HIV poses to men and, hopefully, expand the capacity to respond.

HIV-Related Behaviour and Behaviour Change

We believe that individuals and whole communities have the inherent capacity to change attitudes and behaviours... We recognize that behaviour change at the individual and community level in the present HIV epidemic is a complex and on-going process.... Our experience as affected and infected individuals proves that behaviour change is possible. We believe that behaviour change is the most essential strategy in overcoming the HIV epidemic.[6]

Around the world, many men and women have made dramatic changes in their behaviour and their lives in response to the need to protect themselves and those they love from HIV, as well as to assist those infected to live full and meaningful lives. As HIV has spread across the globe, there has been a counter wave of change in attitudes and practices that has been a source of hope for all who struggle in the face of this epidemic. Yet the virus continues to spread, in large part because many people continue to hold views and engage in behaviours that facilitate its transmission. Hence, while positive changes are occurring, they are not enough.

Given that nearly 90 per cent of HIV infection is attributed to sexual transmission, conditions, norms and practices that facilitate the sexual spread of the virus must be the central focus. HIV is transmitted sexually through unprotected sexual intercourse—anal, vaginal, and oral. Because this is known, behaviours to eliminate or reduce the likelihood of acquiring HIV infection have been fairly easy to identify. People have the options of not having sex, having unprotected sex with only one other uninfected, faithful partner, or engaging in non-penetrative or protected sex (e.g., sex with a condom, dental dam, or female condom). Individuals may choose strategies involving some combination of these behaviours, either concurrently or consecutively, to meet diverse or changing needs.

Early efforts to promote behaviour change in response to HIV focused almost exclusively on identified "high-risk groups." In recent years, the focus has broadened somewhat including increased attention to understand and support change among women. While this expanded focus has been necessary and significant, it has still ignored the development of targeted efforts for most men.[7]

Because men in most cultures dominate decision-making and have greater independent control over sexual relations, it is imperative that efforts to respond to the epidemic and promote behaviour change place greater emphasis on men. As a first step, a better understanding is needed of the process of HIV-related behaviour change among men and the factors that motivate their sexual behaviour, both unsafe and safe.

There are a number of models of health behaviour that provide a foundation for understanding the process of change. All start from the premise that individuals can, and do make decisions about their behaviour and, at least potentially, have the capacity to translate those decisions into action. These decisions and subsequent behaviours are recognized as being influenced by various factors or determinants. Some are considered to be individual or internal (e.g., a person's perception of risk, their view of the costs and benefits associated with changing their behaviour, and their perception of their ability to change), while others are defined as external or societal (e.g., the quality and cost of a product or service, social norms that define expected and appropriate behaviour, laws and regulations).[8]

Behavioural theory recognizes that the determinants of safe and unsafe sexual behaviour will vary by age, culture, relationship status, sexual orientation and general life circumstances. Thc factors that motivate a young man to have safe sex with his fiancee may be quite different from those that motivate an older, married man to do so with a female sex worker, or a school-age boy to do so with a male friend. Likewise, the factors that influence a man's behaviours in a traditional African community will in some ways differ and in some ways potentially be very similar, to those that influence an urban European or Asian man. Adopting new sexual practices and sustaining them consistently over a lifetime are also understood to be distinct behaviours posing unique challenges.

While these theories provide a basis for understanding health behaviour and the process of behaviour change, they seem to fall short when attempting to explain or predict sexual attitudes and behaviours.[9] "As Damien Rwegera, a Rwandan respondent, noted, sex is "the ultimate coded and intimate exercise...."[10] Men and women engage in sexual relations for an array of reasons that range from the pursuit of pleasure, desire for intimacy, expression of love, definition of self, procreation, domination, violence, or any combination of the above, as well as others. How people relate sexually may be linked to self-esteem, self-respect, respect for others, hope, joy and pain. In different contexts, sex is viewed as a commodity, a right, or a biological imperative; it is clearly not determined fully by rational decision-making.

Health behaviour theory is limited by its focus on the individual. In fact, the factors influencing sexual decisions and behaviours involve a complex process that generally involves two people, not just one. How the threat of HIV impacts on people's behaviour is even more complex. It forces people to assess the implications of their own and their partners' past and current behaviours, as well as long-held beliefs, hopes and fears and, ultimately, it forces them to talk about these issues with their sexual partners.

Adopting new behaviours in the face of HIV is extremely difficult. To stay free of infection, individuals must adopt effective strategies and apply them consistently in some form over a lifetime: occasionally failing is only human. As Allan Berube. a historian from San Francisco, writes,

> The tragedy of AIDS. ..... is that so many people are dying random deaths for no other reason than that they took the kinds of risks we all take to lead meaningful lives.'[11]

We must keep this reality in mind as we grapple with the challenge of developing effective behaviour change strategies.

Sex and What it Means to Men

Men who responded to the UNDP request for information provided a number of insights into the meaning of sex in men's lives and the reasons why men engage in sexual relations, both safe and unsafe. There are few surprises, but their input contributes to an understanding of what motivates men to have sex, and factors that might facilitate—or obstruct—HIV-related behaviour change.

Among respondents, sex was noted as being important to men for a variety of reasons. It was mentioned in relation to the desire to love and be loved, connect with others, establish a family and perpetuate lineage, or satisfy a physical or biological need. Sexual relations were also identified as a source of pleasure, emotional bonding, and a means of expressing power, adulthood and "personhood." Respondents also noted that while sex is a commodity for some men, for those who engage in sex for pay, it is part of a strategy to survive.

As would be expected, men noted that sex and reasons for having sex change with stage of life and relationship status. Young, single men tend to have more partners and to view sex as a rite of passage, a way to establish their masculinity, a means of building self-esteem, and a process of exploration. A 24-year old respondent from the U.S. observed of himself and his peers, "We want to explore, we are energetic, and being male, we want to have sex—a lot."[12] In Zimbabwe, researchers found that "boys clearly feel that sexual experience is something of which to be proud. .... to have sex is to be a hero among one's peers."[13] A number of men from diverse cultural backgrounds commented on peer pressure among young men to "keep up" by having sex at an early age and with many partners.

Among older men and those in established relationships, sex was more often linked to the expression of love and intimacy and the desire to procreate and sustain their lineage. Damien Rwegera asserted that one of the most important things in his life is

> to participate in the perpetuation of the human species by siring and bringing up children. .... who are part of a family lineage which descends from a common ancestor and is prolonged from generation to generation. [14]

Other men also noted the continued importance of sex among older men as a means of expressing masculinity and virility. While none of the respondents mentioned it the global pattern of older men having sex with younger women, both consensually and otherwise, may also be tied to issues of prowess and control. Mohamed Osman of Somalia argued that for some older men, success in sexual relations "involves the honour and pride of men." He went on to note that "success" is defined by one's sexual performance, the ability of a man to "show his virility" and "not feel impotent."'[15]

While many respondents noted that the sexual behaviours of some men are changing in response to HIV an AIDS, nearly all felt that changes were not sufficiently widespread or rapid enough, particularly among heterosexual men. The adoption of safer sexual practices was noted by respondents to be frequently tied to the experience of knowing someone infected or affected by HIV. Concern for family members was also a significant motivating factor. Respondents gave more varied reasons for why they think more men are not adopting safer behaviours. They mentioned lack of awareness of HIV, denial of personal risk, fatalism, absence of supportive norms, perceived protection provided bit marriage or a stable relationship, the negative implications of safe sex on intimacy and trust, as well as lack of concern for the effect of one's behaviour on one's partner. Gaining a deeper understanding of why some men are changing gand why others are not is fundamental to addressing the challenge of behaviour change among men.

Implications for Behaviour Change

If uninformed, unskilled, unmotivated, unsupported or simply lacking access to "protection", men will still have sex and, more often than not, it is likely to be penetrative and unprotected. A simple truth is that it is natural to have unprotected sex. This is a fundamental barrier to the adoption of safe sexual practices, but it is important to go beyond it to understand why so many men continue to engage in unsafe sex.

A fundamental premise of most HIV prevention efforts is that understanding the risk posed by HIV and the means of protecting oneself are critical foundations for behaviour change. One respondent, sharing his personal experience, noted that:

> When I had [unprotected sex], I wasn't thinking about what sorts of infections I could get. .... I didn't even have enough information to be able to judge those things. .... it wasn't as if [protected sex] was something that I thought I should be doing and didn't.[16]

This testimony from a college educated man in the United States, reflecting on his awareness of HIV in the late 1980's, is a shocking reminder of how little even those individuals who would be expected to have access to accurate information may actually know.

Despite the efforts of HIV-related education throughout the world, numerous respondents noted that lack of accurate information continues to be a fundamental barrier to behaviour change for many men, especially in the developing world. Because men. (rather than women) generally have greater access to information about sex and assume the more assertive and directive role in sexual decision-making, targeted efforts are needed to provide diverse populations of men with information about HIV transmission and prevention.

Knowledge alone, however, is not enough to influence

behaviour. Health educators recognize that acquiring skills—or perceived skills—to correctly use condoms, say "no" to sex, or negotiate safer behaviours with a partner is also necessary for behaviour change. Studies among men in the Caribbean found that condom skills are relatively easy to teach and skill development can have a positive impact on behaviour.[17] The transfer of negotiation skills has been found to be considerably more complex.[18]

Efforts to transmit information, knowledge and skills are, in essence, designed to change the internal factors that affect behaviour, not the context in which they occur. Yet sex—and safer sex—is inextricably linked to the social and cultural context in which the behaviour takes place. Many of the reasons suggested by respondents to explain men's behaviours reflect social norms related to gender, relationships, power, and sex. Around the world, these norms have been identified as significant determinants of safe and unsafe behaviours, yet there is growing evidence that they can and do change."[19]

In many culture, norms of masculinity encourage men to deny, tear, doubts and any feelings of vulnerability. In some instances, men are urged to demonstrate their manhood by taking risks. Noting the attitudes of homeless boys living on the streets of Rio de Janeiro, Patrick Larvie writes, "the association between heterosexual masculinity and health was very clear: 'real men' do not get sick and do not need to worry about getting sexually transmitted diseases."[20] Denial of vulnerability is a powerful deterrent to implementing behaviour change; as long as men are unable or unwilling to admit that HIV could reach them, they are unlikely to have the motivation needed to change.

As noted by respondents from many cultures, norms of masculinity also encourage men to view sex as a form of conquest and expression of male prowess. According to Ernesto Guerrero of the Dominican Republic, "[i]n some regions, men have been educated under the premise that having many girlfriends (women) is the best symbol of virility and power." At its extreme, sex can become an act of violence with domination or humiliation the apparent goals. Whenever these are primary reasons for engaging in sex, respect for one's partner can be expected to be absent. Without respect, a concern for a partner's health or the health of future children, will have little impact on the behaviour of men.

In many cultures, societal norms (and human physiology) permit men to take little responsibility for the consequences of their sexual behaviour. Generally, women bear the burden of responsibility for pregnancy, often even where they are the result of rape. Because a man cannot be easily linked to his offspring — including a man with HIV — it remains possible for men to deny paternity and any responsibility. A European respondent asserted that in order for behaviour change efforts to succeed, "[w]e need to hammer in [to men] their responsibility for their dependents and themselves."[21]As it is, there are many reports of women being blamed for bringing HIV into a family (generally because their HIV status is identified first, through the illness of a child), in spite of the fact that the socially sanctioned behaviours of their male partners were more likely to have been the cause of the initial infection.

Commenting on these issues, Bob Connell notes:

> In 'Western' culture, the most honoured form of masculinity involves being authoritative. decisive, controlling other people, exerting power. This affects heterosexual relationships in damaging ways. Where sexual conquest is the main goal, a pattern of sexuality can be created where women are repeatedly at risk and have limited resources to resist this.... luntil dominant forms of masculinity are challenged and economic power shifts towards women, this isn't likely to end.[22]

This discussion offers some insights into men's sexual behaviour, and perhaps more than anything. points to its complexity and the need for a greater understanding of how men behave sexually and why.

The Impact of Development on Behaviour

While norms can have an impact on behaviour, so too can their absence. Discussing the challenges facing gay men in Poland, one respondent noted that "there is no model of how to organize their sex lives..."[23] and that this is a factor contributing to men having unsafe sex. This observation may be equally valid for men in a society undergoing a rapid transition, a situation common to many parts of the developing world. If the lifestyle of their parents and grandparent is no longer viable, men lack models of how to organize relationships and other aspects of the sexual life. Regardless of its root cause—whether rapidly changing social mores or deteriorating socio-economic conditions—the absence of viable models is likely to influence men's behaviour.

In many societies undergoing periods of transition, war or economic crisis, men are often forced to travel to other towns or countries in search of work. Male mobility and migration disrupt traditional family relations and influence male sexual behaviours in many parts of the world. One of the primary reasons given by respondents for engaging in sexual relations outside of marriage was physical separation from a spouse, and simple loneliness, both physical and emotional. Research on migrant workers who travel from Lesotho to South Africa, often for years at a time, found that "sex often becomes a source of escape and solace" from what i otherwise a lonely, harsh existence.[24] As Robert Mugemana noted, in Kenya, "[f]or men who leave their wives behind in the rural areas while they pursue employment in the cities, brothels offer an inexpensive source of sexual activity...."[25]

On the flip side of this equation are the men and boys who enter the sex industry to survive. While their numbers are small relative to the women and girls involved in commercial sex work, male sex workers enter this work for similar reasons. K.M Subhan, a Bangladesh respondent, observed that

> men and women are flocking to the cities in search of livelihood, mostly leaving their families behind...There are thousands and thousands of such homeless and jobless women and men who live on the pavements [who] take part in part-time prostitution for just a meal or so. [26]

Similar to migrant workers and men in the military, the men and boys involved in prostitution constitute a segment of the population at increased likelihood of exposing themselves to HTV as a result of their status and consequent behaviour.

Finally, another aspect of development that is likely to affect men's attitudes and behaviours is the changing status of women in many societies, and the consequent changes in relations between women and men. As more women become educated, employed and independent, men may feel that they are losing power. Research on domestic violence in Papua New Guinea revealed that many men saw the growing independence of their wives as a threat. "Men felt both excluded from development assistance efforts and resentful of their loss of dominance feelings that translated into increased domestic violence."[27] Sensitive to the potential for a similar backlash effect, Brendan Bain, a respondent from Jamaica, asserts that behaviour change efforts must be careful not to alienate men and suggests that the success of behaviour change programmes will depend partly on "the degree of care which is taken to preserve male identity and men's feelings of self-worth."[28] In a similar vein, Damien Rwegera from Rwanda asserts that,

> Behaviour change means change in culture, approach and community organization. ... Men must realize that this is a challenge to be met and managed. .... HIV infection will surely upset many commonly accepted values. ... Men must realize this and prepare themselves, not for a retreat, but for an advance into human civilization.[29]

While much of the preceding discussion focuses on why men are likely or unlikely to be motivated to adopt safer sexual behaviours, they must also have the capacity to change. Many of us working on issues related to women and HIV, have asserted that men have the power to change their sexual behaviour—something women often lack. Yet, admittedly, this argument overgeneralizes and oversimplifies the diverse experiences of men. Men—and boys—who engage in sex in exchange for money or goods often have little power in encounters with older, stronger, wealthier men. Other men may lack the power or self-esteem to reject norms and behaviours that are proscribed, in essence, by other men. For many men, the capacity to choose safer sex may be circumscribed in myriad ways depending on the socio-economic circumstances of their lives. Poverty is a recognized barrier to good health. Limited economic resources can put condoms and other services out of reach and the inability to meet basic needs may impede a focus beyond the most immediate future. Illiteracy limits access to information. Lack of intimacy, lack of security and lack of hope may all limit one's capacity to respond to the threat of HIV. The empowerment of men is seldom a topic of discussion, but needs to be considered in the effort to meet the dual challenges of HIV and development.

HIV-Related Illness and Care

The prevention of HIV and the provision of care and support for those affected are overlapping and interrelated issues. Efforts to encourage behaviour change are most effective when they incorporate people living with HIV and those directly affected by the epidemic. For men. who are traditionally less involved in the provision of care. this has significant implications.

Clearly, there are many men — and women — who have responded to those living with HIV and AIDS with compassion and concern. Among respondents who have experienced HIV related illness among their family and friends, feelings shared included deep sadness, compassion frustration, helplessness, anger, fear, and admiration for the courage and perseverance of those infected. While none of these responses are unique to men, some respondents identified factors that may affect how men in particular experience these emotions. Upon learning that his younger sister was HIV infected, Omari Kokole a Ugandan man, noted that he told her "not to worry too much and encouraged her to continue with her education. Reflecting back on that experience after he was tested for HIV, Kokole noted that "despite my external calm, I was deeply shaken.... Rather than pretend not to be worried and sad, I should have helped her to confront and deal with these very painful and unavoidable emotions."[30] While responding to news of the infection of a loved one is difficult for any person, social norms that define an "appropriate" male response may make it even harder for men to show their support and concern.

Men have been deeply affected by HIV-related illness among those they love, yet a number of respondents acknowledged that "men have a bad reputation when it comes to the topic of their support for the sick."[31] Caring for the sick is seen as women's work in most cultures, yet few things take more courage than caring for a loved one who is dying. While many men have provided care in both professional and familial roles, the burden of care for those with HIV in most societies is still being born largely by women. Robert Mugemana from Kenya has written,

> [w]hen a husband becomes ill, it is the woman who nurses him. When a child is ill, it is the woman who nurses it. But when a woman is ill, she nurses herself.[32]

The most notable exception to this pattern has been the response of gay men, initially in the U. S. and Europe, and now in numerous developing countries. As Bob Connell points out, "[h] eterosexual men have a great deal to learn from homosexual men in 'Western' countries. It is the gay communities that have made an immense effort at caring for people living with AIDS...."[33] This observation applies to many gay communities in the "non-Western" and developing world as well.

Even as some men have responded by providing care and support to people living with HIV, in much of the world, blaming and stigmatization have characterized the responses of far too many individuals, communities and governments. Respondents from every region noted the effects of this on the experiences of those living with HIV, as well as on individual and community level efforts to confront the epidemic. Mohamed Osman of Somalia noted that, "[t]he ones affected by [HIV] feel humiliated, discriminated against and abandoned, even by their closest family members, by the doctors, and by the society."[34] According to Godfrey Sealy, a Trinidadian man, "the threat of public disclosure is more frightening than the disease itself." This fear leads many men with HIV disease to deny the nature of their illness, and many friends to void visiting those hospitalized for fear of being associated with the disease.[35]

Fear of HIV-related stigmas have also reportedly had an impact on men's willingness to pursue HIV-antibody testing and counseling[36] or share their test results with others, both of which can be important in stemming the further spread of the virus. Nick Deocampo and Jomar Fleras note that, in the Philippines "[f]ew [young males] will consent to testing and fewer still will acknowledge they were infected for fear of being ostracized by their peers.[37] Describing his own HIV-antibody test experience, Omari Kokole, a Ugandan man, confessed: "I hesitated to confide in others partly because I feared I would be harshly judged and ostracized," noting a tendency in Uganda to shun those with HIV.[38] In 1989, Philly Bongoley Lutaaya, a well-known Ugandan singer was the first public figure in his country to openly acknowledge that he was living with AIDS.[39] What is shocking is she difficulty of disclosure even in one of the countries hardest hit by HIV. Even today in the Caribbean, another region with extremely high HIV infection rates, Godfrey Sealy has written: "[t]he ill and dying are faceless: we do not know who they are and society does not seem to care."[40] In addition to the painful personal burdens of secrecy and consequent isolation, the choice of those infected to remain hidden facilitates misperceptions about who is vulnerable to HIV. The unwary continue to believe that they need not concern themselves with this epidemic.

The increased involvement of men in caregiving is critical. Caring for those living with HIV is undoubtedly the best way to understand who the affected are and what the illness means. The participation of men in caregiving is also essential in allowing communities to respond adequately to the rapidly growing numbers of people living with HIV and AIDS. How people with HIV experience their illness is fundamentally determined by the support they do or do not receive from their families and communities. Martin Suarez, an Argentinean man living with HIV, links his ability to overcome the depression he experienced with his first opportunistic illness to "the affection and care of my loved ones."[41] Without question, men have the capacity to provide compassionate care to those living with HIV. Unfortunately, their involvement remains limited in many parts of the world. Why this persists appears, at least in part, to be due to gendered norms that circumscribe men's involvement in caregiving. However, these norms are being challenged and transformed by circumstances that are forcing men to assume caregiver roles. In Zambia, it has been observed that sons are often called on to care for their father after their mother has passed away. As more responsibilities shift to men and boys, they will need training and support to prepare them to take up these tasks, and enable them to gain a deeper understanding of the realities of HIV in their roles as caregivers.

Death and Loss

Around the world, men are dying from HIV-related illnesses, as well as experiencing losses among family, friends and colleagues. How men and their families and communities experience these deaths cannot be measured. The impact of any person's death will reflect the roles that individual plays in their family and community, as well as their unique experiences, talents, knowledge and skills. The experience of dying of AIDS will be defined, in some ways by both gender and the disease.

Because of the very different roles played by women and men, death is a gendered experience; the death of a man will impact families and communities in very different ways than the death of a woman. As David Nelson, an Alaskan Native man living with

HIV observed, when he dies, his family will lose "a father, a brother, a son."[42] Cheikh Niang of Senegal notes that, in many societies where men occupy the position of head of the household, a man's death "can signify the loss of economic support or a social base...."[43] In societies where women do not have access to paid work or are prohibited from inheriting or owning property, the death of a male partner and provider can have a devastating and far-reaching effect. Reflecting on the death of a fellow Kenyan, Robert Mugemana notes:

> [w]hen a forty-nine-year-old friend of mine recently died of HIV-related illnesses, he left behind two wives, one in the village with six children, and the other in Nairobi with four children. All ten children were in school. He was also responsible for his two elderly parents. ... The entire extended family was dependent on him.[44]

As men die, responsibilities such as these must be taken up by others. Tradition and norms in most cultures suggest that many will be shouldered by other men, leaving those who are healthy with increasing dependents to provide for. And while there is an understandable tendency to focus on the economic and social consequences of men's premature deaths, the loss of love and emotional support they provide will also create voids that cannot easily be filled. As the Somali respondent noted, the death of any person "leaves a great vacuum in the hearts of those who loved him or her."[45]

When AIDS is the cause of death, the impact can be even more painful and complex. In Rwanda, Damien Rwegera notes,

> [w]hen men die, their families lose their honour when the community finds out it was HIV. ... In general, they do all they can to hide the fact that it is HIV because admitting to it equals discrediting the partner and designating oneself as being HIV infected.[46]

Rwegera's comment points to two unique aspects of the epidemic:-the impact on survivors of the stigma and shame associated with HIV. and the harsh reality that. more often than not, more than one member of a couple or family is infected with the virus. Commenting on the situation in Uganda, Omari Kokole writes: "[d]ifficult as it is for a family to discover that one among them has this disease, think how much greater the tragedy when two or more of its members is stricken."[47] Under such circumstances, the impact on the family and the community is magnified, particularly for those survivors also living with HIV. As David Nelson noted,

> I have had some friends die of this illness and I feel a loss and a rip in my heart. [I feel] alone with the feelings that I guess someone who doesn't have the illness can't feel. It's different when you have AIDS and someone you know dies of it.[48]

These sentiments were echoed by Argentinean, Martin Saurez, who commented,

> [t]he experience [of having a loved one with HIV] is much harder when one is seropositive. It produces an identification with the other, which has extremely important emotional implications, since we not only see our loved one as ill, but also see our own possible evolution as sick people.[49]

Those who suffer the loss of loved ones also need to be supported in their grief and given meaningful options for the future. This will require addressing the imbalances of gendered divisions of labour and power that can make the loss of a male partner and provider a devastating tragedy for surviving women and children. Yet this response snould also include efforts to provide men with support and opportunities to acknowledge their grief and move on with hope in their lives.

Men who have lost partners, family and friends to HIV experience sadness, anger, frustration and grief. Numerous respondents argued that men experience the loss of a loved one no differently than a woman, that grief is universal, not gender specific. Others, however, noted that norms that define appropriate male behaviour may make grieving more difficult for men. Juan Jacobo Hernandez asserted that "men are supposed to be strong, stern, they're not supposed to cry or show weakness," and that, "male grieving is scarcely shown."[50] When a European man shared the experience of losing a grandparent (unrelated to HIV), he noted with regret that "...the last time I saw him,...I did not feel able to hug him and tell him I loved him, for reasons of male embarrassment or the traditions of the family and so on."[51] According to Cheikh Niang from Senegal, "[i]n general, men remarry rapidly after the death of their partners and rarely display any obvious expressions of grief."[52] This response could reflect a variety of factors, but may well be connected to social norms that proscribe how men grieve. While it may be impossible to measure. unexpressed or unresolved grief must inevitably impact the health of individuals and their communities.

Death resulting from AIDS can have a devastating impact, yet among the men who provided input for this paper, many credited HIV-related experiences of loss with mobilizing them to do something to respond to the disease. Some noted feelings of frustration and helplessness while others expressed anger at public health specialists and governments and at the "inadequate and insufficient individual and social response."[53] Perhaps most importantly, some credited their adoption of safer sexual practices and/or their decisions to become personally and professionally involved in the broader struggle against HIV to the death of someone close to them.

Allan Berube, who lost his partner to AIDS, eloquently described how the death of community members and loved ones in San Francisco mobilized that community to respond:

> many of us have decided to respond to this epidemic by making changes in our lives. We have taken responsibility for our past actions and accept the consequences without selfhate. We educate each other about safer sex and other safe practices. We ask for help and offer it. We demand the services we deserve from our governments. We learn how to live well in the present. We pay more attention to our health and explore all possible treatments. We celebrate our lives together. We face each other's deaths and our own. We remember, grieve and hope. We respond to AIDS as we would to other lifethreatening situations—by reorganizing our lives and taking care of each other.[54]

This description offers a template for others confronting the many challenges posed by HIV, a way of finding meaning in tragedy, as well as a testimony to the capacity of individuals and communities to change to meet the challenges of this disease.

CONCLUSIONS

How men respond to HIV, both as individuals and as members of communities, has and will continue to have a fundamental impact on the shape and texture of this epidernic. While men admittedly constitute a broad and diverse segment of the world's population, this paper has attempted to focus on the challenges that HIV and AIDS pose to them as a group, the ways they are responding, and barriers to a more effective response.

Profound changes are needed among men at the individual, community, national and even international level in order to respond effectively to the HIV epidemic. At the individual level, more men must adopt safer sexual practices to protect themselves and their sexual partners from infection. Prevention efforts must continue to be built on values that support communication, shared responsibility and mutual respect between women and men. These efforts will radically redefine norms that define masculinity, male sexuality, and the place of women in society.

Prevention efforts must also be built on a foundation of compassion and inclusion of those living with the virus, both because it is their right and because of the benefit it brings to those who are uninfected. Specifically this should include the increased involvement of men in the provision of care. This will help dismantle stigmas and stereotypes about those infected and affected and contribute toward a more supportive and compassionate community response. At the national and international level, policy-makers and programme planners must re-evaluate assumptions about men and the HIV epidemic. With the exception of gay and bisexual men, and some small, select target populations (e.g., truckers, incarcerated men) efforts to combat the spread of HIV have largely ignored the vast and diverse population of men. This lack of attention is intolerable at this stage in the epidemic, and men—as well as women — 2from the around the world are calling on decision-makers to reconsider and redefine their response to include men in both the definition of the problem and part of the solution to HIV.

Men must be involved, together with women, at every level and each step of this process. This Issues Paper is a first step toward soliciting and encouraging that involvement, and is written with the hope that together we can develop more effective responses to the challenges of HIV.

QUESTIONNAIRE

HIV: The Challenges Facing Men

Behaviour and Behaviour Change

1. What is most important in men's [your] lives?
2. How do men [you] experience sexuality?
3. Why do men [you] have unprotected sex?
4. Under what circumstances do men [you] have unprotected sex?
5. Are men [you] changing their [your] behaviour? If so, why? If not why not?
6. Why [or under what circumstances] do men [you] have more than one life time sexual partner?

Living with HIV Infection, Illness and Care

1. How do men [you] experience the HIV infection and illness?
2. How do men [you] experience the infection and illness of those they love [you]?
3 What care and support do men [you] provide those they [you] love who are sick or dying?

Death

1. How do men [you] experience the death of those they

[you] love? What do they [you] do when a partner died.
2. When men [you] die, what is [will be] lost to their [families] and communities?

General
1. What strategies are needed to address the challenges facing men?
2. What other issues need to be explored? What other questions need to be asked?

NOTES

1. Questionnaires were distributed to men know n to the author and staff at the UNDP/HIV and Development Programme or known to their friends. Twenty-three men from 16 countries responded mostly in writing, some via phone interviews. While the process did not involve a random or representative sample, it served to initiate dialogue on this issue.
2. European, whites married male in mid-30's. Response to UNDP request for information, March 1994.
3. 40-year old gay man from Poland. Response to UNDP request for information, March 1994
4. Connell, Robert W. Australia. Response to UNDP request for information, March 1994.
5. The Global AIDS Policy Coalition. *Status and Trends of the HIV/AIDS Pandemic*, Harvard School of Public Health. Francois-Xavier Bagnoud Center for Health and Human Rights: Cambridge, January 1996.
6. Mann, Jonathan, et al. *AIDS in the World: A Global Report.* Cambridge and London: Harvard University Press, 1992, p.29.
7. The Global AIDS Policy Coalition. *AIDS in the World: Redefining the Pandemic.* Harvard School of Public Health. Francois-Xavier Bagnoud Center for Health and Human Rights. Presented at the International AIDS Conference, Yokahama, Japan. August 5, 1994.
8. Helquist, Michael. USA. Response to UNDP request for information, March 1994.
9. The author vividly recalls a conversation with a US government official working in a Central American country who, after I had described the nature of the problem there, said in response, "But when will it hit someone who matters?"
10. Statement of Belief on Behaviour Change: A Central Issue in Responding to the HIV Epidemic. UNDP Informal Consultation on Behaviour Change, Saly Portugal, Senegal, 12-15 December, 1991.
11. The obvious exception are efforts directed toward gay and bisexual men in many developed and some developing countries.
12. See Aggleton, Peter, et al. "Risking Everything? Risk Behaviour, Behaviour Change, and AIDS." *Science.* Vol. 265. July 15, 1994, pp., 341-345; Silven, David. "Behavioural Theories and Relapse." in Focus: A Guide to AIDS Research and Counseling. Vol.8, No 2. January 1993; and Middlestadt.

Susan E. "The Challenge of Changing Sexual Behaviour." in Focus .— Guide to AIDS Research and Counseling. Vol. 7, No. 11, October 1992.

13. See Middlestadt, Susan E. "The Challenge of Changing Behaviour." in *Focus: A Guide to AIDS Research and Counseling.* Vol 7, No 11. October 1992. pp.1-4.
14. Rwegera, Damien. Response to UNDP request for information. June 1994.
15. Berube, Allan. "Caught in the Storm: AIDS and the Meaning of Natural Disaster", in *OUT/LOOK,* Fall 1998. pp.8-19.
16. 24-year old, white male, USA. Response to UNDP request for information, March 1994.
17. Bassett, Mary et al. "Adolescent Sexual Behaviour and HIV Prevention." *Report in Brief.* Washington, DC: International Center for Research on Women. September 1993.
18. Rwegera, Damien. Rwanda. Response to UNDP request for information, June 1994.
19. H.E. Ambassador Mohamed Osman Omar, Somalia. Response to UNDP request for information. March 1994.
20. 27-year old, white male, USA. Response to UNDP request for information. March 1994.
21. Smith. William and Susan E. Middlestadt. "Building Skills for Condom Use." in *A World Against AIDS: Communication for Behaviour Change.* Washington, DC: AIDSCOM/Academy for Educational Development. 1993.
22. Aggleton, Peter, et al. "Risking Everything? Risk Behaviour, Behaviour Change, and AIDS." *Science.* Vol. 265. July 15, 1994. pp.341-345.
23. Smith, William and Susan E. Middlestadt. "Building Skills for Condom Use." in *A World Against AIDS: Communication for Behaviour Change.* Washington, DC: AIDSCOM/Academ for Educational Development, 1993.
24. Larvie, Patrick. A Construcao Cultural dos '*Meninos de Rua' no Rio de Janeiro: Implicacoes para a Prevencao de HIV/AIDS.* Washington, DC: AIDSCOM/Academy for Educational Development 1999, p.40.
25. European. white, married male. mid-30s. Response to UNDP request for information March 1994.
26. Connell, Robert W. Australia. Response to UNDP request for information, March 1994. Research on these issues is summarized in Connell, R.W. *Masculinities.* Cambridge: Polity Press/Berkeley: University of California Press/Sydney: Allen & Unwin Australia, 1995.
27 40-year old gay man from Poland, Response to UNDP request for information, April 1994.
28. Raditapole, Deborah K. "The Impact of HIV and Migration on Women in Lesotho." *HIV and AIDS: The Global Inter-Connection.* Hartford, CT: Kamarian Press/UNDP. January 1995.
29. Mugemana, Robert. "Our Future is at Stake," in *HIV and AIDS: The Global Inter-Connection,* Hartford, CT: Kamarian Press/UNDP, January 1995.
30. Subhan, K.M. Bangladesh. Response to UNDP request for information. March, 1994.
31. Bradley, Christine S. "Attitudes and Practices Relating to Marital Violence Among the Tolal of East New Britain," in *Domestic Violence in Papua*

New Guinea. Papua New Guinea Law Reform Commission, Monograph No. 3, 1985.

32. Bain, Brendan, Jamaica. Response to UNDP request for information. April 1994.
33. Rwegera, Damien. Rwanda. Response to UNDP request for information. June 1994.
34. Kokole, Omari Haruna. "We Are All Vulnerable." in *HIV and AIDS:The Global Inter Connection.* Hartford, CT: Kamarian Press/UNDP. January 1995.
35. Robert, Pierre. Canada. Response to UNDP request for information. April 1994.
36. Mugemana, Robert. "Our Future is at Stake", in *HIV and AIDS:The Global Inter-Connection.* Hartford, CT: Kamarian Press/UNDP. January 1995.
37. Connell, Robert W., Australia. Response to UNDP request for information. March 1994.
38. H.E. Ambassador Mohamed Osman Omar, Somalia. Response to UNDP request for information. March 1994.
39. Sealy. Godfrey. "We Are Our Own Worst Enemies", in *HIV and AIDS: The Global Inter-Connection.* Hartford, CT: Kamarian Press/UNDP. January 1995.
40. Undoubtedly, this can be partially attributed to lack of access to anonymous or strictly confidential testing and quality: non: judgmental counseling services.
41. Deocampo. Nick and Jomar Fleras. "To Meet the Challenge. We Must Overcome Our Fatalism." in *HIV and AIDS: The Global Inter-Connection.* Hartford, CT: Kamarian Press/UNDP. January 1995.
42. Kokole, Omari Haruna. "We Are All Vulnerable." in *HIV and AIDS: The Global Inter-Connection.* Hartford, CT: Kamarian Press/UNDP. January 1995.
43. Kokole. Omari Haruna. "We Are All Vulnerable." in *HIV and AIDS: The Global Inter-Connection.* Hartford, CT: Kamarian Press/UNDP. January 1995.
44. Sealy, Godfrey. "We Are Our Own Worst Enemies" in *HIV and AIDS: The Global Inter-Connection.* Hartford, CT: Kamafian Press/UNDP. January 1995.
45. Suarez, Martin. Argentina. Response to UNDP request for information. March 1994.
46. Nelson, David. USA. Response to UNDP request for information. March 1994.
47. Niang, Cheikh Ibrahima. Senegal. Response to UNDP request for information. March 1994.
48. Mugemana, Robert E.S. "Our Future is at Stake", in *HIV and AIDS: The Global Inter-Connection.* Hartford, CT: Kamarian Press/UNDP. January 1995.
49. H.E. Ambassador Mohamed Osman Omar, Somalia. Response to UNDP request for information. March 1994.
50. Rwegera, Damien. Rwanda. Response to UNDP request for information. June 1994.

51. Kakole, Omari Haruna. "We Are All Vulnerable" in *HIV and AIDS: The Global Inter-Connection*, Hartfor' CT: Kamarian Press/UNDP. January 1995.
52. Nelson, David. USA. Response to UNDP request for information. March 1994.
53. Suarez. Martin. Argentina. Response to UNDP request for information. March. 1994.
54. Hernandez, Juan lacobo. Mexico. Response to UNDP request for information. April 1994.
55. European, white, married male in mid-30' s. Response to UNDP request for information, March 1994.
56. Niang, Cheikh Ibrahima. Senegal. Response to UNDP request for information. March 1994.
57. Hernandez, Juan Jacobo. Mexico. Response to UNDP request for information. April 1994.
58. Berube. Allan. "Caught in the Storm: AIDS and the Meaning of Natural Disaster." *OUT/LOOK,* Fall 1988.

10

Young Women: Silence, Susceptibility and the HIV Epidemic

Gender as an Independent Variable for HIV Infection

There is a critical reality about the HIV epidemic which is yet to be grasped. It can be glimpsed through the following three assertions.

First, women are increasingly becoming infected with HIV. In most of the third world, there are as many, or more, infected women as there are infected men.[1] These women are wives and other partners, daughters and grandmothers, sisters, aunts and nieces.

Second, women are becoming infected at a significantly younger age than men. In areas where the epidemic is newly emerging and in areas where it is deeper, the same pattern is recorded: on average, women become infected five to ten years earlier than men.

Third, proportionally more girls and young women in their teens and early twenties are becoming infected than women in any other age group. A possible exception is post-menopausal women who also seem to be particularly susceptible to HIV infection.

The response to each of these assertions must be to ask why this is occurring.

The implications are that it is plausible that women become infected more easily than men, possibly at all ages and most definitely when they are in their teens and early twenties and after menopause. There appears to be a biological, immunological and/or virological susceptibility in women which changes with age.

Silence

The first diagnosed case of AIDS in a woman was recorded as early as 1982, in the first year of the known epidemic. In 1984, the first joint US/Belgian mission to Zaire clinically diagnosed virtually as many women with AIDS as men. Nevertheless the characterization of the epidemic by gender (male) and sexual orientation (homosexual) remained dominant.

In 1986 two critical studies, disaggregated by gender and age, became available. One from the University Teaching Hospital in Lusaka, Zambia, showed one in ten women attending the antenatal clinic infected with HIV and, amongst the hospital patients:

one in three men aged 30 to 35 were infected:

one in four women aged 20 to 25 were infected.

The other study reported the first 500 cases of AIDS diagnosed in Mama Yemo Hospital, Zaire (Figure 10.1)[2]. This data set was also remarkable in showing:

as many women as men were diagnosed with AIDS;

the diagnosed women were on average ten years younger than the men;

there was a sharp peak in AIDS cases in younger women, 20 to 29 years old.

These data were deeply disturbing yet they did not elicit a particular concern about women and HIV at the international level nor did they challenge and change the dominant discourse on the epidemic and thus the responses.[3]

Now, ten years after the first woman was diagnosed, an estimated three and a half million women are infected, the vast majority through sexual transmission. For most women, the major risk factor for HIV infection is being married.[4,5,6] Each day a further three thousand women become infected and five hundred infected women die. Most infected women are between 15 and 35 years old.

Age as an Independent Variable for HIV Infection

The profile of extremely high rates of HIV infection or AIDS in young women, first seen in the 1986 Kinshasa data set, reappears time and again in later data sets, in newly emerging epidemics, Thailand and Myanmar for example (Figures 10.2 and 10.3), in established epidemics, Uganda for example (Figure 10.4) and in industrialized countries, Europe for example (Figure 10.5)[7].

These data sets dramatically indicate that the patterns are everywhere and over time similar:

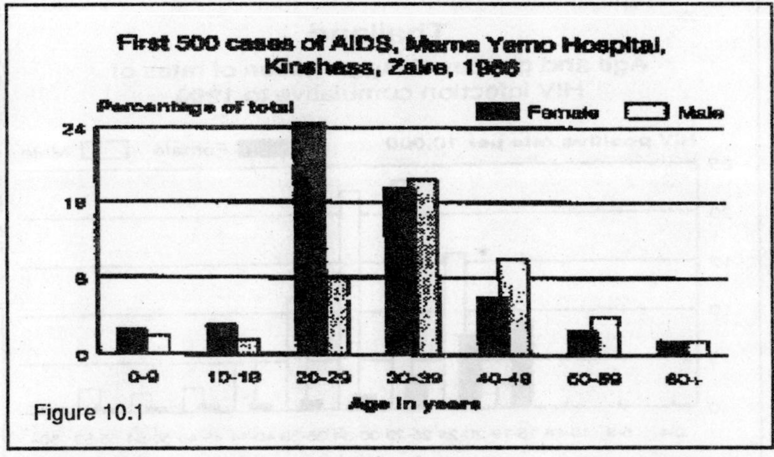

Figure 10.1

the prevalence of HIV infection is highest in young women aged 15 to 25 and peaks in men five to ten years later in the 25 to 35 age groups; and

among women, the infection profile by age has a precipitous peak in the age group 15 to 20 and declines for older pre-menopausal age groups.

Other studies[8, 9, 10] are providing dramatic illustration of the vulnerability of young women when they become sexually active early in life. Anne Chao's data from Rwanda (Figure 10.6) show that the younger the age of first pregnancy or first sexual intercourse the higher the incidence of HIV infection: over 25 per cent of young women pregnant at age 17 or younger are infected and about 17 per cent of those 17 or younger at first sexual intercourse are infected. Infection rates decrease sharply in both categories in later age groups.

It is our contention that the extent of HIV infection in young girls in their teens or early twenties shown in these data sets will be affected by all the contributory factors currently identified in the literature as increasing the rates of infection in women and men but cannot be adequately accounted. for by these factors, even in the aggregate. In the case of young women there would seem to be other influential factors. These need to be identified.

The factors identified in the literature include the incidence of sexually transmitted infections (STIs)[11,12], frequency of intercourse[13], sexual practices[14], and male/ female age differences in sexual relationships [15, 16]. To these may also be added women's nutritional status[17], and the presence of lesions, inflammation and scarification in the female genital tract from causes other than STIs[18]

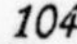

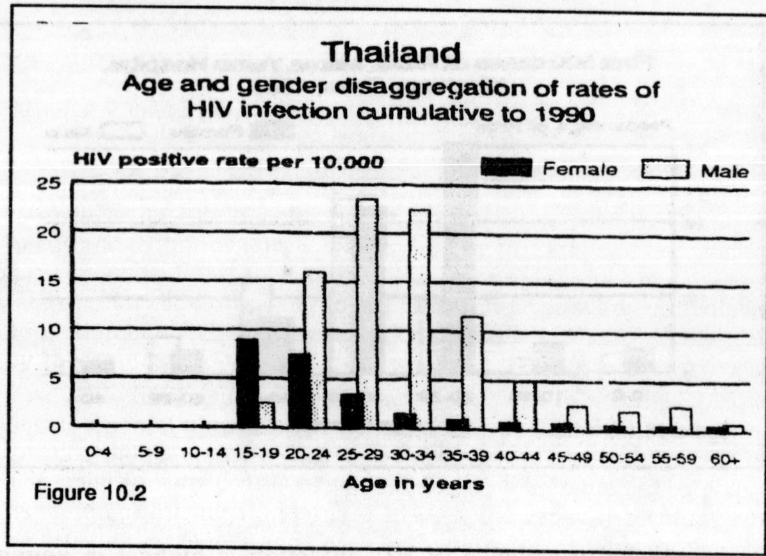

Figure 10.2

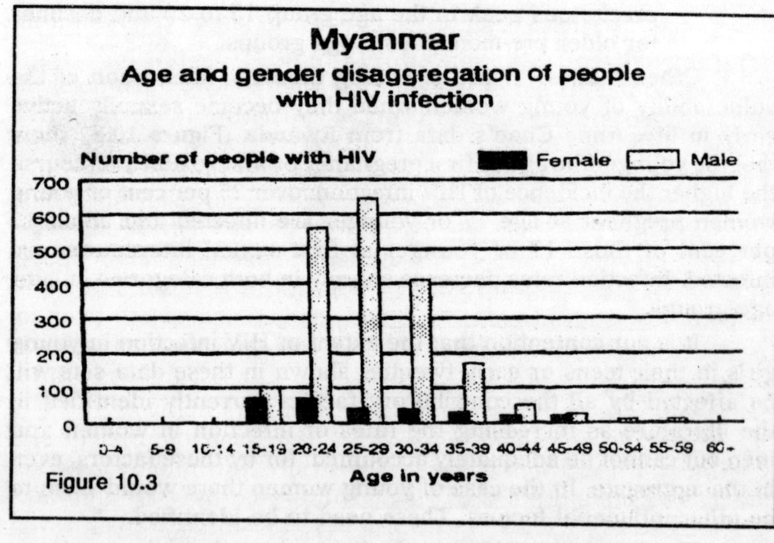

Figure 10.3

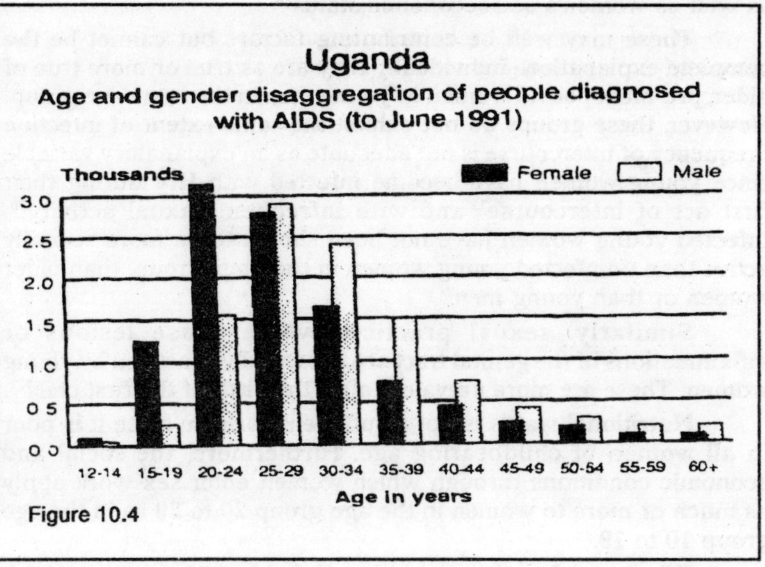

Figure 10.4

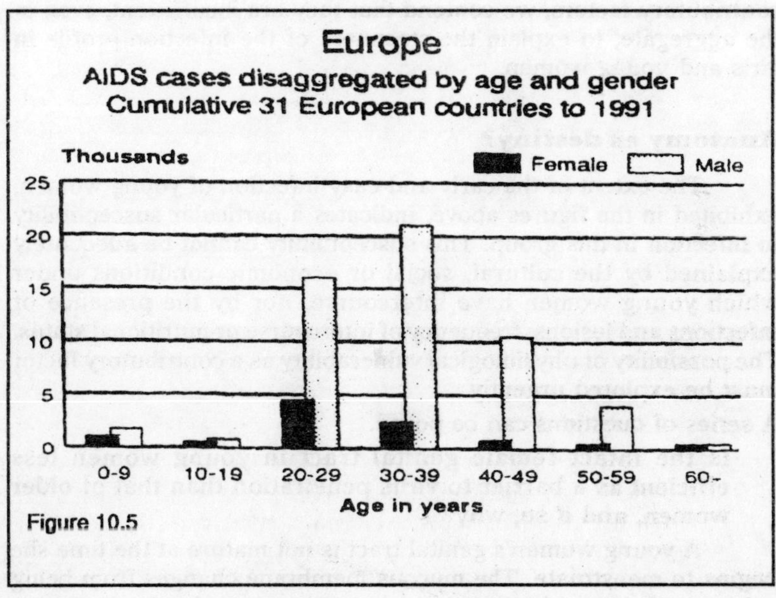

Figure 10.5

as well as women's socioeconomic status[16].

These may well be contributing factors but cannot be the complete explanation. Individually they are as true or more true of older, pre-menopausal women or young men in the same age group. However, these groups do not exhibit the same extent of infection Frequency of intercourse is not adequate as an explanatory variable since young women have become infected with HIV during their first act of intercourse[19] and with infrequent sexual activity[20]. Infected young women have not been shown to be more sexually active than uninfected young women in their age group, than older women or than young men[21].

Similarly, sexual practices which cause lesions or inflammations of the genital tract are not usually practised by young women. These are more prevalent after the birth of the first child[21].

Nutritional status is not a sufficient variable since it is poor in all women of childbearing age. Furthermore, the social and economic conditions through which women enter sex work apply as much or more to women in the age group 20 to 29 as in the age group 10 to 19.

When social explanations are offered for this pattern of high infection rates in young women, they are usually offered in terms of older men having sexual intercourse, consensually or otherwise, with younger women15 . Whilst this and all the above are clearly contributory factors, we contend that they are insufficient, even in the aggregate, to explain the steepness of the infection profile in girls and young women.

Anatomy as destiny?

The extent of the early and easy infection of young women, exhibited in the figures above, indicates a particular susceptibility to infection in this group. This susceptibility cannot be adequately explained by the cultural, social or economic conditions under which young women have intercourse, nor by the presence of infections and lesions, frequency of intercourse or nutritional status. The possibility of physiological vulnerability as a contributory factor must be explored urgently.

A series of questions can be posed.

> **Is the intact female genital tract in young women less efficient as a barrier to virus penetration than that of older women, and if so, why?**

A young woman's genital tract is not mature at the time she begins to menstruate. The mucous membrane changes from being a thin single layer of cells to a thick multi-layer wall. This transition is often not completed until late teens or early twenties. It is

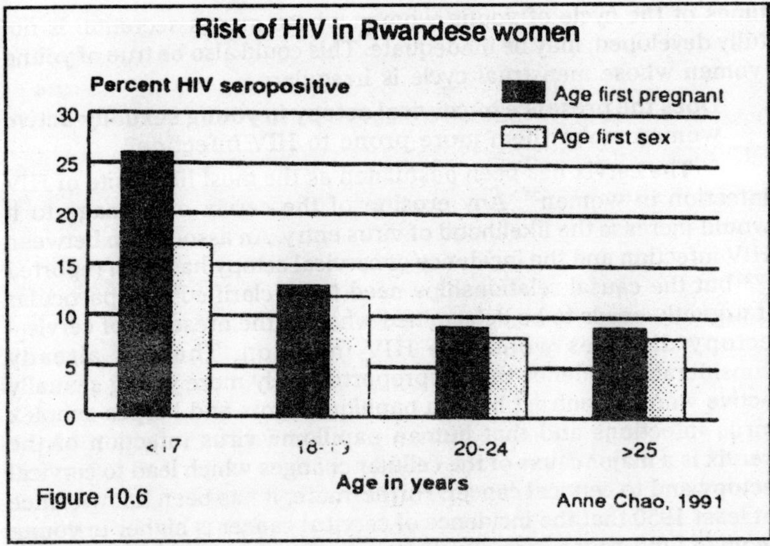

Figure 10.6

Anne Chao, 1991

conceivable there-fore that the intact but immature genital tract surface in young women is less efficient as a barrier to HIV than the mature genital tract of older women. In post-menopausal women, the mucous membrane becomes thinner and so it is also possible that the genital tract wall, even when intact, is less efficient as a barrier.

Is mucous production in young women less proficient than in older women?

Mucus in the female genital tract has four relevant roles. It acts as a physical barrier, separating semen and other material from the vaginal and cervical walls. It is a lubricant, protecting the surface of the vagina from abrasion during intercourse. It flushes the cervix and vagina in the same way that mucus flushes the respiratory tract, removing foreign material. It has an immune function[22], that is, mucus contains cells of a separate immune system whose function is to activate the immune responses of the cells in the vaginal and cervical surfaces.

If mucus production in young women, and postmenopausal women, is less proficient than in older premenopausal women, so too will these protective roles be less effective. There will be less of a barrier to viral penetration. It will provide less assistance in minimizing irritation and tearing of the genital membranes and so facilitate viral entry[23].

It is known that the hormonal fluctuations of the menstrual cycle influence the production of vaginal and cervical secretions[24]. Secretion is most prolific at midmenstrual cycle and so at other times of the cycle of young women whose mucus secretion is not fully developed, may be inadequate. This could also be true of young women whose menstrual cycle is irregular.

Does the presence of cervical,ectopy in young sexually-active women make them more prone to HIV infection?

The cervix has been postulated as the most likely site of HIV infection in women[25]. Any erosion of the cervix or damage to it would increase the likelihood of virus entry. An association between HIV infection and the incidence of cervical ectopy has been reported [20,26] but the causal relationships need to be clarified[26]. In particular it urgently needs to be determined whether the presence of cervical ectopy disposes women to HIV infection. There is already considerable evidence that disproportionately more young sexually active women contract human papilloma virus and herpes simplex virus infections and that human papilloma virus infection of the cervix is a major cause of the cellular changes which lead to cervical ectopy and to cervical cancer. Furthermore, it has been known since at least 1950 that the incidence of cervical cancer is higher in young women who began sexual activity or were married before the age of 17 [27].

Do the hormonal and physiological changes at menopause increase the vulnerability of older women to infection?

There is some case evidence that the efficacy of transmission in post-menopausal women is higher than in pre-menopausal women[28]. However, epidemiological evidence is lacking since the female population most usually tested (commercial sex workers and pregnant women) do not include them. It could be anticipated that post-menopausal infected women would usually die without diagnosis or treatment.

The biology of a woman's genital tract is poorly understood. We know more about the increased protection from HIV infection offered by intact genital mucosae in monkeys[29]. The above analysis, however, does show the urgency of developing an international commitment to providing answers to these questions.

Situational Factors

The influence on vulnerability to infection of these biologically based differences rnay be amplified by the circumstances and situations in which young women have sexual intercourse.

Non-consensual, hurried or frequent intercourse may inhibit mucus production and the relaxation of the vaginal musculature both of which would increase the likelihood of genital trauma. A lack of control over the circumstances in which intercourse occurs may increase the frequency of intercourse and lower the age at which sexual activity begins. A lack of access to acceptable health services may leave infections and lesions untreated . Malnutrition not only inhibits the production of mucus but also slows the healing process and depresses the immune system[30]. Cultural norms may favour early pregnancy, discourage the use of condoms or facilitate intercourse with older men who are more likely to be infected.

The Unheard Scream

These data show that girls and young women are excessively vulnerable to HIV infection. When will the agony of these young infected women press upon us? Anecdotal evidence from one geographic area suggests that one half of all young women there aged 15 to 19 years are infected. In other areas, the figure is one in three or one in four[8].

When will the pain and anger of these young women goad us to action? Or will we be capable of ignoring this too? There is the possibility of a disturbing parallel in the acceptance throughout the world of the loss of women's lives during pregnancy and childbirth. In Africa, as many as one woman in 21 die in the process of bearing a child. In Asia, it is one in 54; in Latin America and the Caribbean, one in 73. The tragedy and suffering of these women is too often unremarked and their deaths unmarked[31]. These deaths are needless[32].

The Prophetic Voice

The growing numbers of women infected and dying bring a deep sadness but must sound an urgent alarm. We must be aware of what the world will lose through the deaths of so many young, and older, women.

Because we live in sharply gender-divided worlds, the impact of women's deaths is different from that of men. Most, if not all, cultures raise girls differently from boys and treat women differently from men. As a result, women bring to daily life different qualities from men. Women tend to be the guardians of compassion rather than ambition, of connectedness rather than control, of healing rather than harming, of closeness rather than conquest, of mercy rather than judgment. They make possible the circle of the dance as an alternative to the ladder.

Women are the creators of new life, the caretakers of daily life and the custodians and transmitters of community norms and social values. However, in some parts of the world, one third or one half or more of all women are infected. How will the loss be borne?

Cabbage soup, writes Helene Cixous, can only warm us

passingly. To live, we need the presence of women who pay attention to life[33]. Yet even soup is usually prepared by women. It is not solely a matter of appeasing hunger of providing shelter, of resolving conflict, of raising, children, of tending fields. Women bring much more to life.

An Action Agenda

We must respond to this tragedy. There are two essential elements in the immediate strategy. First, the silence around the infection of young women must be challenged at every level: individuals, families, communities and organizations, nations and internationally. Second, a new research agenda must be established. The established hypotheses and assumptions about the nature of the epidemic, about research priorities and about gender must be set aside so that the research agenda can be reconceptualized. To do this, those responsible 'or the agenda must also change. The critically important and insightful works of Nancy Alexander[25], Bruce Forrest[22], Elizabeth Duncan[23], Zena Stein[34] and others must be acknowledged, valued and acted upon.

These two elements are necessary but not sufficient conditions for an effective strategy to protect girls and young women from being infected through their sexual and reproductive activities. An effective strategy will need to address all the factors which directly contribute to their susceptibility to infection. It must also address, in the short term wherever possible but certainly in the longer term, the indirect contributory factors[35]. There will be many elements m such an action agenda. Here we identify only a few to stimulate thought and discussion.

Neither the immediate strategy nor the broader response will be effective without political will and pressure for change. Politicians, community leaders and parents will need the courage to speak out to save these lives, to save the continuity of life. We are all responsible.

Breaking the Silence

The silence surrounding the infection of young women must be broken. Girls and young women must be able to speak out, to cease to feel silenced or powerless to change what happens to them. Others, too, must speak out.

It is critical that parents, communities and nations realize that, unless they face this issue urgently, not only will many young women be lost but so, too, will their children and their children's children. Clans and communities will cease to exist and, with them, their ancestors. Pregnancy, birth and nurturing, the continuity of life will all be placed in jeopardy.

If the silence is broken and young infected women begin to speak out and tell their stories, we must have already in place effective programmes to prevent their younger sisters from also becoming infected. If not, the breaking of the silence will add the agony of younger girls who will now know that they face a future of possible, perhaps almost certain, infection, to the agony of the young women already infected. Young girls will feel powerless to avoid the fate of their mothers and older sisters.

The psychological trauma of such a situation is virtually beyond comprehension. If we do not succeed in developing an effective, timely agenda for action, the insight and analysis which demand that the silence be broken will become a curse.

Changing the Operational Research Agenda

The mere possibility of a physiological basis to the susceptibility of infection in young women should provide the impetus for an urgent and significant research effort. Answers to questions about the female genital tract identified here, as well as others, must be found so that protective programmes can be developed.

Those who are undertaking relevant research on the female, and male, genital tracts must be supported and their findings widely and quickly disseminated. A focused effort must be made to bring together the observers of the reality and those undertaking such research and analyses together with research funders so that priorities in the bioscientific research agenda can be reset and financial support be immediately available. Doctors, nurses and social workers who are observant and understanding of the relationship between the condition of young women's genital tracts and their life situations are essential partners in the process of determining the research agenda.

Sanctuaries

Strategies must be found that lengthen the time before the onset of sexual intercourse in young women, increase the age at first pregnancy, and which increase the ability of young girls to control the situations in which they are sexually active.

Spaces must be created within which young girls can be free, and feel free, from the threat of HIV infection, within which they can pass more time before leaving to enter the world of sexual relationship and procreation and within which they can talk to one another about their coping and survival strategies, their difficulties and their successes.

Safe havens must also be found or created which would allow social and emotional interactions between girls and boys, young women and young men, and in which they can discuss and set aside the peer pressures cultural norms and gender archetypes which increase their vulnerability to infection.

The family should be the foremost of these sanctuaries. Young girls should leave their families uninfected and should be able to return to them when in fear of infection. The silence around incest must be broken, above all by mothers and those who minister to and provide service to such families. The direct price of incest is higher than ever now. The collusion of families, whether from greed or acceptance, in customs and practices which threaten the lives of their daughters must cease. Neither young women nor young men should be pressured into child or early marriages or into early pregnancies. Dowry payments or patrilocality should not prevent the possibility of a young woman returning to her family home when in fear of being infected.

Families alone cannot change cultural norms, values and practices[36]. Thus, advocating families as sanctuaries requires a complementary strategy of cultural change. Such a strategy must be led by the guardians and enforcers of culture, influential community leaders, older women, the elders, as well as by those who are now demanding such change, young men and women and their parents.

The school should also be a sanctuary from infection. However, the school is a site of non-consensual sexual activities and of HIV infection. Rape, sexual abuse and coercion by male staff and pupils combined with the exchange of sex with older men for school fees currently make the school a feared and fearful place. Community acceptance of this as normal must change. A policy of providing scholarships would obviate the need for young girls to find older men to finance their schooling. Sanctions enforced by local communities would change entrenched patterns of sexual exploitation of young girls by teachers or male students. These sanctions are now beginning to be imposed in some seriously affected areas as communities strive to keep some of their young girls uninfected.

Organizations and clubs for young women create sanctuaries where young girls can spend time without the threat of infection. They break the isolation of individual women and can lead to the creation of social support networks where young women can seek counsel and be given support to change their behaviour and to create change in their communities.

Groups working amongst street children in Brazil have opened safe houses where the girls can escape from the pressures of the street and regain a feeling of security and control over their lives. One such house is the *Casa de Passagen* (Passage house) in Recife, Brazil[37].

Such groups and organizations can also provide a refuge where infected girls and young women can come together and provide one another with support, exchange information on care and treatment and discuss issues of basic concern such as disclosure, sexuality, discrimination, pregnancy and their children's futures.

It is critical that religious organizations also create such sanctuaries for women and for men, separately and together. This would lend their moral authority to a recognition of the importance and value of young women and would help families and communities to find the courage to change and to provide sanctuary themselves.

These safe havens are critical for young girls to reach the physical maturity and the emotional and social maturity necessary to have greater control over their lives and the situations in which they have sexual intercourse.

Sanctions

The urgency of the situation may well necessitate the use of sanctions. In this respect the law can be used as an agent of social change. For example, the introduction and enforcement of laws in Southern Africa requiring men to provide financial support to all children they father, whether within marriage or outside it, have led to a significant decrease in the number of such children.

Laws against rape and incest and family law relating to the age of marriage or divorce have been less successful where there have not been concurrent changes in social and cultural values. Communities must therefore accept and decide to enforce such laws and place pressure on their members to change.

In Uganda, recent changes in governmental and community attitudes brought about by the epidemic have led to military courts trving soldiers for rape, legal services being expanded for women who have been sexually abused, vigorous reporting by the media of sexual abuse in schools and teachers being sacked for unacceptable sexual behaviour[38].

Safety

For women throughout the world, safety, that is, freedom from physical, sexual, verbal, psychological and other forms of violence, is an issue that dominates all others in their lives. The data on the extent of violence to women is quite appalling[39] but little known or acknowledged.

Abuse in the childhood or early adult lives of young women leads to low self-esteem, little ability for self-assertion and the probability of increased abuse by others, all factors which have been shown to increase the likelihood of HIV infection. In men, childhood abuse also leads to low self-esteem and to an increased likelihood of their abusing others[39].

New women's crisis initiatives exist in at least 35 developing countries[40]. All of these are dependent on external support agencies for their financing. It is vitally important to support and expand programmes to lessen violence to women and to provide refuges for abused women. This can become a significant role for external support agencies.

Restructuring Gender

The ability of young women to protect themselves from infection becomes a direct function of power relations between men and women and, in particular, of men's sexual identity. Gender is formed in families but constructed by societies[36]. Changing accepted patterns of male behaviour and expected patterns of female behaviour requires community organizing and collective action.

Individual families and societies must change how they value girls. The more women are valued, the better they will be fed and nurtured, given access to health services and education, provided with the skills required for economic autonomy and have their rights honoured, in particular to land and property, especially through inheritance.

This valuing of women will make it possible for women to value their own bodies, to improve their genital health and to have their genital infections and conditions diagnosed and treated, for cultural practices such as infibulation which increase women's likelihood of infection to be changed and for women to live through pregnancy and childbirth with minimal risk of death or lifelong disability[32].

Families must also change what they value in boys and men so that men will be less likely to place themselves and others at risk of infection. Boys and men, not only girls and women, must become the guardians of compassion, of respect for others, of healing, connectedness and of mercy.

The Circle of the Dance

For young women to be able to remain uninfected, men and women, their communities and nations must want this to happen and be committed to work urgently towards it. Only then will there be hope. The priorities of the bioscientific research agenda must be changed and knowledge of all the factors which contribute to the susceptibility of young women to HIV infection deepened. Agendas for action must be drawn up locally and nationally. This will best be achieved through the creation of consultative processes which involve all those implicated in the required changes. These processes must be such that men feel able to participate, that women's insights and analyses are valued and listened to and that the external factors, the socio-economic and political climate which creates the conditions which increase women's and men's vulnerability to infection, can be addressed. Such processes are already occurring either spontaneously[41] or set in motion by concerned individuals as in the case of the Women and AIDS Support Network in Zimbabwe. They are critical if the lives of young women are to be saved . The resulting agenda for action will provide the basis for hope.

NOTES

1. Chin, James L. "The increasing impact of the HIV/AIDS Pandemic on Women and Children." Paper presented at the American Public Health Association meeting. Atlanta. November 1991.
2. Quinn, Thomas C., Jonathan M. Mann, James Curran, Peter Piot. "AIDS in Africa, an Epidemiologic Paradigm." *Science.* vol. 234, No. 957. 1986.
3. Reid, Elizabeth. "Gender Knowledge and Responsibility.," *AIDS in the World.* Harvard University Press. Forthcoming 1992.
4. Jacob, May "STDs among seropositive patients of a referral hospital in India and their role in the transmission of HIV." VIII International Conterence on AIDS/III STD World Congress. Amsterdam. July 1992. [Poster Abstract PoC 4334].
5. Hunter, D.S. Kapiga, G. L. wihula *et al.* "Risk factors for HIV-I infection among family planning clinic clients in Dar-es-Salaam, Tanzania." VIII International Conference on AIDS/III STD World Congress. Amsterdam. July 1992. [Poster Abstract PoC 4158].
6. Allen, Susan *et al.* "Human Immunodeficiency Vines Infection in Rwanda." *Journal of the American Medical Association.* Vol. 266. No. 12: 1657-1663. 1991.
7. Sources are respectively: Figure 10.2, Thailand National AIDS Control Programme.1991. Figure 10.3, Myanmar AIDS Control Programrne. 1991. Figure 10.4, Uganda National AIDS Control Programme. 1991. Figure 10.5, European AIDS surveillance. 1991.
8. Wawer, Maria J. *et al.* "Dynamics of spread of HIV-1 Infection in a Rural District of Uganda". *British Medical Journal* Vol. 303: 1303-1306. 1991.
9. Holt, Elizabeth. "HIV seroconversion in Haitian Women." Poster No. MC3010 presented at VII International Conference on AIDS. Florence. 1991.
10. Chao, Anne *et al.* "Risk factors for HIV-1 Among Pregnant Women in Rwanda." Poster No. MC3097 presented at VII International Conference on AIDS. Florence. 1991.

11. Wasserheit, J . "Epidemiological Synergy: Inter-relationships between Human Immunodeficiency Virus Infection and Other Sexually Transmitted Diseases." *Sexually Transmitted Diseases,* 19 (No. 2): 61-77. 1992.
12. Van de Perrey, Phillipe *et al.* "Risk factors for HIV seropositivity in selected urban-based Rwandese adults." *AIDS* Vol. 1:207= 211. 1987.
13. Melbye/ Mads, *et al.* "Evidence for Heterosexual transmission and Clinical Manifestations of Human Immunodeficiency Virus Infection and Related Conditions in Lusaka, Zambia." *Lancet.* :1113-1115. 15 November 1986.
14. Padian, Nancy *et al.* "Male-to-Female Transmission of Human Immunodeficiency Virus." *Journal of the American Medical Association.* Vol. 258, No. 6: 788-790. 1987.
15. Decosas, Josef and Violette Pedenault. "The Demographic AIDS Trap for Women in Africa." Paper presented at the VII International Conference on AIDS. Florence. 1991.
16. De Bruyn, Maria. "Women and AIDS in Developing Countries. *Social Science and Medicine.* Vol. 34 No. 3:249-262. 1992.
17. Bailey, Mike. Report for Save the Children Fund of V International Conference on AIDS in Africa. Kinshasa. 1990.
18. McNamara, Regina. Female genital health and the risk of HIV transmission. UNDP HIV and Development Issues Paper No. 4. Forthcoming 1992.
19. Bouvet, E. "Defloration as risk factor for heterosexual HIV transmission." *Lancet*: 615. 18 March 1992.
20. O'Farrell, Nigel and Isobel Windsor. "Sexual Behaviour in HIV-1 Seropositive Zulu Men and Women in Durban, South Africa." Letter to the Editor, *Journal of Acquired Immune Deficiency Syndromes.* 4: 1258-59. 1991.
21. Nyirenda, Meya. Oral presentation at VIII international Conference on AIDS/III STD World Congress. Amsterdam. 1992.
22. Forrest, Bruce. Women, HIV and Mucosal Immunity. *Lancet.* Vol. 337: 835-836. 1991.
23. Duncan, M. Elizabeth *et al.* First coitus before menarche and the risk of sexually transmitted disease. *Lancet.* Vol. 335: 338-340. 1990.
24. Forrest, Bruce. Personal Communication. 1991.
25. Alexander, Nancy J. "Sexual Transmission of Human Immunodeficiency Virus: Virus Entry into the Male and Female Genital Tract." *Fertility and sterility.* Vol 54, No.1:1-18.1990.
26. Mandelblatt, Jeanne S. *et al.* "Association Between HIV Infection and Cervical Neoplasia; Implications for Clinical Care of Women at Risk for Both Conditions." *AIDS.* Vol. 6: 173-178. 1992
27. Terris, Milton and Margaret C. Oalmann. "Carcinoma of the Cervix: an Epidemiologic Study." *Journal of the American Medical Association.* Vol. 174. No. 4: 1847-1851. 1960.
28. Dwyer, John. Personal Communication. 1992.
29. Miller, Christopher and Murray Gardner. "AIDS and Mucosal Immunity: Usefulness of the SIV Macaque Model of Genital Mucosal Transmission." *Journal of Acquired Immune Deficiency Syndromes.* Vol. 4: 1169-1192, 1991.

30. Chandra, R.K. Nutrition, Immunity and Infection: Present Knowledge and Future Directions. *Lancet* Vol.: 688-91. 26 March 1983.
31. Diallo, A. Boubacar. "A Tora Mousso Kele La: A call beyond duty; often omitted root causes of maternal mortality in West Africa. UNDP HIV and Development Issues Paper No. 5. Forthcoming 1992.
32. UNDP. "Safe Motherhood Priorities and Next Steps: A Forward-Looking Assessment on the Reduction of Maternal Mortality and Morbidity Within the Framework of the Safe Motherhood Initiatives (SMI). April 1991.
33. Cixous, Helene. From "Vivre l'Orange". Excerpted in *Love Poems By Women*, Wendy Mulford (ed). Fawcett Columbine. NY. 1991.
34. Stein, Zena. "HIV Prevention: The Need for Methods Women Can Use". *American Journal of Public Health.* Vol. 80: 460-462. 1990.
35. Hamblin, Julie and Elizabeth Reid. Women, the HIV Epidemic and Human Rights: A Tragic Imperative." Paper prepared for International Workshop on AIDS: A Question of Rights and Humanity. International Court of Justice. The Hague. May 1991.
36. Reid, Elizabeth. "Women and HIV." Editorial in AIDS Health Promotion Exchange. Forthcoming 1992.
37. Baker, G. Felicia Knaul and Ana Vasconcelos. "Development as Empowerment: Brazilian Project Offers Passage to a Better Life for Street Girls." *Passages.* Vol. 10. No. 4: 3-6. International Center on Adolescent Fertility. 1991.
38. Slutkin, G. "What has been Learned in HIV Prevention Programmes." Presentation made at VIII International Conference on AIDS. Amsterdam. 1992.
39. Heise, Lori. "Violence Against Women: The Missing Agenda." in *Woman's Health: a Global Perspective.* Marge Koblinsky, Judith Timyan and Jill Gay (Eds). Westview press, 1992.
40. Heise, Lori. Personal Communication. 1992.
41. Orick, George. Interview with Margaret Mwangola and Rose Mulama. Kenya. UNDP HIV and Development Programme. Reflections on the Impact of the HIV Epidemic Project. Taped 1991.

11

Young Women and the HIV Epidemic

Ms. Elizabeth Reid
UNDP, New York

The HIV epidemic is a women's epidemic: women are particularly vulnerable to infection and increasing numbers of women are becoming infected. It is estimated that one—third of all those thought to be infected—about 2 million —are women. It is also estimated that the number of infected women may overtake the number of infected men by the mid—90s. Already in sub-Saharan Africa there are more women than men infected. Studies in Central African Republic, Equatorial Guinea and Gabon show nearly three times as many women infected than men. In Honduras, Haiti, The Dominican Republic, the Bahamas and Trinidad and Tobago, the male to female ratios of reported AIDS cases, the last stage of HIV infection, have dropped rapidly in the last three years from over 6:1 to under 2.5:1.

It is also an epidemic of youth. At least half of all those infected are under the age of 25 and a large proportion of these young adults were irfected during adolescence. Recent studies indicate that the infection rates in some teenage groups is far higher than that for adults. The number of reported AIDS cases in teenagers has increased rapidly over the last two years.

Data are not available on the number of young women infected. However, women are constituting an increasing proportion of all AIDS cases and often women become infected at a younger age than men. A study from Zaire reported that among young adults aged 15 to 30 years, HIV infection was four times more common in women than in men. These are bleak and disturbing facts. Infection rates in pregnant women in high incidence countries in Central and Eastern Africa range from 10 to 25 per cent. High infection rates in women will cause a sharp increase in maternal and child morbidity and mortality rates. Maternal mortality rates in developing countries are already 12 times higher than in the developed world, the greatest gap in any human indicator.

The overwhelming majority of infected young women do not know they are infected. Most young women are diagnosed during pregnancy or at birth. To the shock of discovering their own infection status is added the fear that their baby might be infected, guilt and grief at having brought all this about and the desolation of motherhood in these circumstances.

Transmission

The HIV virus may be transmitted sexually through anal, vaginal or oral intercourse with an infected person. Sexual transmission can be prevented through the proper use of a good quality condom. Young women in most parts of the developing world are sexually active. Data on adolescent sexuality in developing countries indicate that the initial sexual contact occurs before age 17 for half of that population and by age 15 for one-third of adolescents. In Jamaica, Nigeria and Sierra Leone, more than four out of five single women aged 20 years are sexually experienced. In Mexico and Costa Rica, from about one-fifth to one-fourth of single adolescents are sexually experienced by age 20. Condom use is not common. Studies show that in four countries (Costa Rica, the Gambia, Jamaica and Zimbabwe) the condom was the most frequently used contraceptive at first intercourse. However, in general, use at first intercourse is very low. Condom usage in unmarried women aged 15 to 19 years in 15 countries studies is low but second to the pill in most African countries and in Jamaica, Peru and Thailand. Thus there are, in the developing world, many young women at risk of infection through unprotected sexual behaviour.

HIV transmission may also occur through the sharing of drug using equipment with an infected individual. Protection can be achieved through not sharing needles, through the cleaning of shared needles or through changing the mode of use away from intravenous administration. Fewer young women than young men are at risk of infection through drug injecting since in almost all drug using communities, men predominate. Young women are however at significant risk of infection through an unprotected sexual intercourse with infected current or past drug users. It is virtually impossible to know whether another person is HIV infected, certainly during the long period of infection before symptoms appear. Even HIV testing only tells the infection status of a person at an earlier period of time and not at the present. In the case of sexual behaviour and intravenous drug use, only each individual can take the necessary steps to protect themselves from infection. The responsibility of governments is to make people aware of the epidemic and the modes of transmission of the virus, to ensure that the means of preventing infection—condoms, sterile needles, bleach—are affordable and of easy access, and to minimize the possibility of iatrogenic and occupational transmission.

Young women can also become infected iatrogenically through the medical use of nonsterile needles, through the transfusion of contaminated blood or blood products and, rarely, through the use of infected human tissue or organs in surgical procedures. In many parts of the developing world, needles are commonly used in both the modern and traditional health sectors, without any or sufficient sterilization. Adolescent pregnancy can place young women at further risk of infection from blood transfusion or unsterile needles. The extent of iatrogenic transmission has not been adequately studied, but women and young children are at high risk from this form of transmission.

Vulnerability to HIV Infection

There are many factors affecting the lives of young women which make them vulnerable to HIV infection. While there are few data available to determine the extent of that vulnerability, the following discussion can serve to indicate areas for further research in this area. Prevalence patterns of HIV infection are known to be a factor of poverty, social and geographic mobility, commerce, tourism, social disruption and civil unrest.

Sexually Transmitted Diseases and Adolescent Pregnancy

The presence of sexually transmitted diseases (STDs), particularly ulcerative conditions, increases the likelihood of infection in both men and women when intercourse occurs with an infected partner. STDs are common amongst young women, particularly in Africa, the Caribbean and Latin America. They are not easy to detect in women and so most women remain unaware of their presence. Studies in Central Africa have shown that in some communities up to one-third of women in their child-bearing years are infertile, with 80 per cent of that infertility being caused by STDs. Drug use is also increasing in some parts, particularly in the Caribbean. The incidence may be much lower in sub-Saharan Africa. However, this epidemic carries within it the seeds of violence. Although rape is traditionally uncommon in sub-Saharan Africa, there are increasing reports of the rape of young women by older men in high HIV-incidence countries. This is clearly associated with the belief that the younger the woman, the more she is likely to be free from HIV infection. The raped young woman, however, is at high risk of infection, particularly since reports indicate that the attackers are usually either sexually promiscuous men who do not want to change their behaviour or, increasingly, may be men who have lost their wives, possibly to AIDS, who are fearful of taking another wife.

Sex tourism is an expression of the power of men from rich countries to purchase the sexual services of young women in developing countries. Asia is a favoured destination. The young women and their families are placed at grave risk of infection. Most data from Asia show higher levels of HIV infection in young women servicing this trade than in the general community. Similarly, studies show high rates of infection among prostitutes servicing military bases.

Geographic and Social Mobility

There is a high correlation in men between mobility and HIV infection: truck drivers, soldiers and traders in Africa have extremely high infection levels. Geographic mobility to young girls would also lead to increased risk. Again very few statistics are available but at least one study has shown that 70 per cent of rural to urban migrants are under the age of 25, and 40 per cent under the age of 16. Young girls under the age of 15 seeking schooling and employment predominate in rural to urban migration in many Latin American countries, in some African countries such as Ghana and Morocco, and in Asian countries such as Bangladesh, India, Indonesia and the Philippines. Studies of international migration show the increasing involvement of women, and of young women. A significant proportion of the young women who migrate to European countries from Asia and Africa end up in prostitution. Mail order brides are also another migratory group of young women at risk of infection.

Another particularly vulnerable group are women who live in conditions of civil unrest or war. In parts of Central and Eastern Africa, patterns of infection in women correlate with the movements over the last decade of soldiers and other military personnel.

Increased female education and increased employment opportunities for young women in developing countries have resulted in a trend towards later marriages, especially among urban, educated young women. While this may have the effect of lowering overall birth rates, it also results in an increased period of potential exposure to the risks of pregnancy and HIV infection.

Poverty and Homelessness

The group of young women most vulnerable to HIV infection are those who are homeless or living in poverty. UNICEF estimates that over 40 million young people in the world are living on the streets. Many of those have left home because of sexual abuse or poverty.

Studies from Africa, Latin America and North America show alarming rates of infection in this group. In Sao Paulo, Brazil, nearly 9 per cent of 8,000 children tested in 1988 in states institutions were HIV positive. With an estimate of 7 million homeless children living on the streets in Brazil, authorities estimate that 146,000 children may already be infected. Child prostitution is common and girls of 9 to 10 work as prostitutes, often just for comfort, food or shelter. In New York City one 1988 study of more than 1,100 young men and women aged 16 to 21 living on the street, over 7 per cent were HIV positive. Since almost none of them injected drugs, transmission would have occurred sexually. In Khartoum, a 1988 study of street boys aged 6 to 14 showed 7 per cent of them to be infected.

Increasingly poverty is becoming a female phenomenon. More women are heading households or are their main financial providers: more women and children are living in poverty. The coping options for women, young girls and children living in poverty are few and none rival prostitution as an economic survival strategy. Nowadays, however, it is in many parts of the world a virtual death sentence for the woman and the children they love and support. Levels of HIV infection among women working as prostitutes in some Central and Eastern African towns and cities are as high as 80 or 90 per cent. However there is evidence of a decrease in new infections among these women as they organize to protect themselves and to educate and protect their clients. A growing number of nongovernmental organizations, especially in Latin America, are assisting them with the education of their clients.

Even where women working as prostitutes adopt the use of condoms as a protective measure for themselves and their clients, they often fail to use them in their personal sexual relationships. This failure may arise from a belief that it is romantic love which distinguishes their commercial from personal sexual activities or from the subordinate relationship that so often exists between them and their pimps who are often their lovers.

Infected Young Women

Diagnosis of HIV infection in a young woman means not only the possibility of illness and death but also that choices about sexuality, motherhood, marriage, education and work become fraught with fear and pain. Infection too often means social isolation, loneliness and discrimination. It brings fear: the fear of losing one's job, housing, medical care a dental care; fear of losing family, friends and partner; fear for the future of one's children both infected and not infected. Disclosure of one's infection status has a high price.

For a young woman, a diagnosis of HIV infection brings with it an anguished choice to forego children or to risk giving birth to an infected baby. For young women in cultures where their social identity and acceptability is determined by their fertility, there may not even be this choice. The sexual expression of love may become difficult either for the infected woman or for her partner. Relationships become difficult to enter and to maintain.

Infected young women with an infected child will need to cope with their own fatigue and sickness as well as the child's. It is estimated that infected women in sub-Saharan, Africa have given birth to 600,000 children. Of these, about 200,000 become infected duril pregnancy: the remaining 400,000 children, as well as the others that live, will have mother that will sicken and die early in their lifetimes. One estimate is that, by the year 2000, per cent of children in 10 high incidence African countries will be without mothers as result of this epidemic. Enough is known about the impact of protracted illness and death on households to be able to glimpse the impoverishment and suffering that will ensure for these children.

This is a sad picture and reflects the reality, but not its totality. An infected young woman has years, often a decade or more, of healthy life ahead of her after infection. She and those around her, need to ensure that she can remain an integral part of the communi of social and economic use. She, and they, will have special counselling and education needs and will require supportive programmes including at a later stage child care and household services to assist them.

The Prevention of HIV Infection in Young Women

We have knowingly lived with this epidemic for a decade now. As we look back over our efforts we can identify a number of principles that have shaped our response to it.

Firstly, responsibility for prevention of infection by, or further transmission of the virus through sexual or drug-using behaviour lies ultimately with the individual. Others, family friends, governments, can only provide an environment which may assist individuals change behaviour. They cannot change it for them.

Secondly, community-based organizations, that is, organizations drawn from or based within communities most at risk of infection, have a vital role to play in responding to this epidemic by:

— drawing up education and prevention programmes appropriate and acceptable to their own members;

— providing support, counselling and care to HIV-infected people and their partners, families and friends;
— providing information, support and counselling to communities to assist them to minimize HIV transmission, and lessen discrimination and stigma.

Thirdly, prevention and care policies and programmes can only be effectively implemented where the co-operation and trust of those infected or at risk of infection are maintained.

Our challenge now is to apply this understanding to the young woman of our societies. We must acknowledge their vulnerability to infection. Not an easy task for parents, community leaders or governments. We must ensure that they themselves can acknowledge their vulnerability to infection. Maybe an even more difficult task.

Perhaps the task most difficult of all, once this awareness of vulnerability is created, will be to give young women the self confidence and skills required to change their behaviour and to choose or create relationships based on mutual concern and respect. This freedom of choice is dependent upon improving women's economic independence and upon changes occurring in the ways societies construct gender, both masculinity and femininity, and sexuality. Otherwise, for young women, HIV infection will be a direct outcome of their social, personal and economic subordination.

12

Women, HIV and Development

Ms. Elizabeth Reid,
UNDP, New York

Recognition of the need to reach women with HIV education and prevention programmes and of the need to provide care, support and treatment to infected women and children is viewed by UNDP as a particular aspect of its more general mandate, given to it by its Governing Council of member nations of the United Nations, to ensure that women are participants in, contributors to and beneficiaries from development assistance. To understand this is to understand that we, the development community, are not starting from scratch in this new endeavour within the HIV epidemic to focus attention on women and children.

We have learned many things since the governments of the world first addressed the issue of women in 1975, during International Women's Year. I wish to illustrate but a few areas of growing understanding about women relevant to our response to this epidemic.

Firstly, until data on women is collected and analyzed, women will remain unperceived, unreached and un- or undervalued. Epidemiological data on this epidemic must be desegregated by gender if we are to be able to devise and monitor programmes for women. This is not happening in all countries. WHO staff and consultants must be aware of the importance of desegregating data by gender, and the need to do so should be explicitly stated in their terms of reference.

Secondly, the impact of this epidemic on women is, and will continue to be, different from its impact on men, and different on different groups of women and children and this needs to be understood.

This meeting has been an important stimulus to understanding the emerging topography of women and children affected by this epidemic. Along with HIV-infected women and HIV-infected children, other groups are being identified as in need of understanding and support. These include the wives of infected men, Who are also women with a strong desire for children, children of an infected parent or parents who are not themselves infected, the grandmothers who care for children without parents, to which we should also add the aunts and sisters, children caring for sick parents and the widows of infected men. The differing psychological, social, sexual and economic needs of all of these groups need to be better understood if we are to be able to minimize the adverse personal and social impact of the epidemic and if prevention and care programmes are to be effective.

Understanding the impact of the epidemic on women will necessitate an extensive review of the literature on the social construction of gender and the way it influences women's access to information, services, training, knowledge, decision-making and power; of the literature on women's role in the construction and maintenance of kin and conjugal relationships and how these shape their attitudes to mothering and their economic and social, including sexual, coping strategies, particularly their strategies for caring for their children; and of the literature on women's vulnerability and powerlessness and the means of addressing and lessening these socially induced conditions.

Next, contrary to popular belief, there are fewer women than men in the world. The female to male ratio in Sub-Sahara Africa has been consistently higher than unity. In sharp contrast, in southern and Western Asia and North Africa, the number of women is substantially lower than men in the population. Amartya SEN, the Indian economist, estimates that gender differential mortality rates have created 100 million missing women in Asia. That is, if there were the same ratio of Asian women to Asian men as the African female:male ratio, there would be 100 million more women in this generation.

That the pre-HIV economic, political and cultural factors involved in such gender bias could cause so many women of our generation to be missing indicates the urgency of a better understanding of these demographic dynamics as an essential prerequisite to postepidemic demographic studies. The effect of the HIV epidemic in these cultures may well be to amplify this gender biased mortality and to lead to a disproportionate increase in mortality rates among women. This kind of finding has implications for the modelling of this epidemic since most models have not taken gender specific factors into account. This needs to be addressed.

Further, development studies have shown us just how difficult women are to reach with information, services or programmes. This is for various reasons: women are generally less literate and less educated; they spend less time in schools, work places and public institutions where information is made available; they may be less likely to read newspapers, to listen to the radio or to watch television. This does not mean that women are social isolates. They have their strong social networks but these are very often centered around other women and women's organization and institutions. Such facts must shape and determine the design of HIV education and prevention programmes for women. Furthermore, there is much evidence that many services for women are not effective unless mediated or delivered by women. Mrs. Kaleeba from TASO, Uganda, made this point strikingly yesterday.

Finally, the importance of increasing women's roles in decision-making is widely accepted but has particular implications within the context of this epidemic. Jonathan Mann made a commitment in his opening address to an equitable representation of women within the GPA at Geneva. A similar imperative holds at field level and in the recruitment of consultants. National programmes and committees will need to be reviewed and means found to ensure that women are active in decision-making throughout the programme. If women are active in decision-making throughout the programme, this will necessitate, for exarnple, the re-examination of programmes where women can only get access to condoms if they have a letter of consent from their husbands.

There are many lessons that can be drawn from the past decades of development programmes and research on women. There is an urgent need to draw these lessons together if we are to respond effectively and in a timely fashion to women and children within this epidemic.

The Governing Council of UNDP has given the Organization a strong mandate on women in development as well as a mandate to respond in a timely, effective and humane fashion to this epidemic. The UNDP was established to provide technical assistance to the developing world. It is not a loan facility or a capital development facility. Its primary focus is on human development through expert assistance. It has 113 field officers in all countries of the developing world and certain countries in Eastern Europe.

Within the United Nations system, UNDP plays a lead role at the country level regarding social and economic development. The UNDP Resident Representative in each country is, at the same time, the Resident Co-ordinator of the UN system's operational activities for development, responsible to ensure complementary, co-ordinated and harmonious action at the country level by all bodies within the system.

Because of these roles and responsibilities of UNDP in the field, WHO and UNDP, in March 1988, signed a joint WHO-UNDP Alliance to combat the HIV epidemic. This alliance combined the strength of WHO/GPA as international leader in HIV policy as well as in scientific and technical matters relating to HIV and AIDS with the role of UNDP as the lead agency within the UN system for socio-economic development. UNDP brings to this alliance four decades of accumulated experience in development assistance in all sectors.

This alliance has provided support to developing countries in developing, implementing, monitoring and evaluating co-ordinated, multisectoral national HIV/AIDS plans within the framework of the global AIDS strategy. It has also helped to ensure co-ordinated support for national plans by external agencies and to draw a broader range of expertise into national AIDS programmes.

Between ten and twelve million US dollars have been allocated by UNDP field offices to HIV prevention and control activities and to programmes of support to those infected and affected and this figure is growing. The use of national funds is a demonstration of the importance attached by developing countries to HIV and AIDS and a recognition of this relationship to their development priorities.

One focus of UNDP's assistance has been the minimization of HIV transmission through blood transfusions and through the re-use of unsterile needles in health care settings. UNDP has contributed $3.6 million to WHO/GPA to support the Global Blood Safety Initiative. Women and children have been, and remain, particularly vulnerable in developing countries to iatrogenically acquired HIV infection. Women and children are the major recipients of blood transfusions and the use of injections during pregnancy, immediately after birth and during infancy is extremely common in both the traditional and modern health systems. UNDP has also had an associated concern for the minimization of occupational transmission in health settings.

I would like to end by quoting from the statement by the administrator of UNDP, Mr. William H. Draper, drawn up for World AIDS Day tomorrow:

> *"UNDP has responded swiftly to this epidemic, but, with all that we are doing, I am concerned that much more is required of those active in development if we are to do our part to slow the spread of the virus and to lessen the associated economic and social dislocations. As UNDP approaches a new planning and funding cycle, I have asked our Resident Representatives in every country and those involved in inter-country programmes to include HIV prevention and support measures in new programmes, to measure the impact of the epidemic on their country's development and to propose ways of lessening that impact.*
>
> There can be no complacency. I pledge that UNDP will spare no effort in serving as a partner in all governments to meet this challenge with resources and resolve."

13

Why Women and HIV? It Takes Two to Tango, Safely

Ms. Elizabeth Reid
UNDP, New York

Ho hum, women again. Same words. Same images. Same stories. And, even more alarmingly, same policy and programme responses. We know that socio-economic and cultural circumstances, gender differences and biological realities all influence the length and quality of women's lives. The problem is that this knowledge has not produced the outrage and anger which would force change.

Even the starkness of the insight into women's lives that the HIV epidemic gives us has not stopped us from accepting these inequalities and injustices. We continue to take them for granted. Is the ever-increasing infection of women going to be taken for granted as well?

What is the essence of the issue? Is it a question of condoms and reducing the number of sexual partners? Is it a question of empowerment and economic independence? Or is it the more fundamental question of how we fail to value and treat one another, and women in particular, as human beings.

We should start to look for the answer by talking with women and listening to their stories. These will reveal the insights that will lead us to demand:

why we continue to rely on a strategy of information and education about HIV, AIDS and genital infections which is inappropriate for women;

why we tolerate the fact that more women than men are becoming infected with HIV (and at ages 5-10 years younger than men); and

why the burden of care generated by the epidemic is falling more and more heavily on women.

We should be ensuring that early diagnosis of HIV and genital infections is available to women and men alike and that treatment and care of women who are infected is as efficient and accessible as it is for men. We must no longer accept that women rarely seek treatment for genital infections and injuries because treatment is inaccessible due to lack of time, money and transportation, because women are often prohibited by family or cultural dictates from visiting health clinics or because the treatment available is too impersonal, immodest or threatening for them to pursue.

More than this, we must confront the way our societies and communities regard men and women, how we bring up our children, the expectations we have about the behaviour of our sons and daughters, our husbands and wives, our fathers and mothers.

It seems evident that, given the knowledge and means, men have it within their power to protect themselves from sexual and drug-use infection by HIV and that women often do not. Knowing about safer sex and safer drug use is not enough for women to avoid HIV and genital infections. It is of use only if it leads to strategies women can adopt within their particular circumstances.

Women's lack of autonomy to determine the circumstances of their lives, in particular the circumstances under which they have sexual intercourse, places them in grave danger of infection. Most infected women have become infected during sexual intercourse with their husbands or regular male partners. Men's power spreads the epidemic since it allows them to initiate sexual relationships with comparative ease. The opportunity for sexual relationships is also great for those who have mobile jobs which keep them away from home and family and which may lead to boredom and loneliness.

Women alone cannot stop this epidemic nor care for its sick and its survivors. Women alone cannot bear the burden of its psychological, social and economic impact. Nor should this be expected of them. To do so would be to build in the certainty of failure, not because of any failing in women but because the nature of HIV transmission requires a conjoint, shared response.

This then necessitates the involvement of both men and women in partnership against the further spread of the virus. This partnership can be based on men's love for their partners, children and families but it will only succeed if new patterns of communication and new patterns for the sharing of the present responsibilities and joys of women's lives emerge.

The HIV epidemic and its impact will only be overcome when men and women forge a true partnership of mutual respect and trust and of equitable sharing of the burdens of sadness, pain, care and support created by the epidemic. Men and women must seek to establish the kind of honest communication about sexuality and sexual behaviour needed to prevent the transmission of HIV and STDs in their partnerships, whether hetero- and homosexual. They must work to restructure the sexual relationships in which they take part. As individuals neither men nor women can bear the personal, emotional and socio-economic burdens of HIV alone—in partnerships, they can.

Changes in individual relationships between men and women will occur only in the context of the emergence of a new social contract, not one simply governing men's or women's behaviour but one which changes what it is to be a man or a woman. The social contract must encompass the way in which we nurture and raise our children and the way society constructs its gender archetypes. It must further allow for community explorations of the appropriateness of accepted community values and standards of behaviour. Such a social contract must be supported and reaffirmed by laws, policy, budgetary priorities and programme design and delivery.

The family in all its diverse forms thus becomes the basic nexus of change. For although individual men and women can decide on ways to protect themselves from infection, the likelihood of this happening and being sustained resides in factors which long predate adulthood and sexual activity. They have their origin in how people are brought up in family life.

It is in the family context, from birth, that personalities are formed, gender identity is created and moral values are instilled. We know that self-respect, self confidence for others and an ability to talk about personal and intimate matters are all characteristics which help people to remain uninfected. In particular, we know that it is in families that boys are brought up to be boys and girls, girls, with attendant sexual and social identities, attitudes and behaviours.

Thus it is within families that the basic prevention strategies must be but in to place. Love and nurturing must be given to both boys and girls so that they may grow into independent, confident human beings, able to form respectful and non-violent relationships, whatever their sexual orientation may be. Parental-child discourse must be developed on bodily care and sexuality and strengthened on community norms and moral values, especially with regard to respect for self and others. We must change the ways that girls and boys are raised so that as adults they will be less likely to put themselves and others at risk of infection. This will require significant changes in the social construction of masculinity and femininity.

These gender paradigms must be reconstructed in particular

ways. The new paradigms should lead to the greater valuing of compassion, concern for others and love of family in men and, for women, in a simple recognition of their value and worth. It is hard to reconcile the oft-claimed valuing of women, even as mothers, with the widespread acceptance of female infanticide or the mortality rates associated with pregnancy and childbirth (which are as high as 1 in 21 in some parts of the world: 100 million women per year).

But families individually do not determine cultural meanings, social customs or community values. They inherit, accept, respect and instill them. Thus, for families to change, communities and societies must also change. The new social contract will therefore require a radical reassessment by societies of the very way men and women see themselves and each other, of the way they relate as husband and wife, lovers, brothers and sisters, parents and children, partners, colleagues and friends.

This new social contract will also need to be embodied in law and practice if it is to exist in more than rhetoric alone. It must be reflected, for example, in the attitudes and language of judges as much as in their judgments and the prescripts of the law. Only then will it be reflected in who become the judges, lawyers, police agents and cleaners of floors. Only then will it be reflected in the wage structure, school attendance records, sporting clubs and by those who minister to our spiritual and physical needs.

Thus, changing the way people interact sexually in order to prevent further HIV infection must be a catalyst for quite radical social change. Then may be there can be a choice about who leads in the tango.

14

Women and HIV/AIDS: An Indian Scenario

Geetha Devi Ayappa
Attorney Bangalore, India

INTRODUCTION

Since the discovery of HIV/AIDS in the 1980s, which continues to spread at an alarming rate, debates and research on bio-medical issues and on human rights/legal issues have gained importance. In the popular conception, medicine, and not the law, plays a leading role. But in the absence of a cure, and clear cut medical responses to HIV infection, prevention through education and behaviour modification is the only method for combating and controlling the spread of epidemic. Hence legal interventions, as a mechanism for encouraging social change, occupy the centre stage.

The legal response, which is more moralistic than rational, has paved the way for amendment of public health legislation in order to strengthen the coercive power to deal with people infected with HIV or to find scapegoats to take the blame for society's own inadequacies. However, various studies have proved the fallacy of the belief that this is the disease of 'the depraved and the deviants'. The increasing number of women being infected through hetero-sexual activity proves that the virus is no longer limited to the so-called 'High Risk' category of prostitutes, their clients and blood donors. There are many infected men, who due to their high-risk activity are unknowingly passing on the virus to their wives and partners.

Women and HIV Infection

Various studies in the late 1980s and early 1990s have revealed that HIV/ AIDS is increasingly affecting the poor and women, who by reasons of their socio-economic dependency are unable to take steps to protect themselves against the risk of infection. The race and gender pattern of HIV infection is confirmed in the 1991

WHO estimate that the cumulative total of people infected with HIV worldwide was in the order of 8-10 million. Of this total, more than seven million infections were estimated to have occurred in developing countries of sub-Saharan Africa, the Caribbean, and South-East Asia .

These patterns suggest that the socio-economic factor is a driving force behind HIV transmission. Poverty leads to a breakdown in rural communities and migration of labour. In addition, the lack of alternate economic opportunities often forces women into prostitution as the only available means of economic support.

HIV infection is preventable by all those who have access to information and preventive measures and the means to implement these measures. Hencc, factors such as low level of education and literacy, lack of access to adequate medical care, the low status of women and the corresponding powerlessness to control the basis upon which their sexual relationships with men take place, increase the transmission risk. Women's risk factors include poor health care (even during pregnancy), inadequate treatment of sexually transmitted diseases, lack of awareness or inaccesibility of preventive measures like condoms, lack of power to insist on the use of condoms, and other measures that are exclusively within the control of women.

In India, apart from targeting commercial sex workers, there is a total lack of focus on women in the context of HIV infection. Prostitutes are often identified as the main source for infections. Of late, there is a demand for the legalization of prostitution, not out of concern or compassion to protect such women, but out of concern for public health and as a strategy which provides compulsory health checks and screening of such women to combat the spread of HIV. Though HIV infection has entered private homes, women, due to their easy visibility, are identified as being responsible for spreading the infection.

Women are considered to be the 'reservoir' of the disease, as 'vectors' of transmission to their children and male sexual partners rather than individuals who are themselves infected or are at risk of HIV infection. They are in urgent need of information and education to protect themselves. However, mere knowledge about AIDS and knowledge of law will not ensure security and protection of oneself. Enforcing such measures is difficult in a relationship based on inequality. It is essential to recognise that the policies and strategies for combating HIV/AIDS require considering not only HIV-specific issues but also the underlying structural imbalances and the politics of physical and economic vulnerability which operate to increase women's risk to infection.

Due to the peculiarity of the transmission of the virus through sexual contact, and the moral stigma attached to "promiscuous" behaviour, many women are unwilling to be tested for the fear of being branded as 'Loose Women'. They remain unidentified, suffering silently without any care and treatment. Hence, in addition to the lack of focus on women, it is extremely difficult to ascertain the number of women already infected.

Hence, the issue of women and AIDS needs to be placed in a broader social and cultural context. Women's vulnerability to HIV is enhanced by the inequalities and discrimination they face in the society. Women are the subordinate sex, relegated to second-class status, kept uneducated, dependent, isolated and confined within the four walls of their homes. They are often denied access to education, health, independent income and property rights. All these factors combine to increase women's vulnerability and obstruct any effective prevention campaign. There is a necessity to understand the interaction between HIV infection and cultural values, the rights and needs of women and socio-economic patterns in the society which render women vulnerable to HIV infection.

The dilemma of balancing individual human rights and public rights has clearly established the importance of the legal response to HIV/AIDS. But what should the legal response be? What are the experiences of a decade of different legal response to HIV/AIDS? What are the modules by which law can be incorporated into HIV/AIDS policy? Can law, as a tool for social change, bring about the required changes in the behavioural pattern and value systems? Clear cut responses to many such questions are still evasive. A close analysis of the different roles of the law and the interaction between them is essential if law is to he used effectively to reinforce HIV/AIDS policy.

Analysing the decade's experiences of various countries one could identify three main models:

(a) Prescriptive Model

In this model the coercive laws have proved ineffective and need to be deleted.

(b) Protective Model

Here the focus is on human rights issues where one has to find a balanced approach between individualism and collectivism.

(c) Instrumental Model

Here the law focuses on combating subordination and seeks to change underlying values and patterns of social interaction. The critical point here is to determine to what extent the policies in the public spheres could enter and influence the behaviour in the private sphere of the family to bring about the desired changes.

Very often, laws are enacted in reponse to specific problems, viz. dowry, rape, prostitution, etc. But often it is found that such laws are inadequate to deal with the problem because various social structures and accompanying patriarchial values and attitudes are not tackled and mere cosmetic changes are not an answer to the problem of power structure and gender inequality. Hence it is desirable to bring about a social change in a broader social context. AIDS also presents a unique opportunity for effecting such a change, particularly for women, since it forces society to face issues that had hitherto been largely ignored, such as the relationship between poverty and prostitution etc. AIDS is also providing the impetus to examine issues of sexuality and personal relations, and thus there is potential for women to be able to take a more assertive role in personal relationships, to enable them to establish relationships based on mutual trust and respect. It highlights the need for men and women to take equal responsibilities in their sexual behaviour and concern for their children rather than placing this responsibility on women alone.

The preventive strategies offered to date provide very little protection for women from HIV infection. Enforcement of these strategies (such as monogamy and fidelity, safe sexual practice and usage of condoms) is dependent more on male behaviour. Where discussion about sex is still a taboo, it is difficult to educate women about safe sexual practices, and enforcement of such strategies is practically impossible. Law cannot necessarily resolve this dilemma. Hence, there is a need to address the broader socio-economic structure in the society and to empower women through legal intervention and policies.

Various social structures and cultural factors like religion, type of family structure and the institution of marriage ascribe secondary status to women and influence the perception about women in all other fields. A lack of priority in respect of health and education for women, lack of property rights, lack of access to finance and credit facilities, lack of supportive services in domestic chores, and the existing discrimination in all walks of life, deny women various rights which together form the greatest impediment in access to health care, education and employment opportunities. These, in turn, increase a woman's susceptibility to the risk of HIV infection.

The Indian constitution guarantees liberty, justice, and equality to all citizens of India, and prohibits discrimination on grounds of religion, race, caste and sex. It denounces practices that are derogatory to the dignity and status of women; nevertheless, sexual equality remains a far-too-distant goal. Sexual inequality and the spirit of patriarchy still pervade our personal laws which confer lower status on women.

Indian personal laws are still based on religion, but religion itself is a tool often used to victimise, separate and dehumanise women. Moreover, the diversity of personal laws for different communities is a hindrance for the democratic advancement of the country. Secularism cannot be achieved by recognising a variety of conflicting laws on the same subject. This affects the status of women because many of the reforms and policies are not implemented for fear of annoying communal sentiments.

Many of the existing laws need to be amended to ameliorate the status of women. These include laws regarding marriage and divorce, age at marriage, maintenance, matrimonial home and matrimonial property, inheritance and succession rights, sexual offences under criminal law (such as rape, adultery, prostitution, kidnapping, enticing and seducing a.married woman), employment related laws, etc.

Women perform a whole range of roles in society. They are helped or hindered in these roles according to their status and rights in society and in their family, their literacy levels and access to training, technology and professional activities, their standard of living and access to financial resources. The interaction between law and economic dependency is well established in a legal regime where women are deprived or discriminated against regarding property rights and the right to independent ownership of property. Removal of such legal barriers to economic independence through effective legislative reform can enhance the status of women within the family and in the society.

Law can be used to enhance the status of women within marriage and other sexual relationships. The double standards of sexual morality incorporated in law should be deleted. A woman's sexuality is supressed, and control over her body is denied because she is looked upon as the property of her father or her husband. In many of the Commonwealth countries, fidelity of a woman is a legal pre-requisite for claiming maintenance from her husband. The absence of any criminal sanctions for marital rape further reinforces attitudes about the sexual subordination of women. Similarly, woman do not have any freedom or right to control their reproductive functions. Hence, there is a necessity for enacting laws that ecognise the rights of women to make their own decisions about sexual relations on par with their male counterparts.

Law has a definite role to play even in broad community-based empowerment programmes, especially legal literacy. Legal literacy brings about an increased awareness amongst women and a change in their outlook which may lead to the assertion of their rights.

One effective method to ensure the improved status for women is to involve more women in the political process and in framing policies for women. Though many policies are framed for women, they are lacking in content because they have failed to incorporate women's experiences. Hence, more women should be involved in the process of policy formulation. Further, it is also imperative that more women get involved at the implementation level so as to ensure that the development benefits reach the needy.

In addition, women must form collectives to overcome their individual powerlessness and demand enforcement of their rights and changes in the existing social structures in the society.

In addition to empowering women through law, various other social structures and attitudes in the society need to be reformed, especially literacy levels and the health infrastructure. There is an urgency to ensure the equality of the sexes in the educational process and to prioritise the issue of women's health, often neglected by women themselves as well as by the society.

Women face large numbers of problems that are acute in their own way. The HIV epidemic accentuates these existing problems. Mere knowledge of what has to be done in order to protect oneself from HIV transmission is meaningless if one has no power over the circumstances that give rise to the risk.

Hence the short-term goal is that women should take greater control of their lives and make use of the existing preventive strategies that are available immediately. However, the long-term goal has to be minimising and eliminating women's subordination and to improve the status of women. For this, a fundamental change in socio-cultural values requiring reorientation of the values, beliefs, customs and the law that shape the perception and roles of women within the family and the society has to occur.

It is tme that legislation alone cannot change the values in society. However, an effective legislative policy is a necessary prerequisite for bringing about a change in socio-economic conditions. In order to overcome vulnerability to HIV, human rights considerations must look beyond the immediate concern to minimise and eliminate discrimination for the infected and address the unequal socio-economic position of women.

In this context, support can be drawn from the various international human rights instruments that offer scope to promote the human rights of women which have been neglected so far, and which are clearly highlighted by the HIV epidemic. Formal legal recognition of such international human rights instruments must be attempted by bringing about the necessary changes in domestic laws. And if such rights already exist in the domestic laws, then there is an urgency to amend them suitably so as to make them implementable.

15

Children in Families Affected by the HIV Epidemic: A Strategic Approach

Ms. Elizabeth Reid
UNDP, New York

INTRODUCTION

The concept of families is an important analytical and programming tool which is often overlooked within development theory and practice. Children do not spring untrammelled into the world. They are born with ties of blood, love and law to their families: parents, brothers and sisters, grandparents and other family members. These ties can bind generations together into a supportive and nurturing unit which provides security, care and love to its members. The ties change over time, maturing, strengthening and weakening. Such ties may be created and recreated outside of lineage groups, by street children, by adoptive families and by others.

Many of the most striking images of the HIV epidemic are of families, but of unfamiliar families: a grandparent surrounded by grandchildren, adolescent-headed families, often siblings and cousins bonded together, dying adults tended by their children and communities as families. It is timely to focus on such families rather than on children alone, or youth alone or adults. This allows for an intrafamilial and longitudinal analysis of the needs, skills and resources of families affected by HIV which provides a different basis for determining and ranking the required responses.

This analysis has already been done by a number of organizations assisting adolescents and children whose parents know they are HIV-infected, are ill or have died of AIDS. There is much to learn from them and this paper attempts to draw together some of their insights and knowledge. These programmes teach us that careful attention is needed to understand the trauma of children watching their parents sicken and slowly die and how this experience affects their long-verm development. Attention is also needed to understand how the families and communities caring for these children can be supported in sustainable ways to continue providing care to them and how the capacity for self-support of surviving families of children can be strengthened.

The forms that families take vary within and across cultures and generations. They are affected by increasing urbanization, by poverty, by political and economic migration, by changes in labour market structures, by the changing roles of women and other factors. Superimposed on all these factors now will be the impact on family life of the death of many parents and young adults.

Most of those infected are in the age group 20 to 40 years and the overwhelming majority are parents. Furthermore, the overwhelming majority of all those infected do not know they are infected. Many women are indirectly diagnosed when they are still well through the diagnosis of HIV infection in their children. Many men do not get diagnosed until they have a clinically observable HIV-related illness. In most households where there is one infected person, there will probably be three or more: both parents and one or more children.

WHO estimates that eight million adults in Africa have been infected with HIV and so possibly four million families already know that they are affected or will soon know. Many of these affected families do not cease to exist when the adults die. They live on as grandparent or adolescent-headed families, but many of them are seriously distressed, destitute or scattered. The figures for other developing regions and Eastern Europe are still much lower but in many areas are growing rapidly.

Up until now, many of the policies and programmes addressing the needs of affected children and adolescents have assumed that these needs start with the death of their mothers or parents and consist of predominantly material needs. It is important to broaden this focus. This paper argues that the needs of these young people start with the knowledge that someone in their family is infected and continue on to their social and sexual maturity. Their needs are psychological, emotional. ethical, legal and spiritual; they are for acceptance, nurturing, support, counselling and care; they include financial, material, educational, health and social development needs.

The paper also argues that the needs of these children cannot only be met by policies and programmes addressed to children and youth. There are at least three other types of interventions required: assistance to their parents, to their communities and of their governments. For the well being of their children, parents need to be able to continue working, need to be assisted in planning for their and their children's future and need access to treatment of opportunistic conditions which may lessen their ability to work and parent.

Extended family systems and communities need support in keeping these new family forms in their midst. Governments have a multifaceted role in increasing awareness, establishing an appropriate legal, ethical and human rights framework and in the provision of the required services and support.

This paper is intended to raise a number of issues which can serve as a basis for widespread discussion. It is addressed to all those interested in determining how best to respond to the epidemic. It is not a Manifesto for Children and Youth but rather another way of looking at the complex reality of this epidemic and its exigencies which may enable individuals, organizations and nations to rethink their HIV-related policies and programme priorities. It is now starkly clear in many parts of Africa that, if we do not quickly find appropriate ways of responding to this epidemic, the lives of many future generations will be bleak, anguished and often brutal.

PROGRAMME ELEMENTS

While specific programme components will vary according to the stage, the epidemic has reached and the situation, culture and resources of each country or community, five main strategic programme elements can be identified. Under each programme element, a number of programme components have been identified. These are not meant to be exhaustive nor are they operational in nature. The specific means of addressing each area may vary from one situation to another.

Certain components may already be included in a national response but may not have been seen to have linkages to the wellbeing of children in affected families. Other components may not yet have been put in place. The analysis here can provide a basis for reassessment of programme priorities, both at the national level and in community organizations.

1. Preparing Children for the Future

Most parents come to know they are HIV—infected when one of them or one of their children is clinically diagnosed with HIV related illnesses. The earlier a parent' s infection status is known, the more time he or she will have to plan for the children's future, in particular to find another family or person who can care for and shelter them. The parent will also have more time to pass on their skills and knowledge to them, to help the children be able to support themselves. Knowing their infection status when they are well will help the parents prepare their children and themselves emotionally for their deaths. The longer a parent can work and the longer he or she can be helped to stay well and nurture and raise the children, the less pain and trauma the children will experience.

Components of this programme element could include:

* **Access to voluntary, confidential and affordable counselling and testing for adults and the motivation to use it.** This would allow parents more time to plan for their own and their children' s future. Infected parents often want to seek advice on how and when to tell this to their children. Supportive services and counselling can help parents maintain a nurturing home environment for their children for as long as possible and to find future homes for them. Access to testing and counselling can also assist people in making decisions about whether they wish to have more children.
* **Disclosure with counselling of a child's infection to *both* parents.** The Women and AIDS Support Network Conference in Zimbabwe in 1989 stressed the importance of both parents being informed at the same time if that child is infected and that both receive caring counselling regarding their child's and their own HIV status[1]. In some cases where a child has been clinically diagnosed with AIDS and only the mother has been informed the father has blamed the mother and abandoned her and the sick child.
* **Continued employment.** HIV infected people who remain fit to work have the right to remain employed. If this right is denied them, their children will suffer.
* **Simple treatment of opportunistic infections.** Experience in Masaka, Uganda and Kigali, Rwanda has shown that, for many HIV-infected parents, treatment of conditions such as thrush, skin infection, diarrhoea and fever is important since it allows them to continue to work, to nurture their children and to die with dignity[2]. Providing such treatment can often help parents to remain with their children for a longer period. The parent' s suffering is eased and the children's memories of their parent's dying can be made much less traumatic. Counselling and access to appropriate low-cost or

subsidized medicines may lessen the problem ot families exhausting their resources in a futile search for a "cure".

* **Passing on to children production and income-generating skills.** The Kitovu Hospital home care team encourages parents, once they know they have been infected with HIV, to pass their production- and income earning skills on to their children[3]. In addition to helping the children to become economically independent, it can also be of emotional benefit to an infected parent who, through teaching them these skills, can do something to help their children.

* **Planning for children's future care.** The emotional stress of both parents and their children can be eased through parents planing tor the future çare and support ot their children. The importance ot this has been stressed repeatedly by infected women in all parts of the developed and developing world. Once the future guardian is identified, financial, legal and other arrangements can be made and this person or family involved in planning for the children's future.

* **Protection of children's inheritance and other legal rights.** The children's continuing access to the family house, land and goods is critical to their survival and wellbeing. Specific steps appropriate to traditional inheritance customs and/or national law may need to be taken by parents before their deaths. Discussing inheritance matters with clan elders and/or preparing and registering a will are examples. Parents need to be informed about their legal rights in relation to property ownership and how this can be passed on to the surviving spouse and children.

* **Prevention of infection while caring for the sick.** The experience of the home care and counselling teams of Chikankata Hospital in rural Zambia shows that simple techniques can minimize the likelihood of children or other family members being infected while caring for the sick and dying[4].

2. Assisting Children Whose Parents have Died

Children whose parents have died of HIV—related illnesses have often also lived through the deaths of others close to them: brothers and sisters, aunts and uncles, cousins, friends and increasingly, grandparents. Their very will to live has often been undermined. If they are to grow and develop as human beings and as members of civil society, they need love and care and the opportunity to form and maintain emotional ties with adults. Their material and psychosocial needs will have to be met; their right to remain integral members of their communities and their legal rights may be at risk and need protection. Consideration can be given to the provision of services to all children within an area heavily affected by the epidemic rather than only to those whose parents have died of AIDS. The latter approach may lead to resentment and stigmatization of children who receive targeted assistance.

Components of this programme element could include:

* Minimizing children's psychological and emotional trauma. The grief and loss for all living within this epidemic can be overwhelming but may be particularly so for children who watch their family members die one after another[5]. Such children not only suffer emotional pain but may also experience long-term psychosocial distress. Grief and depression may be evident or they may be expressed through behavioural problems. Children need opportunities to express and come to terms with these losses. Loving care and support can help heal the pain. Play is another important way that children do this. Experience with traumatized Mozambican refugee children. and in villages in Masaka and Rakai districts in Uganda, has shown that community-based activities such as play groups can help children recover. Normalization of daily life, like continuing to attend school. is also important. Teachers, religious leaders, nurses, healers or other adults in the community can be trained to counsel and help children recover from trauma.

Keeping survivors as integral members of their communities. This will necessitate attitudinal change where discrimination and stigma toward survivors exist. It will also require the provision of care and shelter within the children's families or communities. One significant advantage of care within the children' s own community is that relationships can be maintained which will be important as the children grow older. Children cut off from these relationships will have no one to turn to when help is needed. Where discrimination and stigma cause the isolation or rejection of children whose parents have died of AIDS. political and community mobilization for the protection of their

customary, legal, ethical and human rights will be particularly important.

Basic material needs. Direct assistance is often required by affected families. Women in Kigali asked Caritas to help them continue to be able to care for their children as long as possible by providing a nutritious meal for them and their children each day and by treating the opportunistic infections that hindered their ability to care. TASO in Uganda[6]. WAMATA in Dar es Salaam and the Kagera[7] region' provide food and blankets and at times, financial assistance. The basic needs of affected families need to be met on an ongoing basis.

Education, training and employment creation. Formal education, vocational training, nonformal skills training and the provision of necessary tools and equipment can help children support themselves. In addition, such measures as public works programmed revolving credit schemes and other measures to create employment can benefit children directly through the families caring for them. Day care facilities, formally or informally arranged, can free time for work while ensuring that young children are cared for. Young people who have lived through the trauma of this epidemic often have knowledge skills and insights that could help other young people in similar situations. Opportunities could be created for them, for example, by apprenticing them to traditional healers or through working in outreach programmes to newly affected children.

Children's social and adolescent's development needs. To grow and develop into an adult capable of constructive social interaction, children need to be nurtured and stimulated. Younger children, for example, develop best when they have an opportunity to establish an ongoing, caring relationship with one or more adults. Such developmental needs have important implications for the type of care appropriate to provide for children and adolescents whose parents have died. Family-based care in a child's own community generally provides the best opportunities for promoting positive psychosocial development.

Children's and adolescent's sexual development needs. Sexually active adolescents generally lack

access to information services for sexually transmitted infections and to condoms, particularly sizes to fit boys. They also lack opportunities to discuss these issues with each other or others whom they respect. The Anti-AIDS clubs in Zambia or the discussion groups run by the Women and AIDS Support Network in Zimbabwe have shown that providing these opportunities can significantly change peer group sexual norms, expectations and behaviour.

Children and adolescents who have cared for and then watched the adults in their lines die one by one and who know that these deaihs are linked to the expression of sexuality may well experience problems as they move into puberty and into adulthood. There is no precedent for the extent or types of these problems. Community workers, religious leaders and others will need to be aware of these possibilities and keep communities aware of what is happening.

3. Meeting the Special Needs of HIV-infected Children

As with adults, most asymptomatic HIV—infected children do not know that they are infected. They continue to lead their daily lives. Simple infection control procedures can protect all family members or institutional workers from transmission of the virus. Testing has been advocated both mandatory and voluntary to determine the HIV status of orphans. However, there are serious ethical issues involved in testing and disclosure to children. Issues which need to be determined include: Who wants to know and why? Will it benefit the child to be tested and know?

How? Who should determine this and how? Can a child give informed consent to testing? Public policy needs to be drawn up in this area.

Infants and children with HIV-related illnesses may have special care needs. Meeting these is more difficult where one or both of the parents is also infected or has died.

Components of this programme element could include:

Support to families with a sick child. One of the most effective ways of supporting a sick child is by Providing support to the family caring for it, particularly by helping them deal with the trauma of the diagnosis. An infant with an HIV-related condition like many other sick children often suffers from chronic diarrhoea, fever and respiratory infection. As with adults, however the provision of

a healthy diet and basic medications can improve the quality of its life. A child s illness may be the first indication to its parents that they are infected with HIV .

Promotion of non-discrimination policies and programmes. Enforcement of existing laws or establishment of new ones may be necessary to ensure the rights of HIV infected children. For example, inheritance laws, both customary and modern, may have to be reviewed or enforced to ensure that infected children have access to their parents property for support, adoption laws may need to be made more flexible to facilitate care for their children and anti-discrimination laws will need to be established and/or enforced. Creating a community environment where HIV positive children can be placed with families can help reduce discrimination against these children. Families of children with an infected child should be supported if they desire to stay together.

4. Reaching Children and Adolescents who are Especially Vulnerable

Among and within families affected by the HIV epidemic, there will be some children or families of children at particular risk of destitution and of HIV infection: urban families without the support of their extended families, families who for whatever reasons lack the support of their communities, children struggling to survive on the streets, children suffering sexual abuse within families, and others. For many of these young people, survival sex, sex in exchange for money, clothing, affection, shelter, food, etc., is a basic coping strategy.

Components of this programme element could include:

Assistance to street children. Special strategies need to be developed to help children living on the street to have greater control over their lives, to have the means to avoid infection and to seek alternatives to the street. Street children and others living in marginal circumstances may not only be isolated from the wider community, they may be actively persecuted by it. Providing a broad range of measures to help increase their safety, health and well-being may help reduce their social marginalization.

Reducing the susceptibility of young women to infections.[8] Girls and young women may be particularly susceptible to HIV infection not only because they are less able to control the situations in which they have intercourse but also because their genital area provides less of a barrier to the virus and is easily irritated or torn. Communities and families need to assist young women to wait longer before becoming sexually active and to be able to ensure that all their sexual activity is safe.

5. Reducing the Number of Affected Children

This objective can be achieved by decreasing the number of adults becoming HIV-infected. Highest priority must be given to bringing about the attitudinal and behavioural change and the change in community norms and values required to bring this about. Because those with less control over their own lives are at greater risk, efforts to improve the socio-economic status of the most destitute and measures to empower women are critical to reducing the spread of the virus.

PROGRAMME STRATEGY

The breadth and diversity of the interventions required to respond adequately to the needs of children in families affected by the HIV epidemic present particular challenges to programme development and implementation. If the five programme elements just outlined are to be achieved, there must be an overarching programme strategy which is to create an environment that will encourage and support the necessary changes.

In this respect, policies to address the needs of children in affected families are no different from those directed, for example, to adults. Efforts must be made to create an environment that is sensitive to the needs and concerns of all people affected by the epidemic and which expresses care and compassion for these people rather than fear, hostility or alienation.

1. Assess Needs, Monitor the Situation and its Impact

In areas seriously affected by the epidemic, the ability of extended families and communities to provide for the basic needs of children without parents may be threatened. Those from outside the community who wish to provide support should, as an initial step, seek to understand what specific difficulties these children, families and communities are facing and how they themselves are coping with them. Cultural and socio-economic differences will result in different patterns of need as well as different survival and coping strategies both within and among communities and countries. These variations need to be taken into account in planning interventions so that the measures carried out will reinforce and not undermine constructive family and community level efforts.

An inventory and/or needs assessment can provide an initial picture of the situation of children in families affected by HIV. A system for monitoring needs and measuring the impact of interventions over time needs to be established. It can generally best be established by building upon existing systems functioning at the village level and above, such as village health or development committees or health posts. Assessment and monitoring are most effective when they are participatory processes, actively involving people from the communities most affected. Participation in assessing and monitoring needs also creates local awareness and engagement.

2. Create National Awareness and Engagement

There is a need to sensitize the public to the specific needs and problems of children in families affected by the epidemic as well as to promote a national sense of responsibility for responding to these needs. The extent and nature of the situation need to be widely understood and people committed to respond to it. The government, private organizations, nongovernmental organizations, faith communities and international organizations can all help create an environment that will facilitate appropriate responses to these children.

3. Develop a National Policy Framework

The social, legal, ethical and human rights framework of the national response as well as its administrative and co-ordination arrangements need to be in place as early as possible. The national policy framework will guide and support appropriate responses to the needs of children in affected families from the local to the national levels. Policy areas could include: measures to protect the rights and prevent discrimination against affected children and their families; the availability of affordable voluntary counselling and testing; a national drug policy that ensures the accessibility and affordability of the basic medicines needed to treat opportunistic infections; non-discriminatory personnel policies which enable infected persons to continue to work; the rights of affected families to medical benefits and insurance.

The Government of Malawi has developed a policy framework to guide responses to the needs of affected children.[9]

These establish priorities for action and define which types of services are appropriate and which are not. Existing policies and legislation should be reviewed to determine their direct or indirect impact on the well-being of affected children and on the capacities of families and communities to care for them. Some governments have waived school fees for children whose parents have died. In some cases, governments have defined clear policies regarding the kinds of services that can be provided to limit the diversion of resources into well-intended but inappropriate interventions.

4. Create Consensus on the Most Effective and Sustainable Responses

The epidemic is a new and complex phenomenon and the most effective way to respond may not be known or be widely accepted. There could be conflicting and different approaches proposed. It is important that there be widespread discussion leading to acceptance of and support for appropriate initiatives. The affected communities together with other sources of expertise should assist in the development of such a consensus. The process of consensus building will create a broader base of support if all the key actors take part and thereby develop an investment in implementing the agreed upon policies.

External support for initiatives that are not consistent with the agreed approach can be harmful. Families and communities will play critical ongoing roles in meeting the needs of affected children. Well-intentioned agencies can create problems by funding interventions that bypass or supplant these roles. It is much more difficult to try to re-establish spontaneous family and community systems of care than to support them initially.

5. Develop Mechanism to Ensure Resources are used Effectively and Equitably

Mechanisms may be needed to promote the equitable distribution of external support and to ensure that it meets local and national needs and priorities. These may be needed at both the district and national level. One example is the Uganda Community-Based Association for Child Welfare (UCOBAC), which is a consortium of local and international child focused organizations.[10] It has been instrumental in creating awareness of the problem, in facilitating the co-ordination of activities, organizing training for the staff of member groups, promoting appropriate policies and standards of care, organizing research and monitoring children's needs. UCOBAC has also established a grants bank to help ensure available donor resources are used where most needed and in appropriate ways.[11]

6. Strengthen National Capacity to Implement the Programme

Implementation requires adequate expertise, funding and clarity about roles. Governments may find, where resources are limited, that their most effective role is guiding service providers and donors regarding priorities established in the policy framework and monitoring changing needs and programme results. Bureaucratic impediments to supporting needed services should be minimized and interventions inconsistent with the national policy framework should be pre-empted. Raising public awareness and developing a consensus on needed responses can help mobilize local participation, probably the most important resource needed. Training is a crucial element in further developing capacity to respond effectively.

CONCLUSION

The ways in which HIV is transmitted ensure that, at least in the initial stages of its spread in a given country, some communities will be affected earlier and more intensely than others. It is important from the outset that the problems emerging and the services required be seen as national priorities and not just concerns of the localities and groups first affected. Equitable burden sharing is needed. Likewise, within the most affected comrnunities, the tendency is for women to be faced with a disproportionate burden for the care, nurturing and raising of affected children. Encouragement for men to share and alleviate these responsibilities should be built into programmes.

Families and communities are the first to respond to the need of children in affected families. Consequently, government and agency policies and programmes to benefit these children will need to focus primarily on how they can support families and communities to provide for their needs. The emphasis will be on supporting, and where necessary, establishing, sustainable family and community-based efforts. For this to happen an enabling environment is required in which public awareness and government policies and programmes include the full range of children's psychological, social, material, legal and spiritual needs.

NOTES

1. Willmore, Bridgit and Sunanda Ray. Report of the Women and AIDS Support Network Conference, Zimbabwe, November. 1989, Women and AIDS Support Network, Zimbabwe, 1990.
2. Sr. Ursula Sharpe of Kitovu Hospital in *The Orphan Generation.* Uganda, Small World Production, Video, 1991, and Pere Descombes, Caritas Kigali

oral report to UNIFEM on the Bill Pruitt Memorial Fund, 1990.

3. *The Orphan Generation.* op. cit.
4. Williams, Glen. From Fear to Hope, *Strategies for Hope,* No. 1, Action AID, U.K. with AMREF, Kenya, 1990.
5. Mukayogo, Christian and Glen Williams. AIDS Orphans, *Strategies for Hope,* No. 5. ActionAid, U.K. with AMREF, Kenya, AMREF, Tanzania, and World in Need, U.K.1991.
6. Hampton, Janie. Living Positively with AIDS, *Strategies for Hope,* No. 2, ActionAid. U.K. with AMREF, Kenya, and World in Need, U.K., 1990.
7. Kaijage, Theresa .J. in *Women and HIV; an International Research and Resources Book edited* by Marge Berer and Sunanda Ray, Pandora, U.K., 1993. pp. 271-274.
8. UNDP, *Young Women: Silence, Susceptibility and the HIV Epidemic,* 1992.
9. *Policy Guidelines for the Care of Orphans in Malawi and Co-ordination of Assistance for Orphans,* Task Force on Orphans, Minrstry ot' Women and Children Affairs and Community Services, Government of Malawi, July 1992.
10. Information on the Ugandan Community-Based Association for Child Welfare can be obtained by writing to UCOBAC. P.O. Box 7449, Kampala, Uganda or by fax at (256-41) 259149.
11. We wish to record our appreciation of the assistance provided to us in the preparation of this Issues Paper by John Williamson, Consultant. We would also like to thank Prof. Karen Hein, M. D., Adolescent AIDS Program. Montefiore Medical Center, New York: and Dr. Susan Hunter and Jim Sherry of UNICEF. New York for their comments.

SELECTED REFERENCES RELEVANT TO CHILDREN AFFECTED BY THE HIV EPIDEMIC

"AIDS Orphans in Africa," Sub-Working group on Exploited Children of the NGO Committee on UNICEF, meeting notes, January 14, 1992, 9 pages.

"AIDS Orphans: What Can be Done'?" *AIDS Analysis Africa,* Bank, April 1991, 58 pages.

Ainsworth, M. and Over, M., "The Economic Impact of AIDS: Shocks, Responses and Outcomes." *Africa Technical Department,* Population, Health and Nutrition Division, The World Bank, Technical Working Paper No. 1, June 1991, 41 pages.

Ainsworth, M., "Estimate of the Excess Number of Orphans in Uganda Due to AIDS and War." can attachment to a report Africa Technical Department, Population, The World Bank, July 1991, 4 pages.

Ainsworth, M. and Rwegarulia, A. A., "Coping with the AIDS Epidemic in Tanzania: Survivor Assistance," Africa Technical Department, Population, Health and Nutrition Division, The World Bank, Technical Working Paper No. 6. July 1994, 54 pages.

Alden, J.S., Salole, G. and Williamson, J., "Managing Uganda's Orphans Crisis," PRITECH, August 1991, 68 pages.

Armstrong, Jill, "Socio-economic Implications of AIDS in Developing Countries," *Finance & Development,* December 1991, pp. 14-17.

Barnett, T. and Blaikie, P., ***AIDS in Africa: Its Present and Future Impact,*** Belhaven Press. London. 1992, 188 pages.

Barnett, T. and Blaikie, P., "AIDS: Monitoring the Downstream Effect," *AIDS Analysis Africa.* September/October 1991, pp. 8-9.

Children and AIDS: An Impending Calamity," UNICEF, 1990. 24 pages.

Dunn, A., Hunter, S., Nabongo, C. Sekiwanuka, J., "Enumeration and Needs Assessment of Orphans in Uganda: Survey Report," The Children, U.K., April 1991. 152 pages.

Hunter. S. Bulirwa, E., and Kisseka, E., "Report of a Land Utilization Survey: Masaka and Rascal Districts," draft, October 1991, 76 pages.

Hunter. S. The Impact ot AIDS on Children in Sub-Saharan Atrican Cities. draft. 1991, 25 pages.

Hunter, S. "Orphans as a Window on the AIDS Epidemic in Sub-Saharan Africa: Initial Results and Implications of a Study in Uganda," *Soc. Sci. Med.,* Vol. 31, No. 6, 1990, pp. 681-690.

Hunter, S., "The Impact of AIDS on Children in Sub-Saharan African Cities," draft, 1992, 30 pages.

Kaduru, G., Mweige, E., and Nambi, A., "A Preliminary Report on a Needs Assessment of Rakai and Masaka Districts with Particular Reference to the Socio-economic Irnpact of the AIDS Epidemic," March 1990, 25 pages.

Lejune, A., Fogel, M-F, and Walque, E., "les Orphelins de la Ville de Kigali Rwanda." [The Orphans of Kigali, Rwanda: A Quantitative and Qualitative Study] the Red Cross of Rwanda] May 1992, original in French, English translation has been prepared, 50 pages.

Muller, O. and Abbas, N., "The Impact of AIDS Mortality on Children's Education in Kampala (Uganda)," *AIDS Care,* Vol. 2, No. 1, 1990, pp. 77-80.

Mukoyo, C. and Williams, G., *AIDS Orphans,* Strategies for Hope: No. 5, Action Aid, AMREF, and AMREF Tanzania, 1991, 35 pages.

Mulemwa, J. and Badaru, N., "A Report of the Conference on 'Managing Uganda's Orphans Crisis,' held in Kampala April 29 and 30, 1992, sponsored by the Ministry of Labour and Social Aftairs and USAID/Kampala.

Namuli, R.M., "Programme for Orphans and Primary Health Rehabilitation Raika Birungi Byokka Project: Report of the Findings: Orphans and Foster Families Baseline Survey in Rakai District, November-December 1990".

Paloni, A. and Lamas, L., "A Duration Dependent Model of the Spread of HIV/AIDS in Africa," Center for Demography and Ecology. University of Wisconsin-Madison, CDE Working Paper 90 -15, 1989, 31 pages.

Paloni, A., Lee. Y. J., and Lamas. L., "The Effects of HIV/AIDS on Family Organization in Africa." Center for Demography and Ecology, University of Wisconsin-Madison, CDE Working Paper 89-21, 1990, 46 pages.

Paloni, A. and Lee, Y. J., "Families and HIV/AIDS in Africa," Center for Demography and Ecology, University of Wisconsin-Madison, CDE Working Paper 90-32. 1991, 49 pages.

Poonawala, S. and Simenn off, A. Proceedings from NCIH AIDS Orphans Workshop," Nantional Council for International Health. October 17, 1990, 19 pages.

Poonawala, S. and Cantor. "Children Orphaned by : AIDS: A Call for Action for NGO's and Donors," March 31, 1991, National Council for International Health. 27 pages.

Preble, E. A., "Impact of HIV/AIDS on African Children," *Soc. Sci. Med.,* Vol. 31, No. 6, 1990, pp. 671-680

Preble, E. A., "Women, Children and AIDS in Africa: An Impending Disaster," Symposium on International and Comparative Aspects of the AIDS Crisis, *New York University Journal of International Law and Politics,* November 15, 1990, 22 pages.

Preble, E. A., "Pediatric AIDS, Child Morbidity and Child Survival Programmes in Africa: A Complex Interaction," presented at the American Anthropological Association meeting, November 28, 1990 in New Orleans, U.S.A., 18 pages.

Preble, E. A., "AIDS Orphans in Africa," Presented to the Meeting of Norwegian NGO's on AIDS, December 4, 1990, 15 pages.

Reid, E., "Young Women and the HIV Epidemic", Journal of STD, Development 1990:1. pp. 16-19.

Reid, E. and Bailey, M., Young Women: Silence, Susceptibility and the HIV Epidemic", United Nations Development Programme,10 pages.

Reid, E., "The HIV Epidemic and Development: The Unfolding of the Epidemic," United Nations Development Programme, 16 pages.

"A Report of the Conference on 'Managing Uganda's Orphans Crisis' held at Sheraton Hotel, Kampala, 29th-30th of April 1992," Sponsored by Ministry of Labour and Social Affairs and USAID/Kampala .

"Report on a Meeting and Orphans in Africa: Florence 14/15 June 1991," UNICEF, 30 pages.

"Tanzania AIDS Assessment and Planning Study," October 1991, World Bank, 174 pages.

"The Care and Support of Children of HIV-infected Parents," World Health Organization, Global Programme on AIDS, May 1991, 38 pages.

Williamson, J., "Children Orphaned by AIDS: Unprecedented Challenges." Presented to the annual conference of the Institute on African Affairs, Washington D.C., February, 1993. 14 pages.

16

The HIV/AIDS Epidemic in Thailand

Dr. Wiput Phoolcharoen
Director, Division of AIDS,
Department of Communicable Disease Control,
Ministry of Public Health, Thailand.

EPIDEMIOLOGICAL PATTERNS

The first Thai case of AIDS was reported in 1984. The earliest recorded cases of AIDS were predominantly in homosexual men. Three years later, the importance of male to male sex as a risk factor was quickly overshadowed by the rapid increase in infection among intravenous drug users. This was immediately followed by an increase in seroprevalence among female commercial sex workers. Subsequently, the third wave of infection appeared in clients of these commercial sex workers as reflected in an upsurge of seroprevalence among men attending government sexually transmitted disease clinics. A fourth wave reflected a spread of infections among the wives and girl friends of men who visited commercial sex workers. Seropositive rates in women attending antenatal clinics continue to increase, along with an increasing incidence of reported pediatric AIDS cases. This can be observed as evidence of the fifth wave of the epidemic.

With a rather well-developed health care infrastructure, Thailand is in a position to launch and maintain an acceptable system of HIV surveillance. Information on HIV seroprevalence has been collected semi-annually in every province in Thailand since June 1990 by the Ministry of Public Health through the sentinel surveillance system.

The wide regional variations in the epidemic are particularly noteworthy. The north has the highest prevalence, while the northeast consistently has the lowest. Within the north, Chiang Mai, Chiang Rai and Phayao are the worst affected. There has been a rapid increase, for example, in Trat, Rayong and Phetchaburi. This is observed to co-relate with the number of commercial sex workers in each locality.

One of the distinguishing characteristics of the Thai epidemic is that urban and rural infection levels do not appear to be strikingly different as is the case in most African and Western settings This may be explained in part by the high mobility of the Thai population as a consequence of rapid socio-economic changes. It is also notable that the most vulnerable groups are the socio-economically backward and poorly educated labour classes in both the industrial and agricultural sectors.

Political Response

From 1984 to 1990, AIDS was perceived to be a newly-emerging public health problem. Consequently, the Ministry of Public Health was the key player in determining national policies and strategies for its prevention and control. Vigorous promotion of the use of condoms in the commercial sex settings has been an important and reasonably successful programme. Universal screening of blood and blood products was introduced all over the country in 1988. The use of universal precautions was also emphasized from the outset but has been slow in gaining widespread use.

The year 1991 can be considered a turning-point in the evolution of the Thai government's AIDS policies, strategies and programmes. The epidemic had spread to all sectors of the society and there was no sign of abatement. It became apparent that more concerted efforts and innovative strategies were essential. Hence, the National AIDS Prevention and Control Committee, under the chairmanship of the Prime Minister, was established. The Permanent Secretary of the Ministry of Public Health was assigned to act as the committee's secretariat, and the Division of AIDS, Department of Communicable Disease Control, assumed the responsibility of the office of the secretariat.

It was recognized that a multisectoral approach was highly desirable, and efforts were undertaken to involve all government agencies, non-government organizations and the business community. The National AIDS Prevention and Control Plan for 1992—96 was formulated to meet this need. The planning process entailed national level co-ordination under the leadership of the National AIDS Prevention and Control Committee. Government funding was sought to meet the initial needs of the plan. In 1993, all 14 ministries submitted funding requests in accordance with the programmes specified in the National AIDS Plan, amounting to $ 44 million. The National AIDS Programme's budget has been increasing continuously, reaching $60 million in the current fiscal year.

In 1993, the upward trend of the AIDS epidemic continued, necessitating some revisions to the National AIDS Prevention and

Control Plan for 1995-96. The increasing number of the AIDS cases and death signalled a severe erosion of the Thai social fabric. As people with HIV/AIDS began to experience stigmatization and discrimination, families, community and humanitarian aspects needed special attention. Thus, the revised plan gave priority to the following programmes:

1. Programme on Prevention for Behavioural and Social Aspects
2. Programme on Health Promotion and Medical Services
3. Programme on Provision of Counselling
4. Programme on Living with AIDS and Legal Measures
5. Programme on Research and Evaluation
6. Programme on Development of Administration, Organization and Management.

The collaboration among governmental organizations, non-governmental organizations and private sector is the key focus of the plan. There are over 200 development-oriented Thai NGOs participating in the programme against the AIDS epidemic in Thailand. The Thai NGO Coalition on AIDS, a network of 42 NGOs, was established in the late 1990s. The role of Thai NGOs in AIDS has been mainly directed towards developing models of AIDS education and social support services where government services have been relatively weak. NGOs have taken the lead in working among stigmatized social groups; developing participatory forms of AIDS education, client centered counselling and support services, campaigning on social acceptance of people living with HIV/AIDS and their rights to non-discrimination; and in training and employing people to work as AIDS educators and counsellors.

Another step has been the establishment of the Thailand Business Coalition on AIDS in 1993—a non-profit organization providing information, technical support and training programmes to Thai business in the formulation of effective and non-discriminatory measures for AIDS in the workplaces.

The Organization for the Improved Management of the AIDS Prevention and Control Programme, which was at first designed to co-ordinate the multisectoral AIDS policy, has been decentralized to ensure more efficient management. The executive board, chaired by the Minister of Public Heath, was formed in 1994. The permanent secretaries of six ministries have been appointed to lead the work of six subcommittees. These are:

1. Public Relations/ Mass Media by the Office of Prime Minister.
2. AIDS Education by the Ministry of Education.
3. AIDS Programmes for Special Target Groups by the Ministry of Interior.

These three committees will be responsible for reducing risk behaviour through changes in the social environment and community life-style, aimed at achieving both short-term and long- term objectives.

4. Medical and Counselling Services by the Ministry of Public Health
5. Social Acceptance and Human Rights by the Ministry of Labour and Social Welfare.
6. Research and Evaluation by the Ministry of University Affairs.

Achievements of the National Programme

An effective programme to prevent HIV infection must have both universal and targeted components. The universal component includes reducing HIV-related discrimination, removing social and commercial restrictions on information necessary for safer behaviour, and providing information about the risk of HIV. The targeted component involves devoting the limited resources for intensive programmes of behavioural change to situations and groups where the risk of HIV transmission is at the highest. Underprivileged communities should be specially targeted. Social action and educational measures should seek to encourage healthy lifestyles to reduce risk of infection.

Currently, there is some evidence to suggest that the National AIDS Programme has achieved significant results. A continuous decrease in sexually transmitted diseases has been seen during the last four years. Finally, the decline in the HIV seroprevalence rate among the recently recruited military conscripts, which accounts for the HIV epidemic in the majority of Thai youths, explicitly demonstrates the programme's effectiveness.

Legal and Ethical Aspects

As with other communicable diseases, the tragic epidemic of HIV/ AIDS presents the classical public health problem of a conflict between the welfare of the community and the rights of the individual, but with significant differences. Like other sexually transmitted and communicable diseases, HIV/AIDS has called for measures to prevent its spread as for the protection of the privacy and other civil rights of persons afflicted with the disease. But HIV/AIDS poses serious and different problems because as yet there is no cure and no vaccine for prevention; and because the incidence of HIV/AIDS is concentrated in certain high-risk individuals - intravenous drug users, prostitutes and promiscuous males-who are particularly vulnerable to discrimination.

Legislation has been a significant component of the response to the HIV/AIDS epidemic. An early response to the epidemic was to prevent the influx of infected cases through migration. In 1983, under the Immigration Act, the Ministry of Interior prohibited the immigration of foreigners with HIV/AIDS. This regulation was not strictly enforced because of the lack of available tests at the time and pressure from the international community. Consequently, this was revoked in 1991.

Through a public health ministerial announcement in 1984, under the Contagious Diseases Act, AIDS was required to be reported to the health authorities. Six years later, in order to protect the confidentiality of the test results, case reporting was cancelled. Instead, AIDS was required to be notified by using a code for the purpose of epidemiological surveillance. Currently, there is no compulsory notification of those with HIV/AIDS to the authorities.

During 1990-1991, attempts were made to enact a reactionary law. An AIDS Bill which would have adopted stricter measures and punishment against those with HIV/AIDS was introduced. The purposes of this bill were to:

Establish a national committee to prevent and control AIDS.

Compel reporting of those with AIDS to the medical authorities.

Order those with AIDS to appear for a medical check-up.

Oblige those with AIDS to report their movements to the medical authorities.

Compel those with AIDS to be detained in, or to be prohibited from entering, certain areas.

Prohibit those with AIDS from spreading the disease.

Punish those who violate the law by means of imprisonment and fines.

After two years of controversial arguments, the National AIDS Prevention and Control Committee rejected this bill.

Since AIDS related legislation has been controversial and the fact that legislative aspirations may be plagued by poor law enforcement, the current approach towards those with HIV/AIDS should be informed by the National AIDS Prevention and Control Plan with its multipronged strategies. Mandatory testing without informed consent has no place in this plan because it violates the rights and dignity of individuals and is counter productive to control of the epidemic. However, these aspirations are not reflected in the current law and practice in terms of effective redress. A key challenge will be to ensure that the AIDS Control Plan itself is able to be translated into effective remedies.

17

Are Young People in the Philippines Taking Chances with HIV/AIDS?

D. Balk, T. Brown, G. Cruz, and L. Domingo

The first AIDS case in the Philippines was diagnosed in 1984 Since then, the number of AIDS cases and detected HIV infections has climbed slowly but steadily. By the end of 1995, 234 AIDS cases and 470 HIV infections had been reported to the Department of Health Vesting has been limited, however and the number of HIV infections is undoubtedly much larger than reported.

As in most Asian countries, early infections were often associated with overseas travel or contact with foreigners. By 1990, however it was clear that the epidemic was spreading among the Filipino population.

A number of factors contribute to the potential for a serious HIV/AIDS epidemic in the Philippines. For one thing there is a substantial commercial sex industry although the National HIV Sentinel Surveillance System has detected only very low levels of HIV infection among sex workers, the system has found much higher rates of syphilis infection. This is cause for concern because syphilis and other sexually transmitted diseases not only spread through the same routes as HIV but also greatly enhance the chances of HIV transmission between sexual partners. The low level of condom use reported by commercial sex workers heightens this concern.

Secondly reports have sugested that many young men in the Philippines engage in premarital sex with girlfriends and acquaintances. Early AIDS cases were associated with men having sex with men, but more recently heterosexual transmission has increased in importance. Finally injecting drug use may provide an avenue for HIV transmission among a small number of young people.

A national Young Adult Fertility and Sexuality Study (YAFS-II), conducted in 1994, makes a substantial contribution to the information available on risk factors that could produce a serious HIV/AIDS epidemic among young people in the Philippines This issue of Asia-Pasific Population & Policy reports on key finding from the survey. More detailed information will be published in a full report.

ABOUT THE SURVEY

YAFS-II was the first nationally representative survey of youth in the Philippines that covered both men and women. An earlier Young Adult Fertility Survey (YAFS-I), conducted in 1982, included only women.

The University of the Philippines Population Institute conducted YAFS-II with a network of nine regional research centers throughout the country. The project was supported by the United Nations Population Fund (UNFPA). The East-West Center's Programme on Population collaborated in the survey with support from the United States Agency for International Development (USAID).

YAFS-II was a household survey covering men and women we 15 to 24. A total of 10,879 young people were interviewed, with separate questionnaires for men and women and for married and unmarried respondents. In addition to these questionnaires, a sealed-envelop questionnaire covering highly sensitive issues was given to a subgroup of respondents. Screening data were also collected on all households visited and on the 959 sampled communities.

The survey covered many subject areas. Several sequences of questions were designed to elicit information on sexual experience, both directly and in the context of questions about dating. Additional questions explored condom use and attitudes toward condoms, knowledge of HIV/AIDS and other sexually transmitted diseases, and levels of concern about infection.

A LITTLE KNOWLEDGE

Ninety-five per cent of all the young people covered in the survey had heard of AIDS. As would be expected, younger respondents were slightly less likely than older respondents to have heard of the disease. Still, a full 90 per cent of 15year-olds had heard of AIDS. Controlling for age, awareness of AIDS tended to be lower in rural areas, among respondents with less education, and among those with no regular exposure to the mass media. There was no gender difference in AIDS awareness.

Although awareness was nearly universal, knowledge of AIDS was more limited. When respondents who knew about AIDS were asked how it is acquired, 85 per cent correctly identified at least one sexual mode of transmission, and 25 per cent correctly identified at least one non-sexual mode. The most frequently mentioned transmission mode was commercial sex, cited by 66 per cent of these respondents. Twelve per cent could not identify a single correct mode of transmission, and 26 per cent gave at least one incorrect answer, such as having contact with the belongings of an infected person, kissing, or using public toilets.

An overall assessment of AIDS knowledge identified five characteristics associated with a good understanding of the syndrome and its transmission routes. These were age, family wealth, education, being single, and discussion networks.

Discussions about AIDS appeared to be an important factor in promoting knowledge—so important, in fact, that such discussion,s nullified the direct effect of media exposure. Young people who talked about AIDS with three or more different types of people (such as friends, partners, parents, or teachers) had a much better understanding of the disease than those who discussed it with only one type of person or did not discuss it at all. Women were more likely to have discussed AIDS with a variety of people—most young men had only discussed it with their male friends.

Most young people felt that they themselves were at little or no risk of HIV infection. Only 12 per cent thought that they were at some personal risk. Even men who had visited commercial sex workers tended to believe that they had little or no chance of contracting HIV. Among single men who had paid for sex during the 12 months before the survey and had not used a condom, only 29 per cent thought that it was likely or very likely that "someone like them" might become infected.

SOME YOUNG MEN ARE TAKING CHANCES

The risk of contracting AIDS depends largely on two factors—sexual activity and injecting drug use. In the Philippines, sexual transmission is the more serious concern. The YAFS-II survey showed that few 15- or 16-year-olds had engaged in sex, but sexual activity increased steadily with age. Among 24-year olds, 55 per cent of men and 23 per cent of women had engaged in premarital sex.

Most of the men and women who were sexually active before marriage reported that their only partner was their future spouse.

However, men were almost 20 times more likely than women to have had sex before marriage with at least one additional partner.

Reports of premarital sex tended to be higher among men who lived in urban areas and men who were Catholic. Among 23- and 24-year-olds, men with a high-school or college education were more likely to have engaged in premarital sex than were men with only an elementary education.

The survey results suggest that the longer men remain single, the greater their risk of exposure to HIV infection. By age 24, 22 per cent of single men reported having had sex with a girlfriend or acquaintance during the 12month period before the survey, and 8 per cent reported having visited a commercial sex worker. Among all single men, 13 per cent reported having had only one sexual partner, another 10 per cent reported two or more partners, and 3 per cent reported five or more partners .

Modeling studies have shown that even such small groups of sexually active individuals can greatly accelerate the spread of HIV. This is particularly true when men have sex with commercial sex workers and also with other partners. The YAFS-II survey results provide convincing evidence of such overlapping sexual networks.

Thirtynine per cent of married men reported having had at least one sexual partner before marriage other than their future wife. Seven per cent reported five or more premarital partners. As with single men, there was significant overlapping of sexual contacts. Seven per cent of married respondents reported premarital sex with their future wives, other girlfriends, and commercial sex workers Although few married men reported having visited a commercial sex worker during the 12 months before the survey 16 per cent reported having had an extramarital affair at some time during their marriage. Reported levels of extramarital sex were higher in rural areas than in urban areas.

Men who visit commercial sex workers face a particularly high risk of infection Surveys in the Philippines have sporadically detected low levels of HIV in commercial sex workers, but these levels are expected to increase over the next few years.

Eight per cent of the men interviewed during the YAFS-II survey had paid for sex at some time in their lives. The per centage that reported having ever paid for sex increased steadily with age-from 0 per cent at age 15 to 17 per cent by age 24. Men in urban areas were more likely to have paid for sex than men in rural areas, and men with a high-school or college education were more likely to have paid for sex than men with only an elementary education.

Among those who had visited a commercial sex worker during the 12 months before the survey 26 per cent had paid for sex monthly or more frequently 22 per cent occasional and most of the remainder only once. Almost half reported changing sexual partners each time they paid for sex, while another quarter reported visiting the same partner repeatedly. The average number of paid sexual partners over 12 months was 2.5.

Male homosexual and bisexual behaviour has been strongly associated with the HIV epidemic in many countries. Among sexually experienced young men covered by the YAFS-II Survey, 7 per cent reported having had sex with other men, but only 1 per cent reported exclusively male sexual partners. An other 9 per cent gave inconsistent information or failed to answer this question. Most of those reporting some sexual experience with men had predominantly female sexual partners.

Infecting drug use has not yet made a substantial contribution to reported HIV infections and AIDS cases in the Philippines. However 2 per cent of the YAFS-II survey respondents reported that they had tried injectable drugs. This finding probably understates the true level of drug use. It suggests some limited potential for HIV transmission through needle sharing among drug users.

WHEN MEN TAKE CHANCES, THEY POLE WOMEN M RISK

YAFS-II survey results indicate much lower levels of sexual risk-taking among young women than men. Among all single women, only 2 per cent reported ever having had sex unlike their single male counteriarts, virtually all single women who reported any sexual experience had only one partner. Thirty five per cent of married women reported having had premarital sex, but nearly ad of these had only had sex with their future husbands. Only 4 per cent reported ever having had an extramarital affair.

Survey results showed no differences in levels of premarital sexual activity between rural and urban women or women with different levels of education. However, Catholic women were more likely to have experienced premarital sex than were non-Catholics

Given existing differences in social expectations, women are more likely than men to under-report their premarital and extramarital sexual experience Even taking this tendency into account, however results from the YAFS-II survey strongly suggest that single and married women are at risk of HIV infection primarily through the previous and current sexual activities of their partners.

FEW USE CONDOMS

Proper use of condoms can substantially reduce the risk of

HIV infection. YAFS-II survey results showed that knowledge of condoms was high, but actual condom use was extremely low.

When asked about their knowledge of family planning methods, 69 per cent of the men interviewed mentioned condoms without prompting, and another 18 per cent reported that they knew of condoms after being prompted. Among the women,62 per cent reported knowledge of condoms without prompting and another 25 with prompting. Among sexually active men, 98 per cent had heard of condoms, but only 58 per cent of those who knew about condoms were aware that condoms could help prevent AIDS.

Only 23 per cent of sexually active men reported that they had ever used a condom, and far fever [4 %] reported having used a condom during their most recent sexual experience Married men and sexually active single men were equally likely to have ever used a condom. Several other factors were associated with having ever used 3 condom

Residence: urban men were much more likely than rural men to have ever used condoms
Education: among 23- and 24-yearolds, men with at least a college education were three times as likely to have used condoms as men with only an elementary education
Population education in school: classes on family planning and sexually transr..ted diseases had a strong positive influence on condom use.
Regular exposure to mass media.
Knowledge of AIDS: men with the greatest knowledge of AIDS were more likely to have used condoms than men whose knowledge of AIDS was poor or moderate.

Condom use is particularly important for men who visit commercial sex workers. Men who had paid for sex were more than twice as likely as other men to have ever used condoms, but the rates of condom use for this group were still low. Only 27 per cent of those who had recently visited a commercial sex worker reported using condoms all or most of the time, 20 per cent reported using condoms some of the time, and 50 per cent said that they never used condoms at all.

In the Philippines, condoms are available in drugstores, supermarkets, and private clinics. The government family planning programme, however, has an explicit policy against supplying condoms or other contraceptives to unmarried people. When asked during the survey, nearly all sexually active men said they knew where they could obtain condoms. Most mentioned drugstores as a source, but a sizable minority—even of unmarried men—also mentioned government health centers.

Men were asked how long it took to travel from their home

to the nearest source of condoms. Not surprisingly, rural men reported more than twice the travel time (49 minutes) reported by urban men (22 minutes). In both urban and rural areas, men with only an elementary education reported more than twice the travel time (67 minutes) reported by men with a college education (33 minutes).

When asked how they felt about using condoms, 90 per cent of sexually active men expressed some negative attitudes. The most commonly expressed negative attitude (by 58 per cent) was that condoms make sex less pleasurable. Nearly half 147 per cent) said that they would be embarrassed to buy condoms at a store, and sizable minorities stated that condoms were too expensive to use regularly (34 per cent) or that condom use was against their religion (32 per cent).

SUMMARY AND POLICY RECOMMENDATIONS

YAFS-II survey results indicate that a substantial minority of young men in the Philippines are at a heightened risk of HIV infection. By the time they reach age 24, almost 40 per cent of Filipino men have had sex with at least one partner other than their wife or future wife, and 3 per cent have had five or more sexual partners. Almost 10 per cent have visited a commercial sex worker.

Young women appear to be taking fewer chances. Less than 10 per cent of single women have had sex by age 24, and most married women have only had sex with their husbands. If these results are accurate, women in the Philippines are primarily at risk through the premarital and extramarital activities of their sexual partners.

Awareness of AIDS is high, but knowledge of how the virus is spread is somewhat limited. Similarly, the perception of risk is low. There appears to be a strong perceived association of HIV with commercial sex and multiple sex partners. Young people do not seem to realize that sex with a boyfriend or girlfriend also entails a potential risk. Even among young men engaging in commercial sex without condoms, only one-third felt that "someone like them" might be likely to contract HIV.

The low level of reported condom use is of particular concern. Although most young people are familiar with condoms in the context of family planning, only a little more than half of the young men interviewed knew that the proper use of condoms could prevent HIV transmission. Only 23 per cent of sexually active young men had ever used a condom.

The policy implications of these findings are clear. Future efforts in AIDS education need to stress the possibility of risk in any sexual encounter. YAFSII survey results showed large differences in knowledge about AIDS among education groups, suggesting that AIDS information programmes need to target young people who do not have high levels of formal education. The large percentage of respondents who said that they had discussed AIDS with their friends suggests that peer education approaches may be particularly effective.

Young people are not likely to change their Behaviour if they do not consider themselves at risk. Expanded efforts are needed to inform young people of the risks of unprotected sex, perhaps through AIDS education and awareness campaigns. Among those young people who, nevertheless, engage in risky Behaviour, every effort is needed to encourage the proper and consistent use of condoms.

Although condoms are widely available through commercial outlets, the official policy limiting condom distribution at government clinics to married couples may very well be inhibiting their use. Condoms need to be made more widely available in rural areas and possibly in neighbourhoods where the less-educated tend to live. Given reported low levels of condom use among men having sex with men, any programme designed to slow the spread of HIV should also focus on condom use among male homosexuals and bisexuals.

Numerous social and religious barriers remain in the Philippines that inhibit open discussion of risk Behaviours, promotion of condom use, and training in the skills required to protect oneself from HIV. To avoid a serious epidemic, these barriers must be overcome and effective prevention programmes put into place.

18

The HIV/AIDS Epidemic in Uganda: A Programme Approach

Desmond Cohen
Former Governor
Institute of Development Studies

I. HIV AND AIDS IN UGANDA

The HIV epidemic in Uganda has its origins in the early to mid Seventies, although it was not diagnosed as such until 1984. The spread of HIV in the population has been rapid. By the end of 1991 30,190 cases of AIDS had been reported to the AIDS Control Programrne (ACP) surveillance unit, with cases from almost every District in the country. This is thought to be a significant under estimate of the true number of cases as a result of under reporting. Modelling of the epidemic suggests that the actual number of cases of AIDS is some 6 to 7 times greater than reported cases.

In 1987-88 a national serological survey was undertaken to establish the level and distribution of HIV infection in the population. In the event the survey was not fully representative, with gaps in the data for the eastern and northern regions particularly. The survey generated an estimate of an adult HIV prevalence level of 9 per cent, i.e. some 800,000 people were thought to be infected. There were wide variations between regions and between urban and rural areas. In the case of urban areas the rate was estimated to be as high as 29 per cent in some regions; much lower, but still significant, in rural areas. Because most of the population is rural [some 90 per cent] even relatively lower rural HIV rates implies high absolute numbers of people who are infected. More recent data from ante-natal clinics has yielded seroprevalence rates of 27 per cent in true urban areas like Kampala, to as low as 3 per cent in some rural areas [with the possibility that rates are even lower than this in some parts of the country]. Using the national serosurvey as the base, and applying the evidence from sentinel sites, it appears that the current numbers infected with HIV are about 1.3 million.

As noted above, the cases of AIDS which are notified to the Ministry of Health (MOH) are considered to be a massive underestimate of tne true numbers. This reflects the coverage and quality of health care in Uganda, with many persons with HIV related illnesses outside the reach of the formal health care system. Many fall back on traditional healers for assistance, and as such are never reported to the MOH. In part also, the continuing stigma associated with HIV and AIDS leads individuals and families to prefer some other diagnosis. Nevertheless, the data on AIDS as reported has some value in permitting analysis of the sex and age distribution of those identified. About a third of the reported AIDS cases are children under 5, reflecting the frequency of paediatric cases. Otherwise there is a bunching of cases in the ages 15-49, with a mean age for adults of 27 years. The elderly and young adolescents are more or less generally free of infection.

Of great importance are differences in the median ages of infection of men and women; for men this is 30 years, but for women is much younger at 25. Not only are women infected at an earlier age but there is some evidence that infection rates are higher than for men. why this is so is far from clear, and cannot simply be a reflection of males choosing more youthful sexual partners. Many other factors must also be operating, and these require analysis if there are to be effective policies for prevention, for care and for dealing with the impact of the epidemic on the social and economic system. The gender dimensions of the problem need to be constantly at the forefront of analysis and policy, and not simply, although these are important, because of the problems raised for perinatal transmission and for the general health of mothers and children.

A. TRANSMISSION OF HIV

Much is now known about HIV and AIDS and there has been immense progress made in a remarkably short time in understanding transmission of the virus. Nevertheless, there is much that is not known, and there remain major areas of uncertainty. Why women are infected at an earlier age than men is one area where research is urgently needed. It seems unlikely that a vaccine will be discovered, and be available, before the end of the decade, but even then it is improbable that in the conditions which exist in many developing countries, including Uganda, that a vaccine will be sufficient to prevent the continuing spread of HIV in the population. The potential future discovery of a vaccine thus in no way diminishes the need to put in place now effective policies for prevention and care.

Having said this the ways in which the virus are spread are now well understood. In Uganda, as in much of Africa, the major mode of transmission is sexual. Heterosexual transmission is thought to account in Uganda for about 90 per cent of cases, with the other 10 per cent of infections being from mother to child [paediatric] and from infected blood. Securing the blood supply is an important intervention, but given the relative size of the contributing factors in transmission it is of much reduced importance. Thus by far the most significant risk factor in determining the spread of HIV and the resulting size of the population which is infected, are unsafe sexual practices. This is compounded in the Ugandan case by social and cultural factors which lead many men to have multiple sexual partners, and under conditions where neither partner is protected from the virus through the use of condoms. Evidence from Uganda suggests that condoms are infrequently used; and it is reported that only about 5 per cent of women have ever used contraceptives.

There is now a well documented association between STDs and HIV infection, with the probability of infection through sexual activity being sharply increased where STDs are present. The risks of HIV infection are much higher where standard STDs are present. These risks can be substantially reduced, both of HIV and of STDs, where condoms are consistently and properly used. But this requires knowledge on the part of users, a willingness to use condoms, as well as a regular and affordable supply [conditions which are generally not met at present in Uganda]. Studies carried out in Uganda have shown that the presence of STDs in the population has been a significant factor in transmission, as well as confirming the widespread presence in both men and women of standard STDs. It is clear from these studies that STDs are a significant co-factor in the transmission of HIV, and that control of STDs needs to be an important element in any strategy for controlling HIV.

B. TRANSMISSION PROJECTIONS AND SCENARIOS

The major forms of transmission in Uganda are identified under I.A, as also are estimates of the scale and distribution of HIV infection and AIDS in the population. It is clear from these estimates, and from the discussion of the processes of transmission, that very little is known with certainty about conditions in Uganda. Nevertheless enough is known about this issue for it to be possible to model the progress of the epidemic over the next 10-15 years. Bearing in mind that such modelling is bound to be imprecise, and needs to be treated with circumspection. Any predictions have to make assumptions about future behaviour, particularly sexual behaviour, and this is inevitably fraught with difficulties. Changing assumptions does, of course, yield quite different paths of HIV infection and mortality, and quite different demographic outcomes. Of great importance for the future size of the Ugandan population is the response of fertility to rising paediatric and adult mortality, but this is an area where knowledge is very uncertain. Otherwise the most important behavioural assumptions relate to the number of sexual partners, the number of sexual acts per partner, the probability of condom use, the presence of STDs, and the extent of blood screening and blood usage.

Using the national serological survey as the benchmark it is possible to model the future course of HIV infection, and to then vary the important behavioural parameters so as to observe the relative contribution of these to the model projections. Such a set of illustrative projections has been undertaken by the World Bank (WB) [1991] [these are presently being revised to take account of the recent population census which estimated a current population that is significantly smaller than had earlier been predicted]. The worst scenario looked at by the Bank assumes a continuation of present trends, and generates a set of predictions which are highly unfavourable. In this case by the year 2010 there are 1.7 million infected adults; the proportion of adult females infected rises from 13.6 per cent in 1991 to 17 per cent; the number of HIV positive children doubles from 50,000 to 100,000; and AIDS deaths rise from an estimated 34,000 adults and 20,000 children in 1991 to 115,000 and 55,000 in 2010. Whereas in the absence of AIDS it would have been expected that death rates would have declined, in the presence of AIDS the crude death rate in 2010 is predicted as actually higher than in the late 1980s. Indeed if HIV adult infection is as high as 20 per cent then age specific mortality rates are trebled - being higher for women than for men. Similarly for life expectancy, where in the absence of AIDS this could have been expected to improve substantially over the next 20 years, under the "no change" scenario it is actually lower in 2010 than in 1985. In this model run the total population continues to rise but at a slower rate.

The World Bank explores a number of alternative projections so as to identify and quantify the effects of parameter changes. Some of these changes in parameter values reflect the impact of policies on behaviour, and thus allow some estimation of the effects both individually and in the aggregate. Thus a model run which includes changes in sexual behaviour, increased use of condoms and reduction in STDs, generates a set of outcomes for HIV prevalence, AIDS mortality, life expectancy and so on which are much more favourable. What these estimates do is to illustrate the synergistic impacts of multiple policy interventions which in the aggregate are able to substantially reduce the future levels of HIV infection and AIDS. They also illustrate the crucial role which sexual behaviour plays in transmission of HIV, and how critical for the future of Uganda is the development of effective policies in this area.

Epidemiological modelling is in its infancy, and furthermore the Ugandan data base leaves much to be desired. Much, much more research is needed into important relationships of an epidemiological and demographic nature before reaching any firm conclusions. Nevertheless, certain conclusions are more or less well-founded in the available evidence. The present level of HIV infection is high by the standards of anywhere in the world, and there are no signs of it levelling off. HIV and AIDS mortality is much higher than officially reported data would suggest. As the W B model projections suggest theta is the potential for even higher rates of HIV infection and mortality in the future. To levels which will reverse much of the improvement in social indicators, such as in infant and maternal mortality, higher life expectancy, and rising living standards.

Extremely worrying is the evidence which supports the proposition that women are more severely impacted by the epidemic than men, and that in the future this gap will widen further. This means that women will lose more healthy years of life than men; that there will be further deterioration in the rate of paediatric AIDS, and that many of the functions which women are expected to perform as both producers and carers are unlikely to be feasible. As noted above, the gender aspect of the epidemic has received little attention, both in terms of its causes, and in its implications for the development of general policies for prevention, care and socio-economic impact.

C. IMPACT PROJECTIONS

If epidemiological and demographic modelling are uncertain in their methodology and conclusions, and thus need to be treated with care, then this is even more true when attention is turned to the economic and social impacts of the epidemic. What is now generally recognised is that the effects of HIV and AIDS are certainly not confined to the health sector, but rather that the channels of effects are multiple, and the impacts extend throughout the economic and social system. This being readily accepted it follows that the policies called for by the challenges of the epidemic will be complex in formulation, necessarily be innovative both in content and implementation processes, and require a multi-sectoral approach. It is this conclusion which has guided Uganda in establishing its present AIDS strategy.

A taxonomy of the multiple ways in which HIV effects the economic system is not too difficult to construct. These can be stated in a reasonably comprehensive way, and there is widespread agreement about the channels through which HIV will effect the performance of the economy. When it comes to estimating the quantitative size of the economic effects, and the distribution of these impacts on different types of households [and within households], on different sectors of production [and within sectors], on Government as a sector of service supply and production, then there are immense complexities and difficulties. This being recognised as the position it follows that what can he stated as the probable impact both now and in the future is highly uncertain.

For Uganda at the present it is impossible to go much deeper than generalities about the likely economic and social impacts. That these are already substantial, and will become even more so in the future, is nevertheless demonstrable even given the limitations of data, analysis, and understanding. It is doubly unfortunate that these adverse impacts are being imposed on an economy whose structure has been weakened by decades of political, economic and social turmoil, and which is only now gradually restoring its productive capacities.

We have seen above that HIV primarily effects those in the age groups which are crucial in terms of their importance to society as producers, as the suppliers of social and economic support to both the young and the elderly, and as the transmitters of much of the cultural and social values which effectively defines a society. Now in trying to evaluate the economic costs of HIV it is clear that once the full contribution of individuals is recognised that standard estimates are inevitably going to be partial and far too low. It is impossible to place an economic value on the multiple and varied contributions of individuals, other than in the narrowest of terms, and attempts to estimate the economic costs of HIV suffer from major limitations. As we have seen many of the contributions of individuals to society have economic and social value but these cannot be established. Even in the narrowest of economic terms these often cannot be estimated, and many productive activities are often excluded on highly dubious grounds from calculations of national production. This is most obviously true of much of the output and many diverse contributions of women in their multiple social and economic roles.

There is a further major conceptual problem with standard attempts to measure the economic impact of HIV, by for example trying to establish the present value of the output lost through the early death of an individual caused by HIV related illness. This approach in effect assumes that an individual's contribution to output is independent of others, which in the case of an epidemic it clearly is not. The costs, narrowly defined in terms of the measured contribution to GNP, will in the aggregate be greater than the sum of the individual contributions to the national output streams. Overall it can be readily agreed that the economic, social and psychological costs of HIV are likely to be very substantial, and much greater than those which are conventionally identified and estimated.

Persons infected with HIV will experience periods of higher morbidity which will effect their productivity. If they are in formal sector employment they may be subject to discrimination, and possibly lose their job. In any case at this stage of the illness they will have needs which are social—their relationship to their family, and their relationship to the community [defined as overlapping sets of social interactions]. Here support which is other than economic will be essential, and yet every bit as important. How to meet these needs under severe resource constraints is one of the major challenges of this epidemic. In purely economic terms, at this stage of the illness, there will be pressure on household resources, which may be diminishing, at the same time as needs will be intensifying. This stage, and the later one of AIDS, will divert resources to health and care at the expense of other less pressing wants. This increases the probability of worsening nutrition for the household, poorer housing, a reduction of schooling for children, reduced levels of health services for the rest of the family, and so on. All at a time when pressures will diminish the resources available to the household, as labour productivity is reduced, and with the certainty that women will be diverted into caring roles and away from productive activities.

These impacts are happening now in Uganda; probably on a wide scale, but in most districts largely undocumented and not measured. But the tip of the iceberg can be observed in the medical and social support activities of many NGOs, who are tackling as best they can a problem which already exceeds their capacities. Unfortunately, Uganda is only at the start of a process of rising needs, socially economic and psychological, which will inevitably intensify over the coming years as more persons already infected with HIV fall sick and die. The conditions observed in Rakai and Masaka are of massive needs relative to available resources, of intensified destitution, of increasing evidence of family dissolution. of the elderly without support. and large numbers of orphans who have multiple needs for food, housing schooling, training, care and love. Here is the future for Uganda. But the scale of these impacts can still be limited through social mobilisation and more effective policies.

The foregoing can be thought of as the impacts at the levels of the household and the community, but there will also be aggregative effects which will reduce the total output which can be produced. There are the losses due to higher and earlier mortality —the output lost to the economy through death. This will be significant, in terms of the lost contributions of men and women—particularly the loss of the latter, who have such varied roles to play in Uganda. But output will also be reduced through a diversion of savings to "unproductive" uses—particularly into health, and care for the sick. This reduction in the level, and the reallocation of savings to consumption, will take place in all sectors with Government, Business and Households all affected. National output will grow more slowly than otherwise because the savings available for capital formation will be lowered. These negative effects on national economic performance are not yet evident and will take time to come through. At this time it is difficult to predict the size of the losses of potential output, but while these are inevitable as a category, they are not inevitable in their scale. Effective policies for prevention of HIV can reduce the losses of human and non human resources, and thus minimise the adverse general impact on the economic system.

HIV is no respecter of social class, and there is some evidence that infection rises with education and income. This seems also to be the case in Uganda, where reports are now common of losses of highly trained and scarce professional human resources. True both of private and public employment, and doubly serious for Uganda given the thinness of its existing human resource base. HIV and AIDS is eroding an already depleted stock of educated and experienced labour, and as such is confounding present attempts to rebuild national capacity. These losses are not confined to urban areas. but are reported also from quite remote rural districts where HIV prevalence is generally low. The costs are, of course, not simply the losses of human capital that are entailed, but also the losses in terms of management performance as persons fall ill, and the higher health [and other social charges] which fall on employers. But the impacts are much more general than these; HIN and AIDS reduces the quality and the quantity of human resources available to the society in terms of experience, training, knowledge, aptitudes, commitment—across the board, and in all parts of the country. As HIV spreads to previously low areas of prevalence as it is presently doing in Uganda, so also do these costs become more general and pervasive.

No discussion of the impact effects of HIV would be complete without some discussion of the likely consequences for the agricultural sector and those whose livelihood is dependent on it. As noted above some 90 per cent of the Ugandan population is rural; agriculture accounts for about two-thirds of GDP, and for virtually all exports. Most output is produced on smallholdings. and women are responsible for some 80 per cent of total food supply and provide most of the labour inputs. This dependence on women's labour for both food and non-food production, under conditions where higher HIV infection rates for women are observed, is an indicator of the vulnerability of this sector. Women not only account for much of the direct inputs into production but a good deal of indirect ones as well [in marketing, processing, water supply, firewood etc.]. To these functions are added those domestic responsibilities of the household undertaken by women, which are burdensome enough, and on top of these HIV infection and AIDS impose yet further demands.

Since women are disproportionately infected with HIV, and given the dependence of the rural and household economies on their labour, there are inevitably going to be significant and serious impacts. These will not be confined to productive effects, but also extend to those functions which are integral to the survival of households. Under these conditions it is not enough to know that some farming systems are vulnerable to the losses of labour due to higher morbidity, higher mortality, and the diversion of women from productive roles to caring, but also to be able to identify those households which are most vulnerable. There is evidence that some households are already suffering extremes of destitution, e.g., in Rakai, under conditions of high seroprevalence. Other regions of the country, such as Apac and Lira Districts, where poverty is persistent and widespread, will become even more vulnerable if their HIV infection rates approach those of Rakai and Masaka. In part the policy problem is to avoid this outcome through effective programmes of HIV prevention. Whether or not HIV transmission is reduced it is crucial that vulnerable households be identified, their needs be established, and structures be created for delivering the goods and services they will require for survival. This is true both for the urban and rural populations; but in neither case will it be easy to identify the poor and most vulnerable households.

There is rather more information available about farm systems which are vulnerable to labour loss, together with data on particular crops where production is threatened. Tea, which is a minor crop, is especially vulnerable given its need for female labour inputs which are continuously applied. Coffee, which is the main export, seems also to be vulnerable to labour loss. Matooke [plantain], which is the main staple food for most of the population, seems already to be effected by falling labour supplies. Some Districts are especially vulnerable at the present, particularly those with high HIV infection rates, such as areas to the west and north of Kampala [together with Rakai and Masaka]. But all such estimates are based on fairly superficial economic data and analysis, and it would be unwise in these circumstances to base policies on these.

What is not in doubt is that HIV poses a major threat to the maintenance of food and non-food output, so as to threaten much of the rural population. These impacts will extend well beyond the rural sector, given the interactions between the rural and urban economies [in terms of labour flows, food supplies, remittances etc.,], and even into international economic relationships [given the dependence on a narrow range of export crops for the foreign exchange needs of Uganda]. This is an area of so over-riding importance as to be a priority for policy; but policies need to have a firm foundation of factual data on production conditions. It is not presently the case that such information exists; efforts need to be directed now to remedying this deficiency.

One sector is already bearing the brunt of the HIV epidemic; unfortunately for Ugandans the health care system is unable to cope with even the present level of demands. This is unsurprising given the deterioration of the system in the 1980s. Years of neglect and underfunding had by the middle of the decade turned what was once a comprehensive and effective provider of services—with integrated hospital and primary health care—into one of crumbling buildings, weak management, inadequate [if any] supplies of drugs, and a professional and technical staff which in large numbers had deserted both the system and the country. In spite of the attempts made in recent years the health system remains underfunded, understaffed and underprovided, such that rehabilitation will take many years to achieve. Not only is the health care system faced by growing demands from persons with HIV related illnesses, but it is also having to deal with a set of intensified health care needs caused by the collapse of many other programmes over recent decades [such as malarial and TB, where control programmes more or less ceased]. Many hospitals do not have enough beds, drugs and protective equipment to take care of their ever increasing numbers of patients. For example, Lira District Hospital has only 4 doctors to cater for a population of 500,000.

It is natural that HIV infected individuals and their families turn to the acute care system for help, and seek medical attention and drugs which they hope will alleviate their problems. But in doing so they add to the problems of meeting health needs generally in Uganda and in part divert resources away from treatable and curable medical conditions. This is evident from data on hospital admissions, where as much as two thirds of beds are occupied by AIDS patients and/or those admitted with illnesses such as Tuberculosis (TB) [a common opportunistic HIV infection]. This state of affairs is as much true of Government hospitals as it is of the private sector. A state exists where the care of patients with HIV related illnesses, particularly in hospitals, is crowding out other patients in ways which cannot be considered optimal from the national point of view. That this should have occurred is reflective of many factors; a health care system which at all levels already cannot cope with demands and which has been faced over a very short period of years with large scale growth in HiV and AIDS related pressures. Such processes have faced the MOH with problems it does not have the capacities to meet - neither in medical nor non-medical resources. In the event much of the burden of health care has shifted to the private sector, which is itself now overburdened, or is simply not being met at all by the modern health care sector. There is much evidence that many HIV infected persons are in receipt of little or no care from the formal system, and have turned in many cases [and in large numbers] to traditional healers. Although Uganda has been at the forefront of the national response to HIV and AIDS in Africa, it is disturbing to note that there is no STD control programme in place. This is particularly worrisome given the role of STDs as a co-factor in the spread of HIV [noted above]. What is needed is the development of a comprehensive STD programme as a matter of great urgency, but this will require putting in place a complex set of human and non-human resources to be effective.

The present position in terms of health care provision has little to commend it. The system cannot cope with present demands and is therefore double unable to deal with the projected numbers of HIV infected persons. There is no alternative to organisational reforms and the development of innovative ways of meeting the real and genuine needs of the population. To a degree these reforms have already been implemented, in some parts of the private system, where part hospital-based and part home-based systems are already operating. What is needed is an extension of what are currently small scale and pilot community based schemes to a national programme. One which is sensitive to the relative costs of alternative health provision and linking both prevention and care in the community. Here lies the challenge; but it is one which has to be faced sooner or later.

II. SETTING PRIORITIES

A. CAPACITY DEVELOPMENT: GENERAL CONSIDERATIONS

UNDP activities have as their target the building of national capacity, and at first sight this seems to be such an unambiguous concept as to need no further examination. It is as if it is self evident that this is desirable as an objective. But this presumption leaves open many important issues. At the minimum it can be assumed that donor activities aim to strengthen national capacity in ways which permit a country to achieve a preferred [better] level of development. Trying to achieve this objective seems reasonable enough as a guide to the selection of those activities which are desirable and worth supporting, and as an indicator of what ought not to be supported. But there are many problems in practice with this simplistic approach to capacity development.

1. Resources are limited so choices have to be made as to what activities are more or less important. Who defines priorities, and by what criteria are some activities given preference over others? It is unlikely that the exercise of preferences by politicians and policy makers will coincide with the selection of capacity building activities which maximise development. Indeed, and fundamental to conflict between preferences and the selection of activities, will be dispute as to the relationships between capacity building and development in general, and between particular initiatives and the achievement of selected development targets.
2. We have defined in an unambiguous way the recipient of the additional resources as "the country", and in the case of UNDP this is assumed as identical with the government of the day. UNDP deals mainly with governments, and issues of representativeness [how government came to power; does it observe civil and political rights, does it have any or much commitment to developmental objectives, and so on, may not be considered relevant]. What indeed ought to be the attitude of a development agency such as UNDP in its dealings with a government which is terrorising a segment of its population? Destroying national capacity in the process, as well as infringing basic human rights. Or to take the example of Uganda, what is the judgment to be of a government which allocates some 40 per cent of its budget to military expenditure, under conditions where real expenditures on health and education together in 1989 were only a fifth of fiscal allocations in 1970? On a per capita basis health expenditures were only 16 per cent real in 1989 compared with 1970; for education the decline was even worse to 13 per cent. Are such data to be taken as indicators of government preferences; and can it really be the case that internal and external security needs always override social and developmental priorities? Certainly such revealed allocations of budgetary resources against social sector expenditures in Uganda both contribute to the economic and social problems the country faces, and simultaneously constrain attempts through capacity building to ameliorate these.

3. What indeed is meant by "preferred level of development"? Does this mean a higher level of GNP? Is it a matter of interest how this higher level of GNP is achieved [by paying low wages to labour and banning labour organisations]? or through policies which lead to environmental degradation, both short term and long term [threatening the sustainability of the process]? Are the benefits of economic growth fairly distributed or do these accrue to an elite which abrogates the benefits of GNP growth for uses which have low social value? Or is there an acceptable set of development indicators which are the actual and real focii of government activities, with which capacity development can be aligned?
4. Is the discussion couched in terms of the short term, or is it implicit in the process of capacity building that policies are always about sustainability'? But this simply raises a further set of very complex questions. These run like this. Development is a process which takes place over time, and can be judged as beneficial where a set of social indicators can be shown to have shown improvement. There may be problems in getting agreement on what these indicators are, and there will certainly be important issues which relate to the conditions surrounding the achievement or non-achievement of the selected indicators. Also problematic is how to deal with the weighting problem. i.e., achievement of some indicators and non-achievement of others. But it could, of course, be precisely those countries [governments] who are generally non-achievers who are most in need of capacity building activities. It may be the lack of capacities, whatever this means, which prevents development as defined and measured by social indicators.
5. The object of donor technical assistance is to support and strengthen conditions in which a country can develop in a socially acceptable way, so that over time the need for transfers of resources from outside are diminished [not necessarily to zero]. in this case the meaning of sustainability, as far as capacity development goes, is as follows. Resources are made available to a country to meet those needs which are essential for development, but in a manner which over time leads to domestic changes which make the transfers no longer necessary. Transfers which are capacity building do not generate a continuing dependence on external support. This has to be one of the most important criteria to apply to TA. Only if this condition is met can capacity building unambiguously be thought of as desirable.
6. At the core of the problem is not just what is meant by

development and how it is measured, but issues of how best to bring development about. There are only too many theories, too many ideologies, too many special cases - and too many interest groups, both in developing countries, in developed countries and in international organisations [including UNDP]. At any one time there may be a dominant set of beliefs even occasionally some evidence to support these, which sets the agenda for TA and other assistance, such as those policies currently peddled by the World Bank and the IMF. These beliefs will often define what TA is actually on offer, who is delivering it and to whom, and under what conditions. Over time beliefs will be modified, relative positions of governments and organisations change, and with it the concepts and practices of capacity building [note that this is never a single valued construct but is itself one which in practice takes many forms].

B. CAPACITY DEVELOPMENT UNDER CONDITIONS OF HIGH SEROPREVALENCE

Figure 18.1 sets out in a very simplified form a structure for thinking about capacity building in Uganda — a country facing an epidemic with all its consequences [as identified in I.C above]. There are disadvantages in setting out the problem and the choices as in Figure 18.1, not least in that doing so suggests that the relationships are linear and uni-directional. They clearly are not, as will be seen later. Also implicit in this representation is the assumption that we possess sufficient understanding of what is an immensely complex set of inter-actions as to be able to delineate these into separable categories. This is acceptable, perhaps, as a device for assisting exposition of the problems and the choices, but cannot in any way be thought of as descriptive of actuality. What the Figure does is to place the policy problem within a framework which is standard for economics, but this does not prove its suitability for analysing the problem at hand. Time will tell if this way of presenting choices is useful and adds to our understanding.

The issue is that described in II.A, i.e., how to establish a set of activities that will assist Uganda in developing those capacities which will help it meet the severe socio-economic problems raised for the country by the HIV epidemic. Not in any detail, of course, but in very broad brush terms, and building on the description of the present and future position in Uganda as outlined in Section I.

Final Targets

It is perhaps easiest to start with the Final Targets, the

achievement of which is the purpose of development policy. Those which are identified in Figure 18.1 are not intended to be comprehensive, but they are the important ones. These include those targets which are most threatened by the HIV epidemic [both now and in the future]. In the ordinary course of events it would have been expected that various mortality indicators would improve, and in doing so raise life expectancy. The HIV epidemic makes it unlikely that this will occur, and that instead infant and maternal mortality, and adult mortality, will be raised, and life expectancy probably fall. Similarly with poverty, where the probability is for an increase in destitution [with accompanying worsening in other associated indicators of the standard of living, such as housing and nutrition]. The overall rate of economic growth would be lower than otherwise, with significant losses of potential output, and the external position of the economy be weaker—all because of unfavourable impacts on the level and rate of change of labour productivity, and lower rates of capital formation [both in physical capital and in human investment].

All of this was established in Section 1, and in some senses from the viewpoint of meeting the development challenge of HIV and AIDS we are not so much interested in Final Targets as such, but in the complex ways in which these are made unattainable by the epidemic. Rather the focii of policy interventions are what are called in Figure 18.1 Intermediate Targets.

Intermediate Targets

Three categories have been identified as being of over-riding proximate importance; these are the Rate of HIV Transmission, the Care of Infected Persons, and the Mitigation of Adverse Social and Economic Impacts. These are probably not all of equal social weight, and it would certainly be possible to argue that reducing the rate of HIV transmission ought to have priority in the allocation of resources [and in capacity building activities]. It would not be difficult to make this case, given the scenarios outlined in Section I.B. Far and away the greatest benefit in economic and social terms will come from those activities which reduce HIV prevalence, through the minimisation of future social and economic costs. It could also be argued that some of the effects, particularly those on macro-economic performance, will occur later and are thus perhaps less urgent. This is partly true, partly untrue, since some of the adverse economic responses are already being experienced in Uganda.

What is undoubtedly the case is that these Intermediate Targets are interconnected; thus, a mitigation of the economic losses caused by the epidemic will entail a higher level of resources for

Figure. 18.1

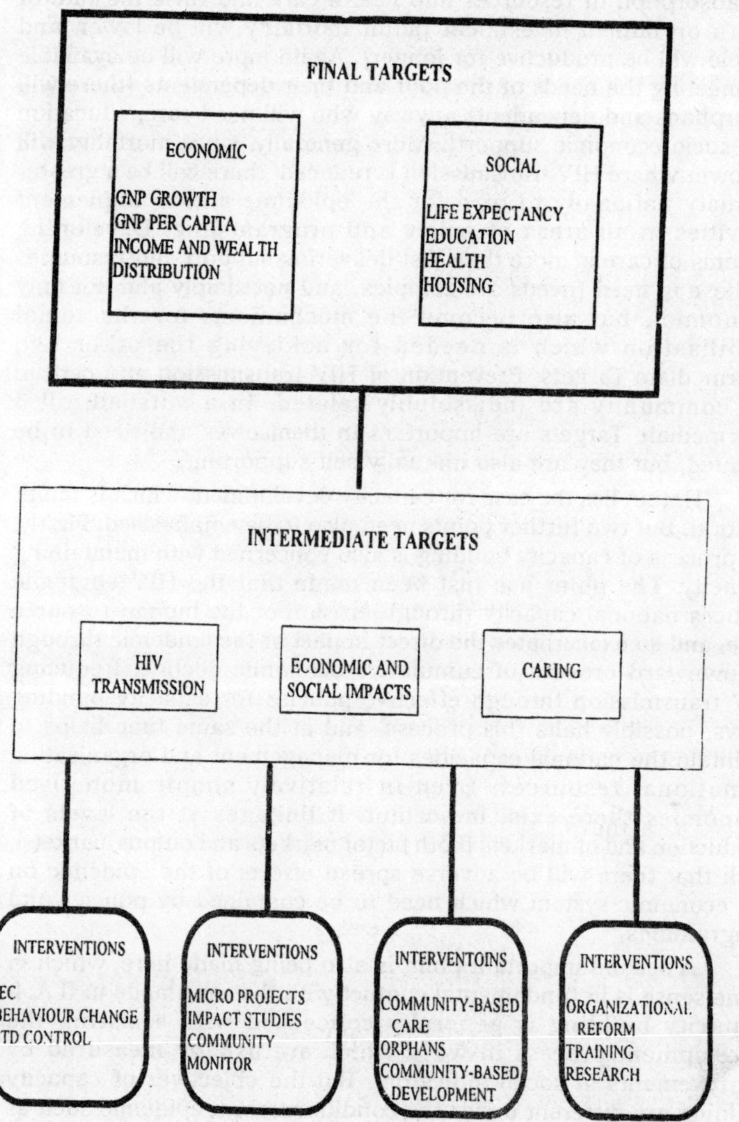
FINAL TARGETS
ECONOMIC
GNP GROWTH
GNP PER CAPITA
INCOME AND WEALTH
DISTRIBUTION
SOCIAL
LIFE EXPECTANCY
EDUCATION
HEALTH
HOUSING
INTERMEDIATE TARGETS
HIV TRANSMISSION
ECONOMIC AND SOCIAL IMPACTS
CARING
INTERVENTIONS
IEC
BEHAVIOUR CHANGE
STD CONTROL
INTERVENTIONS
MICRO PROJECTS
IMPACT STUDIES
COMMUNITY
MONITOR
INTERVENTOINS
COMMUNITY-BASED CARE
ORPHANS
COMMUNITY-BASED DEVELOPMENT
INTERVENTIONS
ORGANIZATIONAL REFORM
TRAINING
RESEARCH

meeting the care needs of the infected and affected populations. Similarly, a reduction in the rate of transmission of HIV will reduce the absorption of resources into health care and raise the rate of return on human investment [adult mortality will be lower, and people will be productive for longer]. Again more will be available for meeting the needs of the poor and their dependents [there will be orphans and dependents anyway who will need care, education and socio-economic support]. More generally, since mortality will be lower where HIV transmission is reduced, there will be a greater capacity nationally to plan for the epidemic and to implement activities in all areas of policy and programming. Developing systems of care is more than just delivering support and resources to those in need [needs are complex, and not simply and not only economic], but also become the mechanisms for the social mobilisation which is needed for achieving the other two Intermediate Targets. Prevention of HIV transmission and care in the community are indissolubly related. In a nutshell; all 3 Intermediate Targets are important in themselves and need to be pursued, but they are also mutually self-supporting.

Herein lies the case for capacity development which is multi-sectoral. But two further points need also to be emphasised. Firstly, the process of capacity building is also concerned with maintaining capacity. The point has just been made that the HIV epidemic reduces national capacity through erosion of the human resource base, and so exacerbates the direct impact of the epidemic through a downward process of cumulative economic decline. Reducing HIV transmission through effective policies for capacity building slows, possibly halts this process, and at the same time helps to maintain the national capacities for management and organisation of national resources. Even in relatively simple monetised economies there exist important. lt linkages at the levels of production and of markets [both factor markets and output markets], such that there will be adverse spread effects of the epidemic on the economic system which need to be contained by policies and programmes.

A second important point is also being made here, which in some sense is in fundamental conflict with the case made in II.A.4. Capacity building is generally concerned with assisting the development process in ways which are usually measured by improvements in social indicators. But the objectives of capacity building are different under the conditions of an epidemic such as that being experienced by Uganda. Here the policy problem is how to prevent, or limit, a deterioration in the level of development, with capacity building objectives seen in an entirely different light. Success may be gauged not by the increment of improvement in social indicators, but by the degree to which deterioration in these has been minimised. In these circumstances the whole process of project design and evaluation needs to be re-assessed. Thus, for example,to see income generation projects as a means of preventing declines in living standards under the impact of immiseration, rather than the conventional approach where projects are selected in terms of their ability to raise factor productivity and incomes.

Interventions

These are multi-dimensional activities which are capacity building. These could be about maintaining national capacity, or its enhancement. Thus a programme of workshops for different professional groups employed both by government and NGOs which aimed to improve knowledge of the HIV transmission process, and/or its social and economic impacts, would generate new insights and improve economic and social performance. These activities could be aimed at raising the efficiency of existing interventions, through for example training in management and organisation, where the aim is to improve the use of resources. Solutions in this area could themselves be innovatory, and at the same time add to domestic capacity. Thus existing NGOs, which are too small to provide internally all the skills and services they need, such as financial control and project evaluation skills, could look to other more specialised institutions. The latter might be in the public or private sectors, and the process of capacity building be about the appropriate development of service institutions where these are currently missing or ineffective. The possibilities for organisational innovation are legion; that these will be important is also self evident. Again we are back with issues of efficient resource allocation, and the need to raise factor productivity—in these cases by removing inefficiency [the failure to maximise use of resources caused by management and other internal practices which are sub-optimal] .

In evaluating national needs for capacity building, it is important not to misread signals which apparently support further allocations of resources to a particular activity. This may be best understood by looking at the example of the Kampala AIDS Information Centre. This was established to provide HIV testing and counselling services. It is about to extend its activities to other parts of the country, in response presumably lo felt needs. Most of its costs are met by USAID, and there is eftectively no cost recovery. An HIV test costs currently some $12 US, at a time when per capita health expenditures in Uganda are presently a mere $3 annually. Under what circumstances can this allocation of resources be defended? A case could perhaps be made, along the following lines. An HIV test and its associated counselling, whether the result is negative or positive, leads to such changes in behaviour as to prevent further infection [of say "n" persons]. If this is so then perhaps a case can be mafe for subsidising HIV tests at the current cost. But the case needs to be substantiated by evidence and cannot be assumed. In this example the existence of unmet demands [indeed any demand] does not prove that creating additional capacity, in the form of testing centres and in training more counsellors. is necessarily justified. Of course other arguments in favour of HIV testing centres can be made which do not depend for their validity on demonstrating any effects on sexual behaviour.

This example raises two important principles. Are resources currently being efficiently used, and does the existence of unmet demand act as an efficient signal for further resource inputs? Both of these need to be considered in decisions on future capacity building activities.

No case can be made "a priori" for or against private of public sector interventions, and in practice there are activities where in particular circumstances either or both are best able to perform. Certainly the effectiveness of certain interventions is constrained by the weakness of public provision, irrespective of whether the intervention is by an NGO or by government. A telling example of this has been the enormous decline in the quality and quantity of public educational provision in Uganda; at the present only about one-third of the relevant age group completes primary education, and very few children proceed to later stages of education. Something like one half of the total Ugandan population is functionally illiterate. This decline in educational achievement over recent decades severely constrains what can be done through policy interventions in the case of all three Intermediate Targets. Such a state of affairs not only constrains what activities can be undertaken but also requires that these factors be taken into account in their design and implementation. Thus any Micro Projects to combat AIDS have to assume as a basic fact that the target population will not be able to meet sophisticated project appraisal and evaluation requirements, and will require intensive assistance by way of training in management skills etc. Similarly with activities for reducing HIV transmission where reaching the population with relevant messages, and engaging them actively in sustained behaviour change, will entail quite different strategies [and be much more complex in design and in processes of implementation].

The final point relating to capacity building, which will repay emphasis, is that most of the population is rural, so that the balance of resource allocation in respect of all 3 Intermediate Targets needs to be focused on this group. All of the forces operating in Uganda will bias programmes against rural populations, for reasons which do not need to be explored here. The potential for disaster, both economic and social if this urban bias is not addressed, is potentially enormous. Similarly, with the gender dimensions of HIV; as we have seen in Section I.B there is an over-riding need to address all issues from a gender perspective. It is perhaps enough to reiterate that the single largest input into agriculture is women's labour, that this is the scarcest factor of production, whose availability for all uses in the society will become increasingly problematic. How to respond to the needs of women must be a major element in any choices relating to capacity building, and to resource allocation generally.

It can be concluded that the overall objectives of capacity development in Uganda, under conditions of high seroprevalence, are.

1. To improve the functioning of existing institutions through raising their efficiency in using resources.
2. To generate new insights and develop new skills in understanding and responding to the challenges posed by the epidemic.
3. To replicate those approaches and institutional structures which are successfully meeting the existing challenges to other institutions and areas of the country.
4. To support innovatory responses to HIV in all of its manifestations, and to strengthen organisational developments, in both the public and private sectors.

Knowledge Base

This is fundamental to any policies of capacity development for any purposes. All countries are resource constrained, and Uganda more so than most. Over recent decades there has been immense deterioration in the economic and social infrastructure, so that effective responses to the HIV epidemic are made doubly difficult. Even more important then in these circumstances to ensure that what is done is well done. Implicit in the approach outlined above is the assumption of known links between Interventions and Intermediate and Final Targets. In part the problem is that these linkages are only imperfectly understood. This may be because a knowledge base has yet to be established, or that where this exists it is not being effectively used.

In part, knowledge and understanding are independent of the activities being followed, and in part these are the outcome of activities. One example will suffice. The focus of much effort presently in Uganda are IEC activities to change sexual behaviour, since this is seen by Government and others as the only effective way to slow transmission of HIV. It would seem obvious in these circumstances to relate IEC programmes to what is already known about sexuality within the cultural context of Uganda. It is in fact the case that Uganda for many reasons has available a good deal of research on these matters, which ought to have informed policies for IEC. But there is little evidence that in fact these sources have been used in the formulation of policies, and in the development of interventions. Much of the IEC activity seems to have been unproductive, in the sense that sexual behaviour has not been changed in appropriate ways. There is some evidence of both poor evaluation and ineffective monitoring of IEC programmes, which has in turn led to weakness in learning the lessons of what works, and what does not.

Capacity building has to be firmly based on what is known about economic, social and cultural structures, if it is to be effective. Where this knowledge of conditions, and structural and behavioural relationships is inadequate for effective policy making then it will need to be addressed. In part capacity strengthening is about developing insights—without understanding there can be no effective policies. Such insights cannot be assumed to be present, particularly as in the case of an epidemic such as HIV, where new analytical frameworks have to be developed and tested against experience. In the case ot Uganda the early learning process is over; and now is the time to ensure the full and rapid integration of experience in policies for capacity development.

III. UNDP PROGRAMME INTERVENTIONS

OPERATIONAL PRINCIPLES

The general principles which should guide UNDP have been established in Section II on Capacity Development. These principles, in conjunction with the analysis of the HIV epidemic and its probable socio-economic impacts as detailed in Section I, set a framework for the general allocation of UNDP resources. But important as these principles are for efficient allocation of resources they are insufficient for the determination of priorities and spending decisions. The definition of operational activities requires the development of additional principles, and the application of these in taking forward a programme for UNDP assistance to Uganda.

The following are important :

* The knowledge base for interventions in many areas is imperfect and inadequate, such that a crucial initial activity will be to establish such a base. It is an important role of the Uganda AIDS Commission to define research priorities, and to direct resources into consultancies, studies, task forces etc. The output of such activities must

then inform policy formulation and the development of specific interventions.

* Policy making is a continuing process. Priorities will change because governments come and go; because the internal and external environments change; and because of learning effects, i.e., the internalisation of experience and the embodiment of this in policy.
* It follows from the foregoing that the establishment of firm allocations of UNDP resources for the period 1992-96 is neither desirable nor optimal. What are feasible objectives at this point in time are broad indications of priority areas, and identification of initial activities. In effect, what is proposed is a system of contingent allocations, where the specific activities should reflect changing needs and improved understanding [what works, what does not work]. It is important to note that a programme for UNDP requires a framework which is more or less determined; it is the activities whose relative balance should be adjusted during the life of the HIV Programme, through a process of consultations, taking into account learning effects, changing needs, and so on.
* UNDP resources are limited so it is vital that these be used to maximum effect. This means, in consultation with the UAC, the identification of the points in the economic, social and political systems where activities can exert their greatest leverage; can induce changes in behaviour and attitudes; shift allocations of resources to areas of greatest need, and support appropriate institutional development. In a word, the activities of UNDP need to be catalytic. Programmes must be concentrated on the essential problems posed for Uganda by the HIV epidemic. In part, this requires a new focus—to see problems and their solutions in different ways—together with an intensification of efforts in respect of all three Intermediate Targets. Critical to achieving a new vision is a more general recognition of the developmental relationships of HIV, and the strengthening of activities for planning for, and meeting, the expected social and economic impacts.

PRIORITISATION OF PROGRAMME INTERVENTIONS

A. PREVENTION OF HIV TRANSMISSION

Certain features stand out clearly in the present efforts to reduce HIV transmission, and there are important matters here which UNDP needs to address. Much has been done to increase awareness in Uganda, and many activities are underway and planned in this area by government, NGOs, UN agencies, bilateral donors, and so on. Three observations merit separate attention.

* The presumption that awareness is generally high is almost certainly unfounded, and the admittedly partial evidence of the Mission field visit to Lira and Apac Districts suggests that there are problems in this area still to be addressed. Regions which currently have relatively low infection rates, and which for other reasons are difficult to access, are in need of communication activities to develop awareness at all levels about HIV transmission and its prevention, and to raise understanding of the deadly nature of AIDS. It is certainly appropriate for UNDP to assist others, such as UNICEF, in the identification of needs in this area, and to collaborate in the development of suitable forms of programme delivery, including strengthening institutional structures, training, etc.
* There is little evidence for Uganda that sexual behaviour has changed in the ways appropriate for a reduction in transmission of HIV. Increasing awareness has not been sufficient to induce sustained behaviour change, so how to bring this about remains the core of the problem for reducing the rate of transmission. There is work proceeding currently in this area, including a Report which is due from AIDSCOM, and there is the development of new approaches nresently underway at Kitovo Hospital. Others, such as UNICEF and DANIDA are active in this field. It is clearly appropriate for UNDP to collaborate with others in identifying why activities for behaviour change have had such little success; to support programme development, probably on a pilot scale, and to then establish joint programmes for gaining and other activities.
* Doing the foregoing would certainly be worthwhile but in crucial respects would be inadequate to meet the challenge. A point which is emphasised in Section I is the absolute need to establish a gender sensitive approach to this issue. Questions were posed above of why women are infected with HIV at a younger age than men, and why apparently there is a higher rate of female infection.

At least three directions for UNDP activities, of great importance, follow from there observations on the roles of gender in relation to the epidemic.

(a) What are the social, cultural and economic conditions which explain the gender biases in HIV prevalence? This requires detailed studies, either separately by UNDP or in conjunction with other agencies with interests in this area. It is obvious that any approach to this question would need to address not simply behaviour change but also, and crucially, the formation of behaviour.

(b) How can women protect themselves from infection? The behaviour change activities undertaken in Uganda have generally not addressed this question, but have concentrated on the ways in which men through their actions can reduce their infection rates. Thus activities have concentrated on matters such as reduction in the numbers of sexual partners, and use of condoms. Whereas most women in Africa have one and only one partner, and have little or no control over their male partner's sexual activities, and so are not able to demand changes in behaviour and insist on the use of condoms. Here there is a major role for UNDP, and one which must have high priority. The issue has received little or no attention from the programmes designed and delivered by WHO, and has been similarly neglected by the Uganda ACP. The development of understanding of the ways in which women can protect themselves from infection; the embodiment of such understanding in programmes for behaviour change, together with the establishment of service delivery activities which make it possible for women to protect themselves from infection. All are absolutely crucial for success in reducing the rate of HIV infection in Uganda.

(c) Unless (a) and (b) are successfully addressed as matters of extreme urgency, then it is difficult to see how Uganda will be able to cope with the immense problems caused by the epidemic. Women, as we have seen in Section-I, are central to almost everything—the care of the sick generally, not just those persons with HIV related illnesses; the maintenance of food and non-food production; the care and support of children and elderly dependents, and so on. It cannot be said that the crucial role of women in the economic and social life of Uganda, and the degree to which they and their contributions are threatened by HIV, have been taken on board.

UNDP has a ensure that in its programme for Uganda, through consultations with the UAC and other partners, that these failures of programme design and delivery are rectified. It follows that not only must the gender biases in transmission be addressed, through changes in analysis, policies and programmes; but that efforts be directed into the assessment of the problems of high female morbidity and mortality for the economic and social system. Both aspects of the issue are important and critical areas for UNDP programme support.

There are four other areas where UNDP could have a role in relation to transmission of HIV, possibly of secondary importance. These are:

(d) In the development of a programme for STDs which, as noted above, have been identified as a major co-factor in the transmission of HIV. Several agencies, including WHO, USAID and possibly the World Bank, are interested in establishing a programme for STDs. There is effectively no programme at present in Uganda. and given the state of general health services in the country it will be a formidable task to set up an effective system for the diagnosis and treatment of STDs. UNDP certainly has an interest in seeing such a programme established, although it would take it away from its developmental concerns, and it would seem preferable to leave the analysis of need and programme development to others. Except for a particular concern which UNDP has and which is not currently reflected in the approach of other agencies to this matter. This relates to the concerns expressed above, i.e., the high level of HIV infection amongst women and the need to reduce it. There is a good deal of evidence that STDs [together with other physiological and culturally determined factors] are important in explaining high infection rates in women. Since most women are never subjected to internal examination by medical practitioners STDs and other infections remain untreated as a consequence, and this raises the risk of transmission of HIV. It is, unfortunately, only too likely that a programme for STDs, if established in Uganda, will neglect the critical needs of women. So UNDP has an interest in being associated with the development of a programme for STDs on these grounds alone, but in order also to enable Uganda to better deal with the economic and social impacts of the epidemic.

(e) There is one important sub-group in the population who are perhaps peripheral to the main concerns of UNDP. This is the military, who may have high levels of seroprevalence and who may play a significant role in transmission. This is an area where other agencies [USAID] are active, and there may be little need for UNDP to become involved. This is, nevertheless, one area where UNDP may want to be involved in the process of training [counsellors particularly], and perhaps in the development of care. The military do have arrangements for those who are infected and who at some stage are retired from the service, but there is a need to look at how individuals and their families cope. There is a complex set of issues here; of IEC activities, STD programme development. HIV testing and ethics relating to it, condom supplies, counselling, care and medical needs. The military are important because of their relationship to the rest of the population; they are a mobile and sexually active group of young men who wield a great deal of power, and as such are in a position to do much harm to the ACP of Uganda. It needs hardly to be added that they are also deserving in their own right of a comprehensive programme for HIV prevention and care.

(f) There are some 150.000 refugees in Uganda who are the responsibility of UNHCR. Some are recent arrivals and others have been long settled in Uganda. They are a particularly vulnerable group for all sorts of reasons, and there is the real possibility that their needs in respect of HIV prevention, care and income support, will not receive the attention these deserve. Many factors are likely to combine to make refugees, and particularly women and young adults, very vulnerable to HIV infection. There seems to be little evidence that their multiple needs are being addressed by UNHCR, who do not have the capacity for dealing with these matters. This is an issue requiring inter-agency discussions and consultations with the UAC.

(g) There is a great deal of IFC activity already, and WHO has an expert in the country and is considering the secondment of another person in this field to the UAC. Others are also active in the area, and UNICEF has announced that this is a priority interest. Other UN agencies, such as UNFPA have activities in progress and planned. Also active in the area are NGOs such as The AIDS Support Organization [TASO], The Uganda Red Cross, Experiment in International Learning [EIL], and so on. There is no lack of activity, but as we have seen above there can be doubts as to its effectiveness. There are general problems here, and they are not only those which are raised above. These include constraints on the local development and production of materials for IEC purposes, and for use in training and counselling. This is raised as a matter of considerable importance at this point in the Report, rather than in the section below which deals with organisational matters. This is certainly an area where UNDP has an interest in the local development of capacity, both of technical skills in developing materials and in production, but only after a capacity needs assessment. A related matter, but one which the mission did not look at, is the role of the Media in IEC. This is certainly deserving of separate study, since capacity constraints in this area are undoubtedly important.

There remain two other areas where UNDP might have some involvement, but which are judged to be of low priority. These are:

(h) It is the case that risks of infection with HIV through contaminated blood and blood products are very high. It is also true that in Uganda only a small percentage of transmission is due to this factor and, as noted above, about 90 per cent is heterosexual in origin. At the present most blood is screened for HIV etc., and the blood supply is considered more or lass secure. Most of the costs of this programme are met by the European Community [ECI] and they are also meeting the costs incurred through the setting up of extra blood screening centres. While the EC has no firm plans for continuing support it is the case that for the moment at least the system is being financed, and is apparently working well. There is some evidence that blood is not reaching hospitals in rural districts, but this distributive problem needs to be addressed by others. The cost of a unit of blood is very high—a unit cost of 42$. This needs to be compared with per capita health costs for Uganda of about 3$, and recent estimates of the World Bank (WB) that the average cost for drugs etc., per AIDS case are approximately 14$. There would appear to be important issues here of the efficiency of resource allocation. One conclusion is that UNDP should not get involved in blood screening activities. With one caveat: the Nakasero Blood Bank hopes to establish a panel of donors [Clubs], which ought to reduce the cost per unit, and act as a vehicle for IEC. This is an interesting proposal and is one which UNDP might well assist. The start-up funding ought to be quite small, and there is the possibility of piggy-backing this activity on more general IEC and behaviour change interventions.

[i] Reference is made above to the AIDS Information Centre (AIC), and doubts were expressed about the scale of resources being absorbed into this activity. It is suggested that UNDP should not support the AIC unless it can be shown that various conditions are being met with respect to behaviour change and other benefits from testing. Carrying out such a Study would be a complex matter, but ought to be a prior requirement for any UNDP involvement. If it can be demonstrated that AIC activities do have significant and worthwhile effects on behaviour change or other important benefits then a case might exist for UNDP support. Possibly UNDP could help with limited finance for any study which is undertaken, although this could perhaps be left to USAID not AIDSCOM.

B. ECONOMIC AND SOCIAL IMPACT

The earlier Section I.C on Impact Projections more or less sets out the agenda for activities, but is no more than a brief summary of possible outcomes. It should also be noted that the WB Study [1991] has value mainly as a general statement of the issues, and does not in any way take the analysis of impacts sufficiently forward. It follows that detailed studies of the economic and social impact of the HIV epidemic are a pre-requisite for policy interventions by UNDP and others. This requirement does not preclude all activities for ameliorating the current impacts on the economic and social system, such as for example the Micro Projects Programme to Combat AIDS, but it does imply that at this stage much of UNDP activity will be preparatory rather than substantive. A constraint, which has to be removed, relates to the national capacity to develop the required insights, and to be able to undertake studies of the multiple ways in which the social and economic system is affected by HIV and AIDS. Developing these capacities and professional skills is addressed below in the Section on Strengthening Organizational Structures. Matters relating to the Health Sector are partly dealt with here but also in Section III. C. This may be confusing, but it seems, on balance, preferably to organise interventions on a functional basis.

1. Micro Projects

The Micro Projects Programme to Combat AIDS [UGAI91/005] is a pilot project which aims to reduce the adverse effects of HIV infection through the provision of financial resources and technical assistance. The target groups are those households and communities considered to be most vulnerable to the adverse impacts of HIV, and the Project involves NGOs and CBOs actively in the identification of appropriate and supportable activities, as well as in their management and evaluation. This is a project which is well deserving of support as an innovatory attempt to meet the needs of vulnerable groups through income generating and other activities. There are various ways of strengthening the Projects, including the following. Firstly it is absolutely crucial that the participation of women be a requirement for both the National Steering Committee and the District Selection Committees. This should be achieved through a minimum percentage of the membership, say not less than one-third of the total. Secondly, the performance of this Project will depend on the quality of the inputs from NGOs, CBOs etc., [the sponsoring organizations], and this is recognised through the provision for some technical assistance to these groups. This does not look as if it will be enough, and provision needs to be made for much more than is proposed. Furthermore, the planned technical assistance is too narrowly focused, and the targeted beneficiaries who are expected to identify projects, formulate and effectively manage these, are going to need much more assistance than is provided for in the Prodoc. It is well known from other income generation projects that weaknesses at the level of operation and control are a major cause of failure. Finally, there are no convincing grounds for the exclusion of Rakai and Masaka from the Project, and given that they are currently facing severe problems caused by the epidemic it is suggested that they be included.

2. Sector Studies

It is urgent that Sector Studies be commissioned on the impact effects of HIV. At present what is available are studies which largely depend on secondary information and the application of intuitive reasoning. This is no substitute for empirical research which directly addresses the important questions raised by the epidemic. There are a number of key sectors where the impact will be severe, which are critical for the performance of the economic system, and including sectors which are important for reducing HIV transmission and for providing care for those affected.

The Sectors identified are :

(a) Agriculture

This supplies most of the food and almost all the exports of Uganda; most of the population is dependent directly or indirectly on this Sector. So far the impact studies which have been done, such as Barnett and Blaikie [1990] and the World Bank [1991], provide little more than a sketch of the probable responses and distribution of effects on Agriculture. There is an immediate need for detailed analysis of the ways in which production will be affected by changing labour supply availabilities, including the effects on factor utilisation, production technologies, crop diversification, food availability, factor and output prices, and so on. In part this means collecting and analysing much new data, District by District. Plus observing the ways in which farm systems are responding already in areas with high HIV prevalence such as Rakai and Masaka. These data are crucial for the formulation of policies for meeting the needs of the agricultural sector—both in terms of production quantities; changing patterns of production [with additional needs for some inputs, such as fertilisers and pesticides]; the impacts on land use [with the possibility that land may be uncultivated and untended causing land degradation]; and the impacts on farm populations. The generation of estimates of the most vulnerable systems of production and most vulnerable households are crucial for effective policies for planning for the impact of the epidemic across a wide spectrum of concerns. The latter include issues of nutrition, food security [and food storagel, the changing pattern of labour use [and the impact of this on households dependent on rural labour markets], changing patterns of land ownership [as assets are liquidated to meet health costs in affected families, and land is redistributed at deaths. What are clearly needed are integrated studies which identify the inter-relationships, and establish the main areas where policy interventions are needed. But time is important, and it will be necessary to use Rapid Appraisal Techniques wherever possible so as to get the information and recommendations to policy makers without delay. The focii for UNDP interventions would be Ministry of Economic Planning and Development (MEPD) and Ministry of Agriculture.

(b) Health

We have seen above in Section I.C on Impact that this sector is already facing intense demands, such that many patients with HIV related illnesses are largely untreated by the formal health care sector. It seems also true that HIV-related illnesses are crowding out other categories of treatment, with results which cannot be considered optimal. This requires a Health Sector Study which looks at the strategic options, and assesses both the needs of HIV infected persons and the best ways to meet these, given the expected resource constraints facing the health sector [both governmental and private]. Inevitably the formal health care sector will be left with important responsibilities for treatment, both in terms of demands falling on different parts of the health care system [particularly on lower level facilities], on essential drug requirements, and on the training of doctors, nurses, etc. There is little point in predicting forward the present state of affairs, in that this would represent an abdication of responsibility. What is needed is a full assessment of health needs and the best ways to meet these, given both human and non-human resource constraints. To this end there will have to be a significant strengthening of the MOH in terms of its planning capacities. It goes without saying that one of the outputs of such a review would be an assessment of the impact of HIV related illnesses on the capacity of the health sector itself, given that human resources will, indeed already are, being diminished through morbidity and mortality. This is perhaps an area where WHO and the WB may be thought to have primary interests, but UNDP certainly ought to be involved both in helping Government in activities aimed at redefining strategic health care policy, and in strengthening the general planning capacity of the MOH.

(c) Education

This sector is facing huge problems and the existing challenges are already enormous. As we have seen above the performance of this sector in terms of enrollment and quality of education leaves much to be desired. Yet, like Health it is a crucial service sector with critical responsibilities for human resource development and its maintenance. As the human capital of Uganda is eroded further by HIV and AIDS the ability of this Sector to educate for replacement of lost skills will become even more important. It will, like Healths be facing the problems of AIDS mortality, so that its capacity to maintain activity will be declining. Furthermore, this Sector has to play a major role in creating awareness of HIV and in the forming of appropriate behaviours amongst a critical segment of the population—the next generation, which is as yet largely uninfected. There are multiple issues here which need attention; some are being addressed by others [such as the programmes of UNICEF], but there are important planning issues which are not. Planning for the Education Sector has to be concerned with, for example. the effects of the HIV epidemic on the school age population [the numbers to be educated], the impact of HIV related illnesses on the supply of teachers [and their training], the need at secondary and tertiary levels to plan for replacement of critical skilled and professional human resources, issues to do with the financing of the sector [under the general impact of HIV on the economy], the particular problems of groups such as children who are infected and affected by the epidemic, and increasing numbers of poor families. There is a range of important policy and programme matters where forward planning is going to be essential, and UNDP should certainly assist both the Ministry of Education and the UAC with technical and planning support.

3. Community Monitoring

Much of the foregoing reflects partial ways of measuring the impact of HIV, and while it is essential to look at effects in this way it is not sufficient to do so. What are also needed are comprehensive methods of recording impacts and social responses, i.e., some kind of cross sectional picture which integrates effects and responses within a defined space. For most households this space is going to be the community, which is itself a concept with ill-defined boundaries. In a largely rural society such as Uganda this will usually be co-terminus with the village, and what are needed are methods for observing and recording the multiple impacts at this level. Only at this level of disaggregation will it be possible to identify affected households with their specific needs, their problems as they change over time; the inter-household relationships and attitudes; the development of social caring processes, including the activities of CBOs, NGOs, churches and the like; and what is happening to rural production and the use and distribution of resources. In short to develop ways of representing and analysing communities who are facing the social and economic impacts of HIV. Since most of the adverse effects of the epidemic are going to have to be handled at the community level it follows that policy has to have detailed pictures of the problems that communities are facing, how they are coping, and what are the effective programme interventions. To achieve this objective UNDP should develop, in consultation with the UAC, a programme of Community Monitoring, with an initial set of differentiated communities as pilot studies. This will require an initial piece of research into the problems of establishing such a community monitoring programme.

C. CARING

This is in many ways the most complex issue to address, and in many ways also the most important. Many aspects of health care have been raised above, particularly those dealing with the formal health care system, both access to it and the quality of care. It is not intended in this section of the report to add further to what has already been written, for it is obvious from the foregoing that, in the case of Uganda, most of the care of the infected and the affected will have to be at the community level. Indeed one of the major challenges policy makers in Uganda have to face is how to ensure that resources do reach communities and households where they can have most impact, and where needs are greatest.

In these circumstances the activities of NGOs, CBOs, churches and other institutions have critical and vital roles to play. These institutions have already proven their value, being active in multiple directions in meeting the needs of society. The objective here is not to review their activities, and indeed much that the Report has to recommend by way of specific interventions is reserved for the following Section, where attention is directed at ways of further raising the effectiveness of the NGO sector broadly defined. But there are three very important areas where NGOs are going to be central to meeting the challenges posed by HIV, and indeed where they are already demonstrating their ability to innovate and be effective.

1. Community-Based Care

In an ideal world it would be possible to wait for the results of any Community Monitoring system such as recommended above, but the problems are too urgent for this. Actions are required now on how best to meet the medical, social and economic needs of households and communities in an integrated and sustainable way. Fortunately there are examples of how this might be done, and these cases might provide the basis for a national programme. The first step would have to be a much deeper evaluation of the two cases to be presented; to identify their strengths, and to consider the problems facing Uganda in replicating these "models" to other Districts. The initial focus of UNDP would indeed be to undertake the commissioning of such an evaluation, with the intention then of directly funding the development of those capacities which are essential for extending the programme to other Districts. This ought to be a major area for UNDP activities in meeting the challenges of HIV in Uganda.

Both of the cases are based on non-governmental hospitals. They are Kitovo Hospital in Masaka, a District of high infection and very severe social and economic problems, and Aber Hospital in Apac District where HIV infection is thought still to be low. Both hospitals have had to face the same problems: patient care needs which threatens to overwhelm the facilities, crowding out other patients; a need to find alternative ways of meeting the medical and social needs of persons with HIV-related illnesses, within the bounds posed by tight resource constraints of beds, drugs and staff; and how to integrate health care and other needs into a community framework. In part because there is no real alternative to doing this, and in part because this is actually better for the infected and affected. Integration of care, the creation of support networks, income generation schemes, IEC and behavioural change activities, support for orphans and destitute families, and mobile tearns of trained personnel [both medical and non—medical] have all formed part of their developing response. What is being achieved is remarkable, but they are of course also resource constrained in what they can achieve, and the numbers they can reach. Their capacities are clearly limited, and the constraints of space, trained counsellors, IEC materials, transport, and the like all need to be relieved. In part capacity building is about relieving these constraints, and doing so for these hospitals and others would in itself be a valuable step forward. But what is being primarily recommended is more than this: it is the evaluation of models of integrated care which have evolved over time in the face of the epidemic, and the replication of these models in their primary elements to other areas of the country, where the model can be effectively applied. This second stage will require substantive capacity building activities by UNDP and others. In a sense, it means using these cases both as models and as centres which could be given training and other responsibilities. In the latter role, they could be seen as "poles of community development", playing active roles in their own replication.

2. Orphans

This problem figures in all discussions of HIV in Uganda and as such can be briefly dealt with in this report. The number of orphans, as defined in Uganda as a child having lost one or both parents, is thought to number somewhere between 600,000 and I million. Many of these are the result of war and other factors, but this in no way changes the scale of the problem which currently exists, and which will become even larger in the coming years. There are many activities already in this area; the UAC sees it as a matter of great concern and a special committee will develop policies and interventions; and there are NGOs such as Uganda

Community-Based Association for Child Welfare (UCOBAC) and Uganda Women's Effort to Save the Orphans (UCOBAC) who have focussed their efforts in this field. The issues are highly complex and the potential solutions by no means obvious. Some of the interventions raised earlier in this Report, such as those for a Community Monitoring System and impact studies of Health Care and Education, will partially address the needs of orphans, e.g., in considering the issue of school fees. Valuable as these interventions and insights might be they are certainly not enough. This is an area where UNDP ought to be involved in capacity building, but what to do and how to do it is by no means obvious. There is a clear preference in Uganda for non-institutional solutions to the needs of orphans, although there can be no reason to suppose that this is everywhere and for all children both feasible and the best option. The national response has so far been ad hoc, and what has been done is an insufficient guide for future policy and appropriate institutional structures for the delivery of support. It is strongly recommended that before UNDP develops a programme in this area that a comprehensive study be made of the whole set of issues raised by the large and increasing number of orphans. Such a study should not focus to any degree on estimating future numbers [having some idea of numbers and their distribution is not the core of the problem], but on identifying needs and the ways in which policies and institutional structures can meet these. UNDP in consultation with the UAC should urgently commission such a study, and then develop with NGOs, government and other agencies, a programme of work.

3. Community Development

This is not a useful operational category, but it is desirable to identify it nevertheless in order to re-emphasise its importance. In practice much of the foregoing is about how to develop and strengthen community involvement in all areas, and the need to refocus the allocation of resources away from urban to rural groups, and away from formalised institutional structures to informal and localised ones. How best to do this, and the identification of priorities, will be the outcome of the recommended studies and policy related discussions in Uganda. There is much already being done at the community level, most obviously by TASO, the Uganda Red Cross and by the churches, which is extremely valuable, but highly constrained in terms of geographic and functional coverage. How to expand these activities, both spatially and in other ways, is by no means obvious. What is presently urgent is identification of needs and constraints, so as to be able, for example, to expand the numbers of trained personnel available for counselling and for behaviour change programmes. This is a matter which is also dealt with below under Organisational Restructuring.

D. STRENGTHENING ORGANISATIONAL STRUCTURES

This is potentially and actually a hugely complex problem and the following should be seen for what they are—tentative recommendations based on unscientific observations. These are thought, nevertheless, to be of value, not least in pointing in the direction of positive and productive change. For purposes of exposition only it has been necessary to identify two categories - Government and Non-Government—but obviously these are in many ways overlapping in their areas of interest, and are and should be seen as complementary. Many of the interventions above entail new functions and changing responsibilities for organisations, and the following should be seen as only a sub-set of these changes which are mainly organisational in their nature.

1. Government

The Uganda Government has recently introduced major structural changes with the establishment of the Uganda AIDS Commission and Secretariat. This signals the commitment of the Government, and its intention that policies for the HIV epidemic be both multi-sectoral and multi-level. However, there remain unresolved issues about structure and function to which attention is turned below. The ordering of the following discussion can be considered as representative of the importance which is attached to particular levels of capacity building activities.

(a) Local Government Structures

It is a historical fact that most UNDP capacity building has been focused at the level of Central Government, to the relative neglect of Local Government. In the case of the HIV epidemic all levels need to be strengthened, but the problems are much greater at the local level. This is scarcely news, and there are many existing proposals of a piecemeal nature which aim to remedy the observed deficiencies of poor policy formulation and implementation at District and County levels. There is generally too little understanding of the developmental effects of the epidemic, and too little integration across programmes—this is the familiar problem of verticality. The UAC is considering the establishment of Field Offices in a limited number of Districts; UNFPA has looked at the desirability of locating Population Officers at the same level, and there are proposals under consideration for economists from the MEPD to be located at the District. There are already many functions relating to health and development located at District level, some of these concentrating on the delivery of medical services and health education. This is also the level at which, at least in some Districts, NGOs are also operating, and need to be encouraged to operate. It is also clear that the Resistance Councils (RC) have, and are expected to have, important functions and responsibilities. but that these are not being effectively utilised. RC leaders in particular need training and especially leadership training. The importance of community action and social mobilisation is at the core of this Report, and for tnis to happen there has to be a major strengthening of LocalGovernment structures. In part this means shifting more resources, financial and human, to the local level which will require different organisational structures with new perspectives and priorities. Effective structures have to be built; in part through a comprehensive evaluation of existing and proposed systems, and support for a process of organisational reforns. UNDP has an important role to play in bringing about these very critical reforms.

(b) The Uganda Aids Commission

The Commission and the Secretariat have been in existence for such a short time that their roles functions, resource constraints needs and responsibilities, are all still evolving. The WB has been involved in needs assessment at the level of the UAC, and in respect of proposals for the setting up of AIDS Units in the various Ministries. In many senses, therefore, this is the wrong point in time for UNDP to assess what its contribution to the UAC and to individual ministries ought to be. The role of UNDP in these circumstances should be to continue with its general support for the Uganda Government's initiative, and to look positively upon requests for assistance. To a degree any response will need to be set within a framework of priorities, which is precisely the purpose of this Report. What has been argued above is that effective programmes across the spectrum of needs have to be concentrated elsewhere, particularly at the community level.

This leaves the UAC with major strategic responsibilities which are important for the development of effective policies for prevention and care, and for responding to the multiple consequences of the epidemic. To perform these functions the Secretariat has to acquire a high level of professionalism in the areas it has already identified as crucial; to utilise consultants where internal skills are unavailable, but generally to keep itself a lean and non-bureaucratic institution. UNDP should, once needs have been formulated in these terms, be willing to provide training and consultancies. For example, assisting the UAC in developing research programmes especially in the social sciences, and in helping the UAC acquire professional understanding in the areas of project development and evaluation. It being understood that these skills are needed at the level of the UAC, but not so that these activities are undertaken by the Secretariat. Thus the UAC has to be able to advise on research priorities, to be able to review research output, and to ensure that this research informs policy formulation and programme development. To become, in short, the centre in Uganda for informed discussion of HIV, and the source to whom those inside government and those outside government naturally turn for advice on policy and programme development.

(c) Ministry of Economic Planning and Development (MEPD)

This Ministry has critical responsibilities and, as such, needs to be informed and to have insights into both the causes and the effects of the HIV epidemic. As a planning ministry it has to ensure that other ministries are aware of the costs, social and economic, which Uganda is both bearing now and will inevitably also have to face in the coming years. Government needs to plan both for the erosion of its own capacities due to HIV and for the changing levels and types of services which will face Departments. As noted above the WB is considering the needs of various Ministries, including those associated with the establishment of AIDS Units. It is crucial that MEPD in particular develop a programme of training for its professionals, especially economists, so that it can modify its internai planning activities to take account of HIV, and ensure that this is also true of other Ministries in their planning roles. Since the MEPD also plays a major role in directing and co-ordinating donor assistance it is doubly important that it be aware of and understand the specific requirements for effective ACPs. To this end it is essential that senior staff and professionals be provided with the opportunity to participate m workshops, etc., dealing with HIV, and to undertake [participate in] studies of the socio-economic effects of HIV.

2. Non-Governmental Organisations

It is now readily agreed by everyone that NGOs, CBOs, churches, etc., are central to policies for prevention, for care, and for activities which aim to limit the economic and social costs of HIV. This is evident from both the analysis and the recommendations made above. Organisations such as TASO have become models for institutional developments throughout the world. An example of what can be done for the infected and affected, for prevention, for income support—across the whole spectrum of activities—by individuals of commitment and determination. Similar qualities are present in other Ugandan NGOs, with the Red Cross, the Catholic Church, UCOBAC, UWESO, and countless others, active in many directions and many areas of the country. A recent UAC inventory of NGO activities is several inches thick—a testimony to their extensive involvement at all levels.

Much has been done, which needed to be done. But the growth of NGOs has been organic, in some directions and not in others, with a regional spread which is very uneven. So also with performance, where it is evident that with growing responsibilities and programmes, in areas such as management and financial control [costing generally], and in monitoring and evaluation, there have emerged real weaknesses. This is unsurprising, and indeed some of the NGOs have already undertaken internal evaluations, restructured management, and considered strategic plans for the future.

The issue for UNDP is how can it help these organisations be more effective in meeting the challenges posed by HIV, and at the same time encourage independence and growth in response to needs. What is undoubtedly a prior requirement is an evaluation of what NGOs are presently doing; in what areas are they strong and effectivc/ineffective; what are the current constraints facing these organizations [of management, of planning, of project evaluation, of research, of cost analysis and control, etc.,] and how can these be tackled [by whom? through collaboration? through establishing specialised service agencies for management training, project evaluation, performance monitoring?]. Where is there a need for rationalisation of activity? Are there activities which are underprovided and, if so, why, and how can obstacles to provision be overcome? This is a major task to undertake such an evaluation, and to ask the questions, "What can NGOs do best?" and, "How can performance be improved?". UNDP should offer to finance such an evaluation, and then develop a programme of support for such institutions through consultative processes so as to improve their eftectiveness. These activities should have a very high priority in any ordering of UNDP activities in Uganda.

IV. OPERATIONALISING ACTIVITIES

A. PROGRAMME APPROACH

The previous Sections have dealt partly with description and analysis, and partly with principles. So far there has as yet been no explicit consideration of operational implementation of the UNDP

Programme on HIV for Uganda. The purpose of this section is to briefly rectify this omission, but to do so in a fairly schematic form. The argument for not dealing in detail with some aspects of the Programme are set out above where it was suggested that flexibility in design and in programme implementation are both desirable. While the details of specific activities remain to be resolved and will have to be established through programme and project discussions, the overall balance of the UNDP Programme—the areas for UNDP concentration of its activities—have been strongly identified in Section III.

It is possible for there to be misinterpretation of what is being proposed by way of a UNDP Programme for Uganda, and it may be useful to state unambiguously what it is, and what it is not. The Programme is not an alternative National AIDS Control Programme (NACP); and it should not be seen as in any sense a parallel programme. Nor is it separate from the NACP, but should be viewed as integral to this, and fundamentally part of the nationally agreed Strategic Plan for responding to HIV. There is certainly no intention of supplanting, or in any way diluting, the authority and responsibilities of the UAC and the MOH [or of other actors such as WHO]. What has been attempted in this Programme is an articulated statement of UNDP's strategic assistance for Uganda which is coherent in its own terms; is founded on analysis of the changing situation in the country; and is the outcome of extensive discussions at the official and non-official levels. But the choices remain those of Government; what fits with, what does not fit with, the National Strategy for HIV and AIDS.

It is in the nature of this approach that not only has coherence been sought, as well as relevance to needs, but that other principles have been applied. These latter have included prioritisation—what are the crucial areas of actual or relative programme neglect, and how can UNDP resources be applied effectively to releasing policy and programme constraints? It is the conclusion of -this Report that UNDP' s contribution should be focused on the developmental effects of the epidemic [and especially the erosion of the human resource base of the society]. Thus activities should be identified, especially at the community level, which address these matters. But not to the exclusion of other important aspects of the national AIDS strategy, and many diverse activities which add to sustainable capacities generally are included in the UNDP Programme.

UNDP needs to see the Programme as serving a catalytic objective—to be partly about advocacy, and in part to be about social mobilisation. In the case of both of these the aims are to improve understanding and to change perception; in part to induce a larger flow of resources, and in part to induce a more effective set of policy and programme responses. To see the Programme as a means of influencing other bilateral and multi-lateral donors in their activities in Uganda. To see some UNDP interventions as "seed corn" which induce further activities by other actors; and at all times to ensure that the relative expertise of different institutions and agencies are exploited. The crucial importance of effective co-ordination of approaches and activities has been emphasised earlier, and this is rightly seen as an important function and responsibility of the UAC. The choices lie with the Ugandan Government. What has been set out in this UNDP Programme is an articulated set of activities formulated within the strategic framework established by the UAC.

Less obviously, but also important for both UNDP and Uganda, is the development of a Programme which is linked to the other priority areas of the UNDP Country Programme, particularly Poverty Alleviation and Rural Development, and Economic Policy and Management Capacity. Both in terms of the foregoing, and in what follows, coherence of the UNDP Programme for AIDS in Uganda has been an important objective; in effect to be programmatic in the many different ways which have been variously identified throughout this Report.

B. ALLOCATION OF PROGRAMME RESOURCES

Section III provides details of the main activities which are proposed, and the rationale for these. Suggested policy interventions are also made in other sections of the report, particularly in Section II. It is perhaps helpful to have more information on the proposed relative importance of different interventions within the Programme, and this is provided by the following schedule. At this stage these allocations should be seen as illustrative, and it is fully anticipated that virement will occur between both the main and sub-categories of expenditure. Nevertheless, the broad balance of expenditure between A-D should be changed only after very careful consideration and through local processes of discussion.

ALLOCATION OF IPF BY INTERVENTION AND BY ACTIVITY *(US$000)*

A. HIV TRANSMISSION

1. IEC; raising effectiveness; capacity building: training	500
2. Evaluating behaviour change; developing new models;	500
3. Low Infection areas - developing and applying interventions.	500
4. Transmission of HIV and Gender; analysis and service delivery.	500
5. STDs; programme development and gender.	200
6. HIV testing policy and behaviour change.	100
7. Refugees; evaluation of needs and HIV transmission factors.	100
8. Other activities Military; blood clubs etc.	100
Sub-Total	$2.500.000

B. ECONOMIC AND SOCIAL IMPACTS

1. Effects of female morbidity and mortality.	100
2. Social indicators; prediction and policy strategies.	50
3. Human resource balance; prediction and policy.	200
4. New approaches to modelling economic and social impact.	100
5. Micro projects.	2,000
6. Community monitoring.	750
7. Impact Studies; agriculture; health; education.	1,000
Sub-Total	$4,250,000

C. CARING

1 Community-based care; evaluation and system innovation.	2,000
2.Orphans; evaluating structures and needs; development of programmes.	500
3.Community development.	500
Sub-Total	$3,500,000

D. STRENGTHENING ORGANISATIONAL STRUCTURES

1. Local Government; evaluation and development.	500
2. UAC; professional development; consultancies; study support.	500
3. MEPD; professional development; new plarming models.	250
4. Private sector; structural evaluation and institutional innovation.	500
5. Strengthening NGO and CBO structures; training; evaluation.	1,000
6. Workshop Programme [ALL — SECTIONS A-D]	1,500
Sub-Total	$ 4,2500000

Total	$14,500,000
Management of Programme	1,000,000
Grand Total	$15,500,000

Figures 18.2—18.7 show the balance of the main programme activities in terms of interventions anal activities .

C. SEOUENCING INTERVENTIONS

It would be possible to set out a fairly precise plan for the ordering of interventions and activities, but for reasons set out above in Section III this would over-determine the content of the Programme. It was argued above that all activities should be seen as interacting and mutually supportive. Interventions, therefore, have to take place on all fronts, but not everything can be seen as of equal priority, nor in the present state of understanding capable of effective implementation. It is critically important for the success of the UNDP Programme that the knowledge base be improved in many areas, and this should be seen as a pre-requisite to policy formulation and programme design. The importance of the learning process cannot be over emphasised; this has been stressed many times in this Report and its significance for effective policy will bear repetition. Cross-learning, from experience internal to Uganda, and between Uganda and other countries, has been a target actively pursued in designing this Programme. The generalisation of the results of activities—building on experience and learning lessons—must be an essential part of the evaluation and monitoring process for all activities. This is true not merely of the Workshop Programme, where the intent will be partly to foster cross-learning, but less obviously also for all activities. It is therefore crucial that the Workshop Programme be established and be set in motion with great speed.

An important task for the managers of the UNDP Programme will be to develop a detailed plan for activities over the next five years, and to build into this plan effective monitoring and evaluation processes. Indeed, one of the activities to be pursued directly and indirectly is capacity building in these crucial respects [partly to be achieved through training, and partly through institutional development]. This has to be seen as one of the important and prior activities of the Programme. Similarly with other areas of technical assistance where it is readily agreed that the human resource base needs to be improved. Two examples of this are Micro Projects and Ministry of Economic Planning and Development (MEPD). But there are many other instances where initial activities will have to concentrate on raising understanding and on developing skills as prerequisites for policy and programme development. This does not mean that everything has to wait on the human resources being strengthened, and many activities can be started now which utilise existing skills and experience. Thus the Micro Projects can begin implementation as of now but will need to be strengthened in terms of TA; as also can some of the HIV transmission proposals, where there are existing plans and operations with which UNDP can collaborate.

As will be seen in the next part of this report there are critical issues of management of the Programme and of its implementation which need to be resolved. In many senses getting these things right will determine how successful the Programme is in meeting the problems facing Uganda. It is worth devoting both time and other resources to resolving these aspects of the problem as an initial activity, and only then to develop the detail of the UNDP Programme. This is an important and cnucial element of the Programme, and one where the UAC, the MEPD and UNDP all have valuable contributions to make in defining effective structures.

D. PROGRAMME IMPLEMENTATION

Section IV.B summarised a complex programme of activities for the period 1992-1996. It is proposed that 19.5 per cent of the Country Programme IPF be allocated to AIDS, i.e., some 15.5 million US. This is a large and very significant proportion of the Country Programme (CP), and it is absolutely essential that in the conditions facing Uganda that these resources be effectively managed. Government has, in agreement with UNDP, an important role in the determination of the implementation process for the Programme. It is an objective of UNDP policy to strengthen Ugandan expertise and increase the use of goods and services supplied by or through national governmental, non-governmental and private institutions in programme development, implementation and management. It is fully recognised that the capacity for government execution has been raised by the establishment of the Government Execution Unit [GEX] in the MEPD.

However, while it is the ultimate objective that national institutions implement both programmes and projects, and the establishment of GEX is an appropriate step in this direction, it is certainly not presently the case that this is feasible. Uganda will continue to need expertise, services and other inputs from external sources during the Fourth CP, including UN system sources. In this respect the Specialised Agencies of the UN system will continue to have a critical supporting role, but with the proviso that over time their contribution will increasingly be in the form of external specialists to complement local expertise. In terms of the UNDP Programme for AIDS it would readily be accepted that ILO, for example, should have an important role to play in the measurement of the erosion of the human resource base caused by HIV, and in the development of policy and programme responses. In a similar way FAO has or ought to have the relevant expertise for assessing the impact of changing labour supplies on agriculture, and in establishing the effects on the level and mix of farm output. It is appropriate that WHO have a continuing and central role in the setting of health policy, and in particular in the development of a multi-sectoral framework for HIV policy. Thus WHO remains the most important technical resource in many areas, most obviously in health.

The experience of the UNV Programme will also be invaluable in the implementation of UNDP's activities. At the national level UNV support can be provided to the UAC, the MEPD, and sectoral ministries, in the fields of monitoring and evaluation, and in research and training. At the District level UNV could assist in training and in planning, monitoring and evaluation and much else. They have particular expertise, technical and administrative, which could be valuable to NGOs and CBOs, particularly in roles

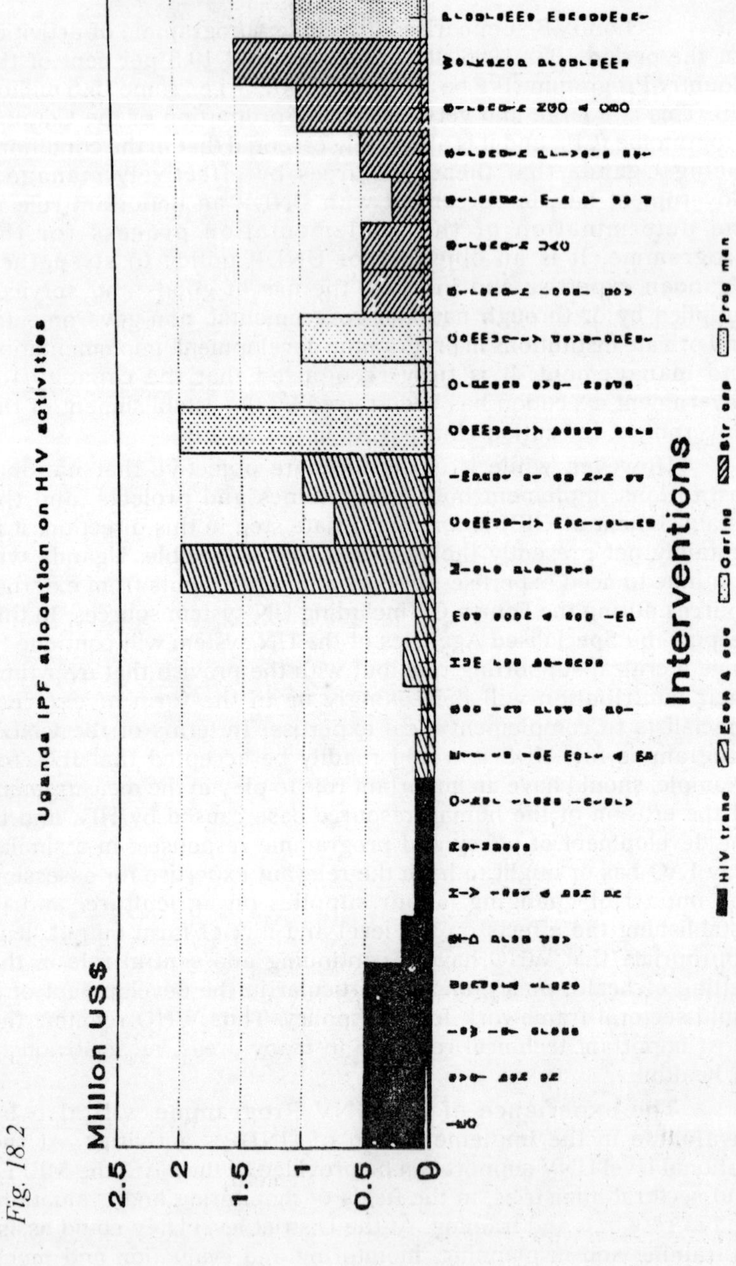
Uganda IPF allocation on HIV activities
Million US$
2.5
2
1.5
1
0.5
0
Interventions
HIV trans
Econ & soc
Str sup
Prog man
UNDP HIV & Development Programme

Fig. 18.2

Fig. 18.3

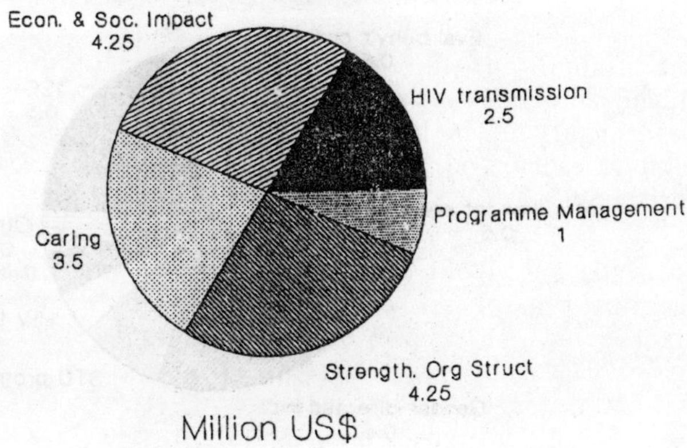

UNDP HIV and Development Programme

Fig. 18.4

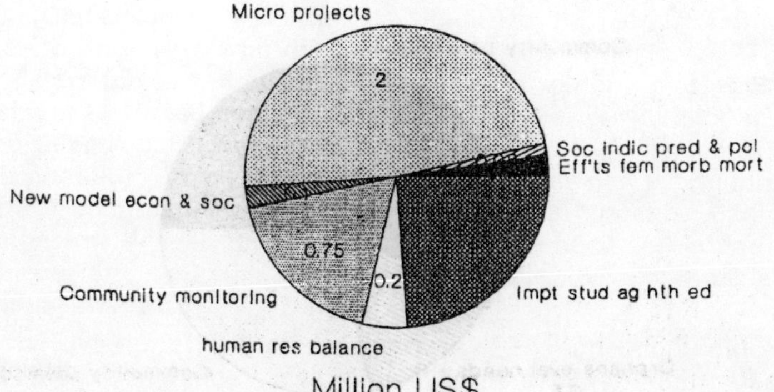

UNDP HIV & Development Programme

Fig. 18.5

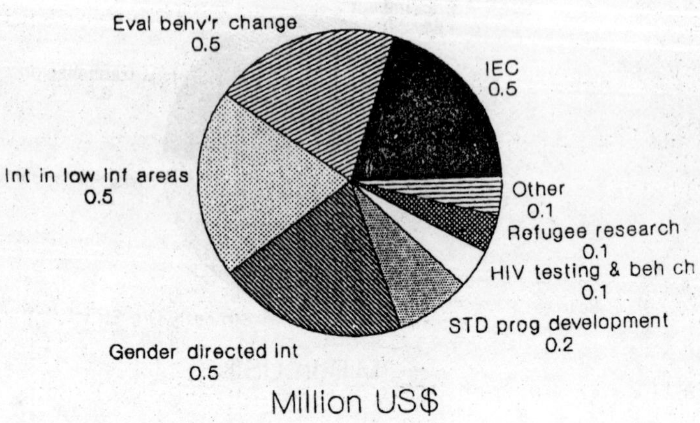

UNDP HIV & Development Programme

Fig. 18.6

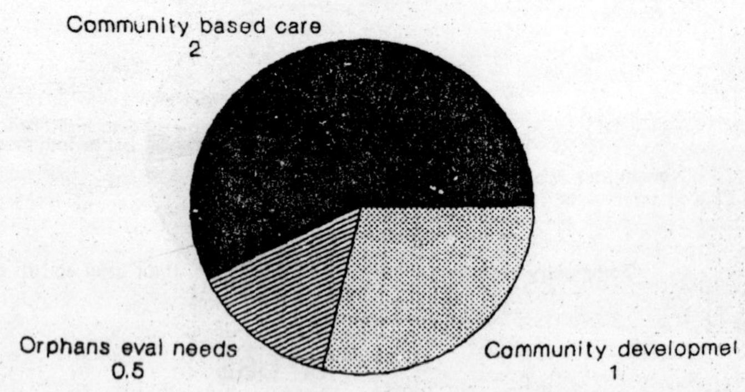

UNDP HIV & Development Programme

Fig. 18.7

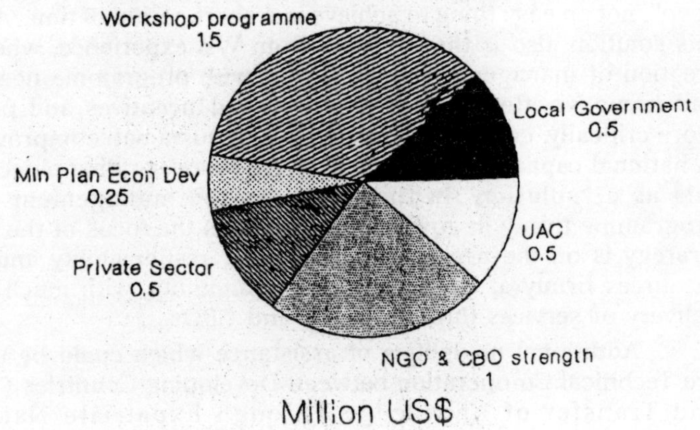

relating to the mobilisation of effective activities at the local level, where technical expertise and experience are major constraints.

The options in respect of implementation are fairly straightforward and in some senses this is not the core of the problem. Some institutions, such as the UAC, are ruled-out by the fact that they are not an implementing agency. For other fundamental reasons to do with the nature of the multi-sectoral approach it would be inappropriate for the MOH to be responsible for overall implementation of the UNDP Programme. One possibility is to lodge management of the Programme with an NGO, which is essentially the option chosen by USAID. But this has its disadvantages too, not least in the high proportion of overheads which are charged by EIL, which substantially reduces the quantity of resources actually applied and available to meet programme needs.

Possibly the best option is to locate a Manager, or Unit, in MEPD, but even this is not wholly optimal. As we have seen above the MEPD has a central role to play in external co-ordination, including planning the use of external resources which directly and indirectly are related to the national AIDS strategy. Its position at the core of Government has been increased by its amalgamation with Finance, so that Planning and Finance functions can now be fully integrated. On the other hand the MEPD has no expertise in the area of HIV and AIDS, and this would have to be created "de novo": not an easy thing to achieve in a short period of time. Against this solution also is the evidence from WB experience, where the creation of management units to deal with programme needs has had disruptive effects on pay structures and incentives, and, perhaps more critically, created no long term and sustainable improvement in national capacities. There is perhaps an over-riding objection to this as a "solution" in that it places the management of the programme firmly in government, whereas the focus of the UNDP strategy is on the need to locate greater responsibility and more resources firmly at the level of the community, with much of the delivery of services through NGOs and CBOs.

Additional modalities of assistance which could be utilised are Technical Co-operation between Developing Countries (TCDC) and Transfer of Knowledge Through Expatriate Nationals (TOKTEN). The challenge of HIV is not confined to Uganda, and it is certainly desirable that it draw on the experience of other countries and institutions through TCDC. There are also additional resources of experience, knowledge and commitment to be drawn on through the TOKTEN programme. This permits Uganda to add to its resources through the repatriation of trained nationals who left the country in the 1970s and 1980s. Their contribution, under conditions of a worsening human resource endowment, has become even more critical in meeting the challenges of the present and following decades.

REFERENCES

Barnett T. and Blaikie P. M. [July 1990]. Community Coping Mechanisms in the Face of Exceptional Demographic Change. Report to the Overseas Development Administration (UK).

World Bank. Uganda: The Economic Impact of AIDS [June 1991].

19

Placing Women at the Centre of the Analysis

Ms. Elizabeth Reid
UNDP, New York

There is a growing consensus in the development assistance world that human development should provide the framework for development assistance in the 1990s. Yet, while this is widely welcomed by women, there are few, if any, grounds for assuming that this ideology will benefit women any more than any of the previous development assistance ideologies, be they economic growth, growth with equity, basic needs or whatsoever.

The literature on women and development extends back almost as far as the literature on development itself. The mandates and directives have long been in place. Yet, the success stories are anecdotal rather than systemic and this is causing a growing questioning of past approaches.

There are those amongst us, serious but with a sense of humour, who, in response to this chronic failure, are now proposing two new but linked approaches: the radical procedural approach and the radical analytical approach. The first approach consists in developing a set of procedures that might better bring about the achievement of our women in development objectives. For example, all missions that are responsible for programme or project formulation, implementation teams and evaluation missions must be predominantly or exclusively composed of women. All hose consulted during such missions must be predominantly or exclusively women, and so on. Such procedural directives, if issued by UNDP or CIDA, for example, would undoubtedly be greeted by great discomfiture if not outrage. But it is interesting to note that the obverse, which is the present situation, is not.

The radical analytical approach places women at the centre of the analysis; that is, in any development-related activity whatsoever, the analysis should begin at where women are, whatever they are doing, and should aim to get them (women) where they want to be and bring about the changes they want the rest of the world (men, children, social institutions, financial institutions, economies, etc.), are to be drawn into the analysis primarily on the basis of how they relate to women or how they can contribute to achieving women's goals. Again, radical only in that the obverse is the accepted modus operandi.

Today is not the occasion to elaborate on these approaches, but it is the occasion to understand the cost if we do not place women at the centre of the HIV analysis. The failure to do so has already brought an immense cost in women's lives, a cost which is forcing an understanding that, for the 1990s and beyond, human development will be conditional upon human survival; that is, human survival, not human development, may well become the primary focus of our development assistance.

Let me elaborate on this, taking the example of HIV/AIDS. The main focus of HIV/AIDS programmes to date has been the prevention of the further transmission of the virus. I will focus on sexual transmission since, for women, this is the overwhelming way in which women become infected.

The three main prevention strategies for sexual transmission that are being advocated, particularly in developing countries, are: one, the reduction of the number of sexual partners; two, condom usage; and three, faithfulness in relationships and celibacy and abstinence outside of them. To these, a fourth has recently been added, namely, the treatment of STDs.

I do not wish to discuss, today, the merits of these strategies, per se, bur rather to look at their adequacy as prevention strategies for women and those who people women's world.

Let's take the first, reduction of sexual partners. Preliminary data from African studies indicate that 60 per cent to 80 per cent of all infected women have one and only one sexual partner. Therefore, this strategy has no relevance to their lives. Nor is it relevant to the lives of those women who, because of economic circumstances, are forced to sell or exchange sexual intercourse. Thus, for the majority of women this strategy is inapplicable, irrelevant strategy.

Secondly, condom usage. Men use condoms. Results from programmes with sex workers have clearly shown that some women can successfully negotiate condom use. However, this remains a rare skill among women. Most men do not use condoms, and most women do not have the ability or the leverage to protect themselves in this way. This is a strategy for men.

Thirdly, faithfulness, abstinence and celibacy. At the current stage of the epidemic, it can be estimated that every day, each day now, 1,500 faithful women are infected. That is, every day, just now, there are 1,6500 women who have no sexual partners other than their husbands who are becoming infected. This number will increase as the number of infected men increases. There are some indications that the incidence of rape, particularly of young girls, has increased and there is no reason to believe, in fact, on the contrary, that this is not also true of incest. For most women, abstinence and the faithfulness of both partners in a relationship is not within their power to bring about. For a growing number of girls and women, sexual assault is a reality. So this strategy is inapplicable.

These are grim facts. But they are the realities that lie hidden behind the epidemiological data. The strategies that are being advocated are strategies that men, now women, have under their control. This is the area why one in every 40 adult women in Africa is infected. It is the reason why there are as many or more women in Africa that men as infected. It is also the reason why, in the Latin American and Caribbean regions, the male/female infection ratio has dropped so precipitously over the last couple of years.

Is there no hope for women? In the longer term, the power imbalances in relationships and society which create women's subordination must be changed. But what, in the short term, can women to do save their lives and those of their children?

If one lays aside for the moment the current strategies and begins the analysis with the reality of women's lives, then the first question is: Is there any protective measure that a woman has under her own control which will offer her protection from infection?

Protective measures can be divided into two types: those which prevent contact with an infected person and transmission of the virus and those that decrease the efficacy of transmission when unprotected sexual contact occurs. The first, for example, includes condom usage, faithfulness and abstinence. Then measures are much more efficacious than the second type. However, the second type may overall be just as effective, or more effective, if more people can act upon them.

There are, in fact, in each of these two categories, some measures that an individual woman can use. It is important that we start naming them.

One of the most efficient know means of reducing the efficacy of transmission of the virus, that is, when you have unprotected sexual intercourse with an infected person, is unbroken genital skin. This is the advice we give to health workers: The most effective barrier is unbroken skin. If you are covered in blood, wash it off. In the genital area, unbroken skin is also protective.

Transmission of the virus can be facilitate by the presence of genital lesions, inflammation, secretions and scarification. The causes of these conditions in women include genital urinary tract infections, STDs, sexual practices and traditional infibulation practices. All genital conditions which may facilitate transmission should now become a focus of attention. Not all of them do women have the power to change. A number are treatable. Others, in particular, sexual and infibulation practices, will require longer term solutions. However, there are many conditions that can be improved, through improved hygiene or through treatment.

Women may be culturally or socially constrained from using STD-dedicated services, or even from seeking treatment for a genital condition. This is often not culturally or socially sanctioned. If we want to enable women to avail themselves of this means of protection, it becomes important to know whether the diagnosis and treatment of these conditions can be combined, for example, with other consultations requiring an internal examination. That is, if women cannot go to be treated for these conditions, can we locate services where they are already being externally examined.

This analysis will lead to a broader emphasis on, then an exclusive focus on improving STD services. STD services are mainly used by people, men and women, with multiple sexual partners. Most women do not use these services and most women suffer from genital conditions other than, but also including, STDs. Thus, a woman-centred analysis in this area would focus on the diagnosis and treatment of those genital conditions in both men and women which place them at increased risk of infection and would focus on the delivery of services at points where these people go.

Another strategy for reducing the efficacy of transmission may be to ensure that the change sin a person's infectivity over the course of infection are widely known. A person's infectiousness, the ability to infect someone else, increases as he or she progresses from asymptomatic infection to symptomatic infection. Whereas an individual woman may not be able to refuse sexual intercourse in general, she may be able to find a way if her partner were ill. In other words, she may be able to do this in a short period of time although not over a long period of time. This knowledge about infectivity is an important element in the counselling of discordant couples in our societies. In societies where the virus is diffused throughout the population, this information should be widely known so that those who can, can use it as a protective measure.

Apart from the above, there are at least two strategies for preventing contact with an infected person, the first type of measure, which are under a woman's control.

Little attention has been given to barrier methods which, unlike the condom, are under a woman's control. The literature on the sexual transmission of diseases other than HIV to women indicate that diaphragms protect women from, for example, gonorrhoea, to the same extent that condom usage does. There is no reason to assume that condoms protect women more than diaphragms do, with or without a spermicide, in the case of HIV. Yet, no attention has been given to determining the adequacy of diaphragms as a protective measure.

The second strategy under women's control for preventing contact with an infected man is, in the absence of any known alternatives, becoming more widespread in high incidence areas. This is desertion, that is, just moving away, walking away from home and relationship. It is an option often with tragic consequences for the woman who may well find herself unable too support herself and, when she is able to take them, her children. In such cases, prostitution, and so infection, may be her only coping strategy.

There is a pressing need to further explore and identify the strategies which a woman may have under her control. However, at the same time it must be understood that the most efficient and effective prevention strategies are those that men have under their control. Thus, every effort must continue to be made to change men's behaviour.

In this area, also, there has been a great neglect of a woman-centred analysis. There are at least two very powerful instruments that have not yet been fully identified in the efforts to change men's behaviour the first is women's collective action. The second is the law.

While women individually may feel and be powerless to change men's behaviour, women collectively can effect extraordinary changes. The literature on the global movement of women over the last couple of decades abounds with examples. The women of Maharastra who decided to no longer tolerate drunkenness in men, in their husbands, formed themselves into vigilante groups. As a group, not individually, the went out looking for the stills and for drunken men. They changed drinking men's drinking patterns. The Chipko women tied themselves to trees to prevent environmental degradation in Nepal. Mexican women in the mid- to late seventies formed an alliance across all types of women and women's groups to bring down the incidence of rape and sexual assault of women. Kenyan women, also tired of drunkenness in their husbands, came together to devise strategies for stopping that behaviour. And the models go on and on.

There is a need to look for models of women' s collective action which have changed men's HIV-related behaviour. The collective voices and actions of women to be called upon can range from the national machineries for women and national women's organizations, all the way to groupings of women at the village level. We learnt in Kenya that if you wish to increase women's income, you cannot give a goat to an individual woman.

Traditionally, goats are owned by men. If you give a goat to a woman, the man will slaughter it when he chooses and take the money. What the women did, then, was to come collectively together. If women collectively owned a goat, no individual husband could make such a decision. We need analogues to face this epidemic.

The second instrument is the law. There is now an extremely effective and very active Women and Law in southern Africa project. At the initiation of this project and for quite different reasons, it was decided that one important area of study would be the newly introduced laws relating to child support. These laws required men to pay for the upkeep of any children that they fathered. What the women and law project has found is that there have been striking changes in male sexual behaviour. Men are now fathering fewer children. Now that they are required to provide for and support those that they father, they father fewer.

This provides an important model. We have tried for a long time through direct legal intervention in the area of rape and incest to change men's behaviour but with varied success. Here is an example of the use of the law to bring about behaviour change which has been extremely effective.

While the primary analysis so far has focused on prevention, a similar analysis is needed to determine the potential impact of this epidemic on individual families, communities and economies and, hence, to plan effective and timely responses. Even in, so to speak, the malecentred analysis, we are not very far along the road to understanding, describing and finding effective strategies. But the point I am making is that what we need to do is to start elsewhere, in this area too, to start in women' s spaces.

Let me give you some glimpses of what a woman-centred analysis would reveal.

Firstly, most women do not know that they are infected. Most women do not want to know. Infected or otherwise, they must still continue with their daily lives. There is no one to take their place.

For many women who know that they are infected, there is no privacy, no confidentiality. Disclosure is not in their hands. Most women find out that they are infected during pregnancy or when a young child falls ill and is diagnosed. The diagnosis of the child makes public the women's infection status.

For women who know that they are infected, what dominates virtually every minute of the day are two primary emotions: anger and guilt. Anger towards the person, usually their husband and the person with whom they have so often infected one or more of their children.

The reality of the lives of these women is that, although, as stated above, probably up to 60 or 80 per cent of infected women were not infected though their own behaviour, they are blamed as the source of the transmission. The stigma and the discrimination associated with this disease rests too often with women.

Next, the supportive services required by seropositive women will be more than drugs and medical care. They will range from household care for ill women, child care for their children, emotional support to lessen discrimination, and financial support, as so often they will not have an income coming into the house. The dominant concern for many infected women is the present and future support for and care of their children, particularly since the fathers of those children will often be sick or dead.

The displacement of women's work from patenting, from productive activities and from community work to care for the sick will have immense consequences within those families and communities. This deplacement, coupled with the high mortality rates in women, could well lead to the disintegration of family structures. This can be seen already in parts of Africa. It will lead to changing patterns of agricultural production and the possibility of decreased food production, and to a decrease in informal sector trading where women trade mainly food. It will lead to shortage of personnel in those formal sectors where women predominate, which still include health and education.

If one includes in one's analysis of the HIV epidemic an analysis centred on women, whether it be with respect to prevention or with respect to developing strategies for minimizing the impact of this epidemic. It is my contention that different strategies and priorities will be identified which may end up being more effective than the present strategies. This is not an academic or a feminist exercise. For women it is a matter of life and death.

Putting women at the centre of the analysis leads to quite different approaches and strategies. For women today, the lack of this analysis for the HIV epidemic has already cost perhaps millions of lives, their children. The price is too high to continue with the blindness of the past. We must change.

20

Creating the Possibility: A Movement for Social Change

Ms. Elizabeth Reid
UNDP, New York

For a movement for social change to come about, there has to be a shared cause or vision, a collective will to change and a sufficiently large group of people as its base. In Africa today, one of the most important challenges is to bring about a will to live, a will to live as an infected person, the will to remain uninfected and the will to live with and despite this virus which is silently and invisibly invading its communities.

This first meeting of the network for African people with HIV and AIDS is the kernel of this social movement, embodying individually and collectively this will to live, a will to live the life that one has richly and fully, the collective will to bring an end to the stigma, rejection, discrimination, neglect, isolation, pain and fear that each of us has had to bear.

The question I would like to pose is: how can we turn this gathering here today from a meeting into a movement, a movement for the changes that we talk and dream about, a movement of activism, of solidarity, of empowerment, a movement sweeping Africa, changing the fatalism and indifference to passion and concern?

There are, perhaps, 220 million adolescents and adults in Africa today living in fear, the fear that they may be or soon will be infected. This is an awful lot of fear, a fear that need not be there. Among the 220 million, there are only, perhaps, at a guess, a quarter of a million who know their infection status, perhaps, only one-tenth of a million. Yet there are at least 8 million people in sub-Saharan Africa who are infected. Among those who know that they are infected, there are even fewer who have come to live with that knowledge.

Most people in Africa die without knowing whether or not they are infected, even if they silently fear so. Reflect upon how you yourself came to know that you are infected. Few men get diagnosed as being infected. Some young men and women get diagnosed, still too often without their consent, when they are granted scholarships for overseas study, when they enter certain professions or vocations or donate blood. A number of women get diagnosed indirectly through a diagnosis of AIDS in one of their children. Most of the few men and women who know that they have AIDS are diagnosed clinically when they are quite close to death.

Very few people in Africa have access to voluntary testing and counselling services. Very few people who know that they are infected have access to counselling, peer groups and other support services to help them learn to live with this knowledge. Very few countries have created the supportive ethical, legal and human rights environment required in order to be able to provide such services.

Programmes of care and support are, for the most part in Africa, programmes for the terminally ill. They are to assist with the dying with HIV, not with dle living with HIV. They are emotionally draining for the counsellors and carers since they work almost exclusively with the dying and those close to them, people often rendered destitute by illness and with few or no coping strategies. The kind of care and support that they can be given is limited. Most people are too sick to take care of themselves or their families. to provide for them or to feed them. They are too ill to be able to do anything to prepare their children for the future, to set their affairs in order, to pass on their knowledge to their families or colleagues or to be activists for change.

Assistance to the dying is not widely balanced by assistance to those living and well with HIV, by programmes to assist people to live with the knowledge that they or someone they love are infected, yet well. There are so few people who have access to voluntary counselling and testing services or who wish to find out. Thus few National HIV/AIDS Programmes achieve the synergy and the energy which can arise when the infected well are included. Furthermore, those that are struggling to learn to live with this knowledge, to become the activists, are too rarely the politicians, the church leaders, the educated or the articulate. This epidemic requires a seemingly rare form of courage, a form of courage which each of you has. But there are too few people yet to create the base of a movement for social change.

How can we change this, break through the stifling silence that has wrapped itself around Africa? Is this silence and paralysis inevitable where people cannot find out their infection status and do not even want to? Does it increase the fear, the anguish and the apathy? Do others feel like the women farmer in Uganda who described herself as "crippled" by not knowing? Does not being able to find out increase an individual and collective sense of powerlessness?

Why might a person want to know their infection status? Statements glibly made that people in Africa do not want to know their infection status have made me think back over my own experience. My husband, Bill, and I were living in Kinshasa, Zaire, when we began to suspect that he might be infected. He had grown up in rural Zaire and had spent much of his life in Zaire or elsewhere in Africa. We had been married less than two years and we had a baby son, John-William. Bill was a fine and much loved person. He was my companion, colleague, lover and husband. We had a very close and loving relationship. It was 1983 and there was no test and, in Kinshasa, virtually no access to information about progression, symptoms or treatment and little, mostly wrong, about life span.

We lived with fear as a constant companion. Which means to say that we lived as if it were not true that he might be infected. We went about out daily lives as before the fear. Except in our lovemaking where the fear that he might be infected haunted us. Except in our love for each other where this fear kept confronting us with the possibility of the loss of this deep and satisfying love. Except that we would look at our little son and wonder how, if true, this might affect him. Except that we had planned to have more children.

To others it was as if nothing had changed. They could not see the fear and we certainly could not have shown it or spoken about it without losing everything we valued outside of ourselves: our work, our friendships, our dignity. And anyway we lived in the hope that it might not be, that the fear was ungrounded. Fear and hope were tangled up inside us. It was a terrible time, living as if he were infected and as if he were not, unable to speak about these fears, dreading and hoping. We were in the same position as about 220 million Africans are today. It was cruel.

As soon as he had begun to fear that he might be infected, Bill went out and bought condoms. I did not have to suggest, beg or negotiate and I may not have been able to if it had been left up to me. I have not been brought up to do such things easily. But, fortunately, I did not have to struggle with the fear of death in the act of love. Neither the knowledge that he might be infected nor the possibility of condom breakage had any place in our lovemaking. I was not making love to a virus, or to an infected person. I was making love to Bill.

Yet sometimes the fear of pain and loss was unbearable and

it was I that drew back his hand as he reached for the condom.

I can understand those who have said to me that the condom becomes a symbol and a reminder of the death to come. I can understand those who have said: "I love him. What does it matter if I become infected too?" Or those for whom the edges blur, who sometimes, living so much within the epidemic, feel that they are already infected.

Finally, a test became available and we decided to challenge the fear, to allow for the possibility that the hope might be justified. We wanted to know.

In those parts of the world where testing and counselling is widely available, many people will choose not to know. Their right to this knowledge is respected, they could know if they wanted to, but they choose to live protectively of themselves and others, without this knowledge. This is a different psychological setting from a world where few, if any, can gain access to this knowledge. For many years after Bill's death, I choose not to know. I knew that I could not live with the knowledge that I was infected and facing the same future. I feared that I would give up, even take my life. But I had a son to raise who had already lost his father. I chose not to know.

What happened when we found out that Bill was infected? The finding out was brutal. No counselling. No support. Just the result. There was no more hope.

The feeling of hopelessness was overpowering. Bill was infected and there was nothing we could do about it. We were left with a sense of deep bewilderment, of absolute powerlessness.

We struggled, mainly separately and alone, the only time in our life together that we were so far apart, to learn to live with this knowledge.

Eventually it became clear to us that the only way to live with this knowledge was to go on living. We had stumbled through helplessness, distress, turmoil, impotence. We stumbled into living.

How did we make that transition from the trauma of the diagnosis to living? Much of it had to do with the sort of person Bill was. He believed that life was worth living, that we together had much more happiness to find and that we had worthwhile work to do. He realized that not taking his life into his own hands was leading to a death wish, a sense of helplessness and hopelessness. It also had to do with my family and our friends. They too had to learn how to live with this knowledge and so they understood what we were facing. We helped each other.

The living we found was simple enough: we did those things that we would have been doing anyway. We led full and happy lives. The reality of his infection had been acknowledged but placed in its proper perspective. And life continued.

We had come back to living but our lives had essentially changed.

I was never again to be without the knowledge that Bill was infected. It was not incapacitating, just constant; not a fear of death, not an anticipation of death, not any state of mind with respect to death. Just something intractable inside me as I went about living my daily life, a constant call to courage.

We had made the journey to living within the epidemic. Pity had no place there. It is an emotion from outside looking in. We were involved, absorbed, challenged, laughing, learning, bickering together.

Bill is dead and has joined the ancestors. His son and I keep him living with us, in our memories, in our hearts and in our lives.

This is just one story of moving from the cruelty of fear to knowing that someone one loves dearly is infected, to learning how to live with that knowledge. It is a story of the will to live, of the ability to influence the quality and, perhaps, the length of one's life, of activism, of solidarity and of sexuality.

The more stories we have the more we will know about the critical questions facing us: why would a person want to know their infection status? What happens when they find out they are infected? How can they be supported in making the transition to living with that knowledge? How can the group of people who are infected, active and well be expanded? And how can it be formed into a movement for social change so that we can all, the infected, the uninfected and the affected, live peacefully with this virus and with each other?

These stories must be told but will not be if the story tellers or their children or families are rejected or in any way harmed by their telling.

These questions are a part of what you are here to talk about: the processes of empowerment and change through solidarity, activism and self-organization.

Thank you for the honour you have given to me in inviting me to be with you on this momentous occasion, the birth of this Africa-wide movement for social change, a movement towards living with HIV and AIDS.

21

Breaking the Silences

Ms. Elizabeth Reid
UNDP, New York

A blanket of silence has wrapped itself around Africa, smothering the voices, the fear, the pain, the cries for help. There are some brave voices, including those of a number of courageous women who are with us today. But, still, few couples are talking to one another about staying uninfected, few parents are talking to their children, few colleagues are talking about the future management of their work places, few leaders about the future of their countries.

Why this blanket of silence? Is it because there seems to be a difficulty in living in a present where people do not themselves know whether or not they are infected, where they can only watch to see if those they love - spouses, daughters, parents, siblings—start growing thinner, where each day there are more funerals?

There is even more silence surrounding the future. Few seem to be willing to address the question of how they will live in a future, perhaps only five to ten years away in some countries, when they will be surrounded by people dying, where the normal expectations of daily life will be more and more disrupted, where the devastating impact of this epidemic will be more visible in the faces of children on the streets, in the empty seats in offices, in the scarcity of public services.

Yet if people do not begin thinking about and planning for the future now, the impact of this epidemic could cause civil and economic disintegration as people flee or turn against their leaders or turn against each other. Just because the pain and the silences are no longer bearable.

To prepare people for a less bleak future, a future which could mix pain with hope, grief with love, today's silences must be broken and people start talking about HIV in the way they talk about the effects of devaluation on their lives, or who will win the soccer or when the rainy season will come.

Breaking the silence is critical for keeping families together. Without couples and families talking, there could be a breakdown in trust between men and women, a reluctance, particularly on the part of women, to marry, to have sexual intercourse or to have children. Many women and men may decide not to marry, not to establish families.

Breaking the silence is critical for preventing more people from becoming infected. Experience in responding to this epidemic has taught us the profound importance of dialogue, of discussion between sexually interacting people.

Such a dialogue presupposes a desire to remain uninfected and not to infect others. Thus it presupposes not only awareness but also self esteem and mutual respect. But it requires something more. It requires a capacity to talk intimately about sexuality, desire and protection from infection. Seemingly, and for different reasons, talking things over, breaking the silence, is not easy either for women or for men.

There is also a need for greater insight into, and discussion about, why and how men and women enter into sexual relations.

For women, this may have to do with cultural imperatives which place high value on motherhood and on the continuation of the lineage. Or the reason may have to do with economic imperatives, an inability to survive economically without the support of a man or except by commercial sex work. Or with a need for protection, a critical social role that men play.

For both women and men, factors which are causative or contributory include:

— the impact of poverty, particularly as women seek to care for husbands and children;
— the impact of the structures of the labour market on family structures through, for example, mobility and migration;
— the impact of a lack of employment opportunities, including for the young and for women;
— the incidence of war, civil conflict and violence;
— cultural practices such as child-brides and female infibulation;
— the impact of an upbringing centered around relations of authority, control and coercion on male sexual practices;
— the cultural role of sexual relations, particularly as a cleansing of the past, or a freeing of a person's spirit or as a safeguard against bad luck; and
— the influence of alcohol or drugs on sexuality.

All of these factors have to be discussed in the context of national HIV/AIDS programmes if the spread of the virus is to be slowed.

The second programme focus of most national HIV/AIDS programmes is the care and support of those infected and those who care for them.

Most people in Africa die without knowing that they are infected, even if they fear so. Those who do know, particularly if they are men, know because they are diagnosed with AIDS when they are quite close to death. Some women get diagnosed indirectly through the diagnosis of a child with AIDS. Few blood donors choose to know their results. Few people in Africa have access to affordable voluntary testing and counselling sites.

Thus programmes of care and support are, for the most part, programmes for the terminally ill. They are to assist in the dying with HIV, not in the living with HIV. They are not programmes to assist people to live with the knowledge that they or those they love are infected.

Many counselling, care and concern programmes are volunteer based. They are built on the widespread concern and commitment that exists in African communities towards those who are experiencing misfortune. Most but not all those who volunteer are women who are already burdened by their other roles and responsibilities. Many of the men who volunteer know themselves to be infected with the virus.

Home-based care programmed in particular, play an important role in breaking the silence around this epidemic. They lessen fear and stigma in communities. They help men and boys learn how to care for the sick and the dying. They help protect those for whom they are caring from abuse and neglect. They help in making AIDS a part of everyone's daily life. However, their effectiveness and sustainability is often limited by a lack of integrated planning. There are often no associated systems that guarantee the timely provision of basic necessities such as soap, food for starving households, protein supplements for the sick, simple medicines, especially for the treatment of opportunistic conditions, transport to and from the hospital or health centre or services for children.

They are also emotionally wearing for the counsellors and carers since they are working almost exclusively with the dying and their families, often rendered destitute by the illness and often with few or no coping strategies. Assistance to the dying is not counter balanced by assistance to those living and well with HIV.

Further, because on the whole these programmes are for the terminally ill, the range of support and counselling that can be given is narrow. Most people are too ill to take care of themselves or their families, to provide for them or to feed them. They are too sick to be able to do anything to prepare their children for their future, to set their affairs in order or to pass on their knowledge to their families or their colleagues.

Thus most national HIV programmes are stretched between prevention and the care of the terminally ill and few achieve the synergy which can arise when the infected well are included. Most programmes do not reach the majority of those affected by this epidemic—the infected well and those who love them. These people remain untouched, unacknowledged and without help. In some countries they constitute 20 or 30 per cent of the adult population, in some communities 40 or 50 per cent.

In Africa today there are possibly seven or eight million or more HIV-infected and well men and women who do not know their infection status. The majority of them are married and supporting families. Most are productively active. Most do not want to know their infection status. However, a number of studies are now showing that a significant exception to the latter statement are widows and many youth.

The questions I want to pose today are: Is it in the national interest to motivate people to know their infection status? Could it be in people's own interest to know? If these questions are answered in the affirmative, then there will be a need to radically revise national priorities and donor policies.

What happens when people do not know their infection status and do not want to know? Is this a significant contributory factor to the blanket of silences? Does it increase fear, anguish and apathy? Do others feel like one rural woman in Uganda who described herself as "crippled" by not knowing? Does it increase an individual and a collective sense of powerlessness? Do all these essentially psychological conditions prove a serious constraint to behavioural and attitudinal change? As of yet there are only partial answers to these questions since few studies have raised them. But those that have would seem to indicate that they may be answered in the affirmative by many people.

However, a number of studies have shown that not knowing and so not talking has meant that children are unprepared for the loss of their parents and that parents have not planned for their future. Studies recently carried out by FAO in Eastern and Southern Africa have shown that where people do not have access to this information, where they feel unable to talk about the eventuality of their deaths, whole bodies of knowledge relating to agricultural practices and agricultural processes can be lost. Anecdotal evidence from a number of countries have shown that fear of their status coupled by a reluctance to speak has meant that skills and experience relevant to industrial and financial management of firms and government departments have been completely lost and the opportunity for training of replacements missed.

Thus, particularly in more seriously affected countries, it could be in the national interest to create a milieu in which people Would be able to find out their infection status and feel able to discuss this with their colleagues. This would make it possible to train replacements for those infected, to create opportunities for them to pass on their knowledge and experience, to restructure workplaces to make them less dependent on the skills of particular individuals. Furthermore, if there were evidence that knowing one's infection status could make it possible to live longer as a well infected person, this would assist in increasing their productive lives, increasing the return of the investment of their parents and the State in their education and training and, equally importantly, decrease the likelihood of future civil unrest, since these people could remain caring and providing for their families longer.

Should the State decide that it wishes to motivate people to know their infection status, it would have to ensure that those who knew and were prepared to disclose this information were protected from stigma and discrimination before ensuring widespread access to voluntary testing and counselling sites.

Why might a person want to know? For many women and men the overwhelming reason is a desire to stay alive and well as long as possible to care for, raise and support their children, to plan for their children's future and to provide for their spouses. In Uganda, men and women have used the time while they are well to pass on to their children their own income generating skills: subsistence or cash crop farming, beer brewing, weaving and cloth making, carpentry, and so on. Parents, particularly in urban areas, have opened bank accounts for their children and both men and women have made wills, often discussing their wishes with village or political leaders or with their family elders. They have taken the time to put their affairs in order before God and men. They have also used the knowledge of their infection status in sexual and fertility decision making.

Often knowing one's infection status creates a will to live as long and as well as possible, particularly when one knows others who are living well and happily and as these long-term survivors of HIV infection become more known and studied. The creation of this will to live well and long is, perhaps, one of the greatest challenges that this epidemic offers to Africa.

The length of time a person will live after infection is also influenced by whether or not they prevent themselves from being reinfected and by nutrition, exercise and lifestyle, including alcohol and drug use. It is directly influenced by the support and care they receive after being tested from their families, their carers, their friends and from other infected people and by whether they are in productive employment. Often HIV-infected people become HIV educators and counsellors.

The length and quality of their lives will also be dependant on whether they have access to the treatment of common infections such as pneumococcal pneumonia, salmonella and TB. Hence their ability to live long and well as HIV infected, to continue in productive employment and to care for their families is directly dependent on the health care sector and its priorities.

There are very few African studies on the impact that being tested for HIV has on people's lives. But a small recent study in Zimbabwe showed a gender difference in the impact, in particular in communication with one's partner after getting a positive HIV result. All the men who were married and living with their wives informed their wives of their results. All of their wives accepted their diagnosis, that is, accepted that their husbands were infected. All of the wives then went, themselves, to be tested. Both the husbands and the wives reported consistent condom use after diagnosis. Only those marriages with a previous history of marital discord broke up.

All except one of the married women in the study informed their husbands of their diagnosis but only half of their husbands accepted the diagnosis and only half of the husbands went to be tested. Less than half of the husbands consistently used condoms after the diagnosis. As with the men, almost a quarter of the marriages broke up. Almost none of the single women tested told their partners since they were afraid of being stigmatised and of having their infection status known all around town.

Less than five per cent of the women in the study earned enough money to support themselves.

Tnis small study would seem to show the importance of motivating men to be tested and counselled. Their wives are more accepting of the diagnosis and there is more consistent condom use after diagnosis.

Thus, creating a desire among people, and perhaps especially men, to know their infection status could help break through the barriers of fear and denial, could decrease the powerlessness of women to prevent themselves from becoming infected, could make people more active participants in national HIV/AIDS programmes and could lead to their greater empowerment, whether their results were negative or positive.

In breaking the silences that surround this epidemic, families may better survive and cope and nations better control their destiny.

22

A Call Beyond Duty

Mr. Alpha Boubacar Diallo
Co-ordinator, UNDP's Regional
Project in Sub-Saharan Africa

It is one of the merits of the Nairobi (1987) and Niamey (1989) conferences on Safe Motherhood to have brought to the attention of the international community the true dimension and nature of the long neglected and tragic problem of maternal mortality. Their call for action has produced an encouraging mobilization of international and national institutions and organization, with new studies of the problem being undertaken and new national programmes being developed.

While there is a consensus that the most appropriate approach to solving the problem of maternal mortality has to be multisectoral and multidisciplinary, most of the strategies developed so far have put the major emphasis on a medical solution, with sometimes limited socio-economic supporting interventions. By contrast, the socio-cultural dimension has so far received very little attention in both referenced studies and in the development of national programmes. In most cases, socio-cultural conditions have been lumped in with the socio-economic factors.

One of the reasons for this situation could be the bias of research towards quantitative methodologies. Another reason is the understandable caution required in handling cultural values, together with a judgment that these are difficult to change.

Is the omission of the socio-cultural dimension justified for any understanding of such a sensitive, intimate, complex but also important phenomenon as is human reproduction? In doing so, are we running the risk of overlooking some key primary causes in the pursuit of symptoms and secondary causes? This has serious implications for the effectiveness of strategies designed to bring about the conditions essential and necessary for assuring safer motherhood for millions of women, particularly in the developing world.

It was during a 6000 km journey through rural Senegal in 1989 to collect data for a study[1] on maternal mortality that the importance of the socio-cultural dimension was clearly illustrated. We were privileged to a wide spectrum of rich experiences. Some were unusual, many were dramatic and most were deeply moving. From this mass of data, impressions and feelings, two critical impressions stand out.

First, a strong connection was established with the women we met. The success of our approach was thus predicated on an ability to explain the purpose of the study, and consequently to gain the active support of the host community through an equal partnership. One outcome was our strong sense of moral obligation to improve the fate of these women, and to help them avoid the tragedy of maternal mortality, a risk they face during each and every pregnancy.

The second observation is that, while the team felt that the findings of the study had made some significant contribution to the understanding of factors affecting maternal mortality through a systematic investigation of factors contributing to maternal death in both the health system and the community; including the modelling of demand and supply for obstetric services; the development of an index of obstetric risks; the correlation between risk and knowledge; the distance from a health centre, etc., our Report could only capture a small fraction of the reality that we had experienced.

Beneath the reality open to study with the tools and methodologies generally used to analyze the phenomenon of maternal mortality lie other crucial determinants. Understanding these could be essential if one is ever to develop effective strategies which reduce rates of maternal mortality in West Africa.

Let us explore the nature and consequences of these determinants and their implications for the development of effective strategies for substantially reducing maternal mortality.

These determinants are best summarized by the expression: *"a tora mousso kele la"*, which in Bambara is an expression used for the loss of life of a woman in childbirth. The equivalent is: *"she fell on the battlefield in the line of duty"*.

The internal logic and corresponding concepts embodied in this expression are an integral part of a larger reality, namely a system of societal beliefs developed through the ages to manage a major event: the procreation process. As with any such system, society also develops a related set of practices, customs, and normatively sanctioned behaviours within its accepted values which become elements of its culture.

From the onset and throughout the field trip we were to discover the importance of the socio-cultural dimension.

The initial indication came from our first community

interview. To compensate for the small size of our sample and improve the reliability of our results, we chose to collect the data from three independent sources. For data on maternal deaths we used the local government official census documents, the health services statistics, and the community official records, and then carried out our indepth interview of community leaders. We then checked for inconsistencies and discrepancies.

We soon discovered that for the collective memory of the community[2] that maternal death was a "non event". We could not get data from a direct question such as, How many maternal deaths occurred during a given time period? We had to devise a four-step approach. We started with the total number of deaths for the period. From this total we got the number of deaths to women. Then from the latter the number of deaths within the age bracket 15 to 45. Finally we correlated this number to known pregnancies and births.

Many significant determinants of maternal mortality can be attributed to a large extent to the "logical" implications of the Bambara expression.

Let us examine some of these implications and their consequences for maternal mortality. Finally we can see how these elements will affect the choices for an effective set of strategies for the development of programmes for safer motherhood.

The implicit assumptions underlying the Session are:

(1) Childbirth is assimilated to a battle.

(2) Any battle, in essence, has inherent and unavoidable associated risks. Among the risks are casualties and deaths.

(3) It is the duty, not to say destiny, of women to have to go through this battle in order to achieve the ideal family size required by the norms of society.

(4) As a "warrior", the pregnant woman is valued for her bravery, expressed in terms of stoicism.

(5) In preparation for the battle, the major emphasis is centered around psychological coping strategies for achieving the stoic stance.

(6) Society, for its part, develops strategies to transcend the adversity of an eventual casualty; in this instance, maternal death.

(7) The phenomena of both is beyond our power to understand: being supernatural.

(8) It is also beyond our abilities to defend ourselves against this phenomenon through ordinary measures.

(9) Thus traditional interventions will be on the plane of metaphysics.

In most of West Africa many key issues related to the ways devised by society to manage the phenomenon of reproduction have serious impact on a number of determinants of maternal mortality. A fuller understanding of the problem would thus require consideration of the socio-cultural context. From this perspective, a key cultural parameter is the importance given to the continuation of lineage. It is deeply rooted in the world view of the society and shapes its value system.

> **Using a battle as a metaphor for childbirth emphasizes the recognition by society of the high level of risk associated with giving birth. The women are called upon to fight this risky battle as a matter of DUTY. The fate of women is thus subordinated to the realization of the requirements for the continuation of the lineage.**

The first requirement for the continuation of the lineage is the value placed on childbearing. In the scale of social values childbearing is elevated to a virtue which confers high social status. On the other hand, a stigma is attached to a childless woman who is often regarded as tainted with sin and, at worst, with evil. In parts of West Africa, where funeral rites play an important function in social relations, the ultimate punishment is reserved for barren women and for those losing their life in childbirth They are denied normal funeral rites and are buried secretly at night outside the village. It is a case of the society reserving it harshest punishment for its innocent victim.

By focussing on fertility to satisfy the continuity of the lineage, women are under strong pressures to bear children. Most studies have shown that it is only after 6 to 8 surviving offspring that a substantial majority of African women wish to stop childbearing. But under prevailing conditions of high infant mortality, to insure the probability of survival of the desired optimum family size condemns women to repeated and frequent pregnancies. In part, this may explain the high fertility rates still observed in most of Africa and the associated high maternal mortality.

I was recently alerted to the strength of the value attached to childbearing even in a non-traditional urban environment. A well traveled and western educated professor of social sciences at an institution of higher learning, out of sympathy for the "desperate" situation of her sister who has been unable to bear children, decided to get pregnant for her sister. This is viewed as a proof of deep love. Her sister will raise the child as her own.

The consequences of numerous and frequent pregnancies in order to attain a socially determined ideal family size expose African women to a higher lifetime risk of maternal death (1 in 21) compared with women in northern Europe (1 in 9.850).

The responsibility for the fulfillment of the requirements for the continuation of the lineage is vested in the clan. This exclusive social organization is characterized by a strong interrelationship of mutual support and obligations binding the members together. It is governed by the principle of subordination of individual interests to those of the group. The notion of duty is toward the group: the extended family. The role of women in the reproduction process is subordinated to the requirement of maintaining the "viability" of the extended family. She is a passive actor called upon to fulfill with "dignity" and "modesty" her ascribed duties.

I have often been baffled by the extravagance of naming ceremonies in West Africa. Even in periods of deep economic crisis, these are grandiose festive events requiring lavish expenditure way beyond what the majority of the population could afford. In this always well-attended event, the mother of the newborn is conspicuously anonymous in the group of women. What is being celebrated is not even the newborn but first and foremost the lineage and, secondly, its strengthening through the name given. This is amplified by the *"griot"*[8] in his litany on the pedigree of the extended family. This glorification calls for lavish rewards to the benefit of the griots.

While preparing this paper, I had a discussion with a medical doctor friend. She related a recent incident and how hurt and angry it made her. While recuperating from a cesarian section in a private clinic, the aunts of her new-born burst into her room. She was barely greeted and all the attention was focussed on the baby. They had come to take the baby for the naming ceremony. She was left by herself to endure both physical and emotional pain. *"She was only doing her duty"!*

One consequence of this subordination of the individual to the "greater good" of the group, the extended family, is that the major decisions during the reproduction process which affect the whole life of women are outside their control. Society is depriving them of the authority for autonomous decision making in this vital event in their lives. They are *powerless* in making the decisions that shape their fate. During our field trip we came across over and over again cases requiring an urgent medical evacuation to a nearby health center being unduly delayed or not acted upon because the husband, whose consent for such a decision was required, was either working in the field or absent.

While this could be expected in a traditional social setting, women do not fare better in the modern health delivery system. Here they are subjected to mutually reinforcing sets of unfavour able circumstances. While the health providers have acquired the medical skills based on scientific knowledge, their behaviour is shaped by the prevailing traditional social values that they have retained. They operate in a health structure model inherited from the former colonial power in which the decision making process is the exclusive, unchallenged privilege and prerogative of health providers. It should be remembered that the bulk of expatriate medical personnel was then made up of military health providers. Finally the maze of bureaucratic hurdles with unpredictable rules changing according to the mood, personality or personal interest of each agent can severely limit the access of health services in emergencies for those without connections or wealth.

It has been estimated in a major urban center that in the great majority of the SMI (MCH centers) it took only six minutes for most of the midwives to conduct a normal prenatal consultation with a predominance of one-way communication[1]. It is also not uncommon to see visiting teams being taken through the delivery room while a woman is in labour without ever seeking her prior permission or consent.

The study project offices were located in a major urban SMI. I once witnessed the heroic efforts of a caring resident doctor to secure admission for an emergency case patient into the hospital. The patient had been shuttling back and forth between health facilities. Finally, as a last resort, the supervisor advised the doctor to deposit the patient at the entrance of the hospital and hope for a miracle, so that she could at least attend to her heavy case load at the SMI.

In order to fulfill their ascribed "duty" to the extended family, the whole life cycle of women is affected. From childhood she will be prepared to play her roles of wife and mother. At a very tender age she will be initiated to demanding domestic work while her brothers are spending most of their time playing children's games. In any compound it is common to see little girls helping their mothers while the little boys are roaming free of responsibilities. In most cases she will be eating with the women. A well-bred wife is expected to reserve the best portions for her husband. The little girl will share the meals with the women and most probably receive less in terms of nutrition than her brothers. Because her destiny is first and foremost to be a good wife and mother, she will have less chance for formal education or training than boys. In our study, only 7 per cent of the women could read. Because of the very strong social stigma attached to the status of unmarried women, the family is under strong pressure to marry her to the first convenient party. In most cases, this will be at an age when her body is not yet ready for childbearing. In our study, 7 women out of 10 had their first birth before they reached 17 year . Because of the dishonour on the family name attached to pregnancies outside marriage, unwanted pregnancies are kept secret and preferably terminated through clandestine abortion under less than optimal sanitary conditions — a major cause of maternal deaths.

The preparation of young women for safe motherhood is totally inadequate. In terms of acquisition of a useful knowledge base, this is most often limited to reassurances about the menstrual process along with advice on personal hygiene. Pregnancy, delivery and care of the newborn is seldom explored in detail. If it is, it will be in the form of metaphors requiring guesses at the true meaning. Further, the code of behaviour set up by society does not allow for frank discussion between a mother and daughter on reproductive matters. Even if this was possible, its usefulness would be limited because the society does not seem to have accumulated a practical knowledge base to systematically pass on from one generation to the next. The information transmitted takes the form of "stories" among peers or parables from the older generation which are very difficult to decipher for a young woman with little life experience.

In our study we attempted to determine the knowledge base of our target population on indications of a normal pregnancy, complications during pregnancy and delivery. On the scale of the knowledge index we developed, 58 per cent scored low, 36 per cent average and only 7 per cent high. We did find a correlation between a higher score and having experienced the event themselves and also being at a greater distance from a health center. When presented with facts indicating a probability of a severe hemorrhage some of the women we interviewed indicated that they believed this to be a good sign because the body was eliminating the bad blood to be replaced by new blood.

Contrary to the inadequacy of preparing young women for safer motherhood in terms of useful factual information, the psychological preparation receives a major emphasis. The desired outcome is to increase the threshold of tolerance to physical pain. This is to be demonstrated through stoic behaviour. A common example is the advice given to young women to be prepared to endure a level of effort equal to that which would be required to produce water by pressing hard enough on a stone. The pains of delivery are endured in expectation of harder moments to come. One is surprised and relieved after delivery not to have gone through the dreaded anticipated level of pain. The desirable heroic stance is usually rewarded by lavish praise for the demonstrated courage and admiring compliments from the women attending the new mother and also from the family members and the community. A less than "heroic" behaviour is the subject of verbal abuse and scorn. At this point a paradox is worth exploring. The midwives in maternity wards are notorious for their ill treatment of their patients. One would have expected a more supportive behaviour because of their training, the ethics of the medical profession and the fact that they also are mothers. On close examination one can see that their behaviour is quite similar to that of the traditional birth attendants when confronted with similar situations. Their behaviour is culturally determined and is guided by the norms requiring the mother to maintain a stoic stance. Because of this stoicism, vital life threatening signals that require urgent and immediate action are suppressed and not communicated until too late, leading to tragic loss of life.

In place of a body of practical knowledge capable of insuring safer motherhood, traditional society has developed a supernatural set of explanations for the phenomenon of reproduction. This has led to the attitude that the phenomenon is beyond the power of rational understanding. This being so, there are no concrete steps that can be taken to modify a predetermined outcome. The interventions to secure a favourable outcome will be in the realm of metaphysics and call for traditional para-psychological therapy.

The consequence of these attitudes is a large number of non-assisted births. Our findings indicate that only 2 out of 5 women received assistance from a qualified birth attendant during delivery. It is worth noting that traditional birth attendants usually intervene only during the last phase of delivery — the expulsion. Further if they intervene in case of complications, they are more likely to increase the risk to the life of the mother and baby by ill-timed, unsafe and intrusive interventions to speed up the process.

Society has developed coping strategies of *"denial"* for dealing with maternal mortality which is treated as a "non-event" in the collective memory of the community. This attitude of *"denial"* is also found among health providers at all levels of the health services. As pointed out by Pr Fadel Diadhiou of the Dantec Teaching Hospital, maternal death is too often viewed as "daily occurrence dramatically common".[5] He has been working with great dedication to bring about a change in this prevailing attitude. He keeps emphasizing to his students and staff that each maternal death should be regarded as a dramatic event which should mobilize the conscience of each health provider so as to make it an event as rare as possible.

Those who are advocating caution on the ground of sensitivity or respect for the integrity of the host culture have to weigh this against the fact that any delay in ACTING NOW is to condone the avoidable cruel and unjust death of millions of innocent women (one death every minute).

A closer examination will show that methodological considerations are not a real obstacle to the inclusion of socio-cultural variable in our study of maternal mortality.

These quantitative methodologies do not necessarily always lead to effective policies and programmes and qualitative methods can yield valuable results in terms of effective strategies. While quantitative methods demonstrate possible relationships between dependent and independent variables, as well as the strength or significance of the relationship, qualitative methods allow a more general understanding of the phenomena under investigation by analyzing it within the sub-system of which it constitutes an element. This requires first an understanding of the internal logic of the sub-system along with its relation to the larger system. Only then can the logical sequencing of the chain of causality be established. From this chain the key variables can be identified along with their relative significance in explaining phenomena. In our case study, we focussed on the dominance of the centrality of the continuity of the lineage in the socio-cultural value system as a key element in understanding maternal mortality.

The results of our analysis of the system can be used for programme development. Identification of key parameters permits the design of effective strategies so as to affect events along the chain of causality in order to achieve desired outcomes. Programme effectiveness will be enhanced by testing the consistency of a selected strategy with the internal logic of the system.

For example, in the case of socio-cultural values affecting some important determinants of maternal mortality in West Africa, we can for the purpose of programme design consider two enabling factors. These are the moral duties of children toward their mother, and the web of mutual obligations required from the members of the extended family.

While society in West Africa confers status to women bearing children, this translates into worship of mothers by their children. As a rule of thumb, insulting a peer could lead to a quarrel; if it is someone's father, this could escalate to a serious conflict. Insulting someone' s mother, he will have to fight if he is a man of honour, even if he is sure of loosing the battle. The implied moral foundation of mother worship is the debt of gratitude owed to the one who has given us the gift of life. Mother worship is an important element of the values system. Since society requires a fight to preserve the honour of one' s mother, to be consistent it cannot require less to preserve her life particularly when she is giving the gift of life. Therefore, society will have to promote safer motherhood. This, in turn, implies the need to remove the *"denial"* surrounding the tragedy of maternal mortality. This will necessitate that society finally come to terms with this tragedy and give it the too long overdue priority it deserves. Only then can we have genuine community mobilization of conscience, will and resources to address the problem.

This would be a major area of strategy design for programme development. Some immediate outcomes of this social mobilisation would be a substantial reduction in the workload presently required from pregnant women, the removal of food taboos for better nutrition and reallocation of financial resources from name giving ceremonies to pre-natal and natal care. An example is the practice on the island of Goree for friends and family to contribute for every pregnant woman toward acquiring a layette. The island is linked with the mainland by a ferry boat only during the day. The maternity is lacking the bare essentials, as is often the case. The layette is meant to solve these problems; it will usually have the minimum required supplies for safe delivery and post natal care for the newborn. As far as accessibility is concerned, the great majority of the rural population in West Africa lives on "islands".

The web of mutual obligations characteristic of extended family translates in the area of health into a system of continuous support through physical presence of relatives and friends. In sharp contrast to the western need for privacy in such circumstances, in West Africa this would be perceived as a form of punishment through isolation and exclusion from the group. With some exceptions, the layout of health services has not yet come to terms with the reality that the family will move in with the patient.

Curiously, a notable exception to providing this network of support through physical presence is with birthing. Tragically it is when the woman is most in need of physical, material and emotional support that she is left by herself to cope with the challenges of childbearing. This is even more tragic with the case of a large number of inexperienced young women with their first child.

A second major area of strategy design for prograrnme development could be the extension of this support system to childbearing. Again, society, to be consistent with the value accorded to childbearing cannot deny the necessary support required to achieve the desired outcome. To this end, two basic premises in the belief system which hold that—the phenomenon of childbearing is beyond our understanding and, secondly, that it is beyond our power to modify the course of events, have to be shown to be no longer valid. The realization by society of the possibilities for ACTION which would enhance favourable outcomes will give the necessary purpose to extending the support system to childbearing and safer motherhood.

This new knowledge and understanding of the attitudes of the community could impact now on several determinants of maternal mortality. Thus, identifying the web of the family support system could promote a more systematic follow-up of each pregnancy and an earlier identification of problems. It provides a mechanism for more rapid decision making in case of emergencies, even in the absence of the husband. Most importantly, it could drastically reduce the number of unattended deliveries. Finally, the positive psychological impact on pregnant women cannot be underestimated.

A major element for the success of the extended support system would be the role to be played by traditional birth attendants since they are already an integral part of the community. The experience of Professor Fall in Khombole, Senegal has shown that trained and supervised birth attendants over a period of years have achieved significantly better results in reducing maternal mortality than midwives in the formal health service. This opens up the possibility of solving the problems resulting from unattended deliveries in a very short time period. The role of traditional birth attendants in this strategy should not be one of an inexpensive substitute for para-medical personnel but should be that of an active agent of social change within their community.

One important result of the Nairobi and Niamey conferences is the Safe Motherhood Initiative. Since then, there has been an increase in interest for the problem of maternal mortality. More research has been undertaken. Some countries have initiated programme development activities. A broad approach was recommended in recognition of the fact that a combination of factors: medical, socio-economic and cultural, affect maternal mortality.

So far, most of the studies and corresponding programmes have put most of the emphasis on strategies based on medical solutions. This bias can partly be explained by the choice of variables. These studies are centered around intermediate and proximate factors affecting maternal mortality but underlying factors such as socio-cultural parameters have been notably neglected. This approach has serious shortcomings and inevitably limits the effectiveness of the corresponding public policy strategies. Analyzing only some elements of a phenomenon in isolation can lead to erroneous conclusions when used as a basis for decisions affecting the whole system.

An illustration is the study by Harrison in Northern Nigeria[6] on the effect of the health care and intensive nutrition programme for pregnant women in relation to operative delivery due to fetopelvic disproportion. He concluded that, for a generation or more, for small women (150cm or less) there will be a rise of the-operative delivery rate for fetopelvic-disproportion due to gain in weight of the foetus. The absence of a programme to treat the increase in obstetric complications could lead to an increase in maternal mortality.

For programme development does this mean that health care and intensive nutrition only benefit the foetus? Unless there are adequate health services capable of treating the obstetric complications, should the nutrition programme be abandoned for small women?

Another shortcoming of an exclusively medical solution is

an implicit assumption that an effective demand exists and that the problem is primarily from the supply side. This is often not verified by the field realities. In our study, the analysis of demand and supply for obstetric services gave the following results: 83 per cent felt the need for the services, 79 per cent wanted them but only 39 per cent actually sought the services.

We visited 43 health facilities, including a newly built regional hospital. None could compare in cleanliness and comfort for the patient to a community built health post run by a dynamic group of women' s organizations but we were surprised to find out that it was seldom used. The reason was that the door was in full view of a regular meeting place for men. This lack of privacy discouraged many women from using the facility. After a meeting of community leaders, it was decided to move the meeting place.

This is not to imply that the medical solution is not essential to the solution of the problem of maternal mortality. It is a necessary but not sufficient condition. Medical and non-medical solutions are not mutually exclusive; in fact, they are complementary and allow synergy among activities. Without strategies dealing with the socio-cultural constraints and involving the active partnership of the community, health services even if they are appropriate and adequate, which is often not the case, will continue to be overwhelmed by the scope and complexities of the problem. For any programme to be effective, there is need for an optimum mix of strategies taking into consideration all the major factors in the chain of causal events that affect maternal mortality.

In the West African context, the problem of maternal mortality is deeply rooted in the socio-cultural value system of society. Since along the path all the factors that contribute to maternal health are interrelated, a viable programme has to take these into consideration for strategies to be effective. It is therefore essential not to omit the root causes. As one moves down the path, opportunities for effective interventions are missed while the probabilities of unfavourable outcomes increase. Unfortunately, this is too often the case with a great number of women reaching the health facilities too late to be saved, as is shown by higher maternal mortality ratios from most hospital service statistics.

"A tora mousso kele la"! If society is going to send the women to battle, then it must remove the mines from the battlefield. The necessary knowledge about the nature of the mines, their location and how to remove them is now available. It must also provide full support: material, physical and emotional. Finally, it should honour those who have been willing to give the precious gift of life sometimes at the risk of their own. It is a moral obligation for society to minimize casualties on the 'battlefield' of motherhood. One fundamental human right is the right to life. Safe motherhood is a

fundamental human right. There is no democracy without fundamental human rights being respected. The new hope for democratization in Africa will never be fulfilled as long as half of the population is denied a fundamental right: *safe motherhood.*

AND THE TIME FOR ACTION IS NOW!

NOTES

1. DIA, A., et a.l., "Rapport de la Deuxieme Mission D'Identification Pour la Reduction de la Mortalite Maternelle au Senegal".
2. The collective memory of the community is significant, particularly in societies with oral traditions. It constitutes a driving force of most social events.
3. Griot: Caste of traditional musician-entertainers of West Africa. They have an uncommon mastery of the spoken word. They are the depository of the history and traditions of the clan as well as the genealogies of important extended families.
4. Aissatou Lo, "Impact of Surveillance of High Risk Pregnant Women in Urban Areas".
5. Dia. A. et al. op. cit.
6. Harrison, K.A. "Predicting Trends in Operative Delivery for Cephalopelvic Disproportion in Africa". Lancet, April 7, 1990.

23

Behaviour Change: Some Analogies and Lessons from the Experience of Gay Communities

Adam Carr
Journalist and
HIV Consultant, Australia

1. The Gay Community and Behaviour Change

The HIV epidemic first made itself known to the world when it appeared among gay men* in the United States in 1979 and 1980: the first published account of the disease, in July 1981, described cases seen among gay men in Los Angeles, over the following three years AIDS appeared in the gay communities of all the developed countries. Although as early as 1982 cases of AIDS were seen in people other than gay men (male and female injecting drug users, recipients of HIV-contaminated blood products, heterosexual men and women including female sex workers and infants born to HIV-infected women), the great majority of diagnosed AIDS cases in most of the developed countries during the 1980s were seen in gay men.

The appearance of the HIV epidemic had an enormous impact on the gay communities** of the developed countries, and

* *The term "gay men" is used here to mean all men who have sex with other men, regardless of whether they identify as homosexual, bisexual or heterosexual.*

** *The term "gay community" referred originally to the community of gay men and lesbians. Lesbians increasingly do not accept that they share a community with gay men, and the term "gay and lesbian communities" has been adopted. Accordingly, I use the term "gay community" here to refer to the community of gay men.*

organisations to respond to the epidemic were formed in most countries by 1985. One of their most urgent tasks was to advise gay men how they could avoid contracting the disease. Before the discovery of HIV as the cause of the disease in 1983/84, the reason gay men were developing AIDS was unclear. It was therefore very difficult for gay men to protect themselves from it. Since, however, it was evident that HIV was sexually transmitted, gay community organisations (and government health authorities) recommended to gay men that they reduce the number of sexual partners they had. Many gay men followed this advice, some to the extent of ceasing to have sex at all.

In retrospect, though, it is evident that this advice was ineffective. Reducing the number of sexual partners does not significantly reduce the risk of contracting HIV infection in a population where infection is already widespread. It just slows the process down somewhat. In any case, men are extremely reluctant to accept advice even at the risk of their own lives. In this respect, at least, gay men are no different from man in general.

The discovery of HIV and the subsequent determination of the exact mechanisms of HIV transmission during sex between men enabled gay community organisations to make more specific recommendations to gay men. It became clear that unprotected anal intercourse was responsible for virtually all HIV transmission among gay men, and the correct and consistent use of condoms and water-based lubricant during anal sex would reduce the risk of HIV infection for gay men to close to zero.

These discoveries made it possible for gay community organisations to make recommendations to gay men which were both effective in preventing HIV infection and capable of being adopted in a sustained way by the majority of gay men. Few men enjoy using condoms, but the use of condoms for anal intercourse was a compromise between fear of HIV infection and fear of giving up sexual gratification which most gay men were prepared to accept and able to implement. While compliance with even this fairly minimal modification of sexual behaviour has been far from universal, it has been sufficiently widespread to reduce greatly the incidence of HIV infection among gay men in most developed countries.

I have referred to gay community organizations making "recommendations" to gay men about changes in sexual behaviour. In fact, of course, the process of bringing about behaviour change among most gay men was vastly more complicated than simply issuing recommendations. The populations of gay men in the developed countries are very diverse, and include a significant group of "submerged gay men (few of whom actually identify as gay) who are not in contact with the organised gay community. The gay communities are divided along lines of race, ethnicity, age, place of residence, educational level and social/economic status. Patterns of sexual behaviour among gay men differ considerably along these lines, and are further complicated by issues such as injecting drug use, use of alcohol and other recreational drugs, the sale of sex for money, trans-sexualism and other behavioural influences.

These considerations made the task of bringing about sustained and appropriate behaviour change among gay men an extremely complex one, and a task made more difficult three further factors: the great urgency imposed by the rapidly expanding number of gay men acquiring HIV infection, the lack of previous research into the sexual behaviour patterns of gay men, and the lack of models of successful campaigns to bring about rapid and widespread changes in personal behaviours. When gay community organizations undertook in the early 1980s the task of bringing about rapid, radical and sustained changes in the sexual behaviours of a large and diverse population of sexually-active men, they undertook to do something which had never been done before, in a very short period of time, and bereft of the usual resources, research data and analytical tools which usually accompany such major campaigns of social engineering.

2. Factors Influencing Behaviour Change Among Gay Men

By the late 1980s, however, these deficiencies had to some extent been addressed. A number ot major research projects had been carried out among gay men to find out more about their patterns of sexual behaviour, to monitor the speed and extent of behaviour change, and to determine the social and cultural factors which facilitated or impeded the process of behaviour change. One of the most far-reaching of these projects has been carried out in Australia. This is the Social Aspects of Prevention of AIDS (SAPA) project, a joint undertaking of the AIDS Council of NSW (a gay community non-government organization) and the School of Behavioural Sciences of Macquarie University, Sydney.

In 1986 and 1987, SAPA researchers conducted extensive interviews with 535 Australian gay men, and have been analyzing the results since, issuing their findings in regular instalments since 1988. Report No. 7, The Importance of Gay Community in the Prevention of HIV Transmission, appeared in April 1990. The report consists mainly of a statistical analysis of the relationship between the interviewees' attachment to the gay community (measured by several criteria) and the degree, appropriateness and speed of the changes in their sexual practices in response to the HIV epidemic.

The report's conclusion is worth quoting at length.

"In general, gay community attachment and locale are important predictors of change. These data speak to the importance of informed social support. It appears that educators who stress the need to address communities from the point of view of the communities themselves are correct. Gay community and locale are also implicated in the relationship between knowledge and change. Knowledge of "safe sex", something that to some extent only the gay communities dealt with in their media and educational campaigns, is also implicated in change.

This study does point to the importance of gay community attachment to sexual behaviour change ... sexually-confident, well-educated (about safe sex) gay men ... who are sexually and socially engaged with gay community ... are more likely to have changed their sexual behaviour than gay men who are not attached to gay community.

It is evident that education campaigns should continue to be informed by gay communities and that the men who perhaps are most at risk are those who are not reached by gay community campaigns. Men who for whatever reason are separate from any form of attachment to gay community need special attention.

In general, men who have contact with others, via attachment to gay community, sexual, social or cultural/political, are most likely to have changed their sexual practice. They have the informed social support necessary to modify their behaviour. Men who are isolated from others like themselves and (who) are unattached to gay community in any form are those least likely to change."

The SAPA research demonstrates that the most important component of preventing HIV infection among gay men is their willingness to identify themselves as gay, and to become "sexually-confident, well-educated gay men, who are sexually and socially engaged with community". Other Australian research has supported this view. Sinnott and Todd (1988) found that the most important source of accurate information about HIV transmission and prevention available to men who have sex with men is the material produced by gay community organizations and distributed within the gay community. Bennett et al. (1989) found that men who find male sexual partners in public places such as parks ("beats"), and who have a low rate of self-identification as gay and a low level of contact with the gay community, also have a much higher rate of unsafe sexual practice and therefore a higher risk of HIV infection.

The conclusion of this research seems clear. Men who identify as gay, who are confident in that identification, who are socially, culturally or politically active in the gay community and who find their sexual partners in the gay community, are much more likely to have accurate knowledge about HIV infection, than are men who have sex with men who are not attached to the gay community. They are also much more likely to act on that knowledge by making appropriate and sustained changes to their sexual practice.

It is therefore clear that bringing about appropriate and sustained behaviour change among gay men has not just been a matter of producing information about HIV and safe sex and distributing it to individuals. Behaviour change among gay men has resulted from a community wide response to the epidemic, which has sought to use the existing communication networks and value systems of the gay community to influence the collective behaviour of that community. New community values about acceptable and unacceptable sexual behaviours have been established, and have been enforced by community opinion, a far more effective way of enforcing standards of behaviour than coercion by the state.

The experience of the gay communities in the developed countries is not uniform. The Australian gay community, on which the SAPA research is based, has had certain advantages not enjoyed by some other communities: a high degree of racial and linguistic uniformity, concentration in a small number of cities, government funding, a supportive social and political environment to carry out prevention work, and access to a cadre of skilled community activists to design and carry out both the programmes and the research which has guided them. But in broad terms the experience of the Australian gay community has echoed those of the other developed countries. Rapid and massive behaviour change can be brought about through community-based programmes.

Since 1985 or so a number of studies have been undertaken, in the United States, Australia and other developed countries, to determine the reasons why some gay men have adapted to the demands of behaviour change in response to HIV and AIDS more readily than others.

The SAPA studies have cast some light on this subject, as have American studies such as the Multi-Centre AIDS Cohort Study (MACS), which has followed thousands of gay men over several years to monitor their behaviour and the factors influencing it.

The findings of these studies and others like them, taken together, show that a number of identifiable groups of men are at continuing risk of HIV infection. These are:

- # men under 25
- # men with low educational and literacy levels
- # men from non-English-speaking backgrounds

men who use alcohol and recreational drugs while having sex
men who do not identify as gay or as part of the gay community (this factor has already been discussed above.

An additional, perhaps more surprising, finding was that gay men in relationships were more likely to be at risk of infection than were men who were not in relationships.

These groupings reveal distinct social co-factors for HIV infection among gay men.

Age is clearly one of the most important of these factors, because it relates to several of the others. Many younger people are likely to use alcohol and "soft" drugs while having sex. Many young gay men have low incomes. Young people of all sexual orientations are prone to the opinion that nothing bad can happen to them, and this is aggravated in the case of HIV risk by the fact that, because of the eight to ten year incubation period of HIV, few gay men under 25 have many friends with diagnosed AIDS. Young men are also less likely to have formed firm sexual self-identifications or to have developed strong gay community links, which are important in building a sense of the immediacy of the HIV threat and of responsibility for one's own and one's partner's health.

The issue of the relationship between social and economic status, of which educational levels and literacy skills are generally assumed to be indicators, and sexual behaviour among gay men is a complex and controversial one, and has been bedeviled by a politically-motivated preoccupation with identifying (or creating) a category of "working-class gay men". Gay men have a peculiar occupational structure, heavily weighted to white collar and service occupations, with many transient, part-time and shift workers. This blurs traditional distinctions of class. In addition, many young gay men from working-class backgrounds find that the gay community offers contacts and opportunities, and a ladder to higher-status occupations and incomes.

Nevertheless, many gay men still have limited educational levels and poor literacy skills, partly because of the alienation that many gay men feel from their peers during the period of accepting a gay identity, which coincides for many with the years of higher secondary education. Low literacy cuts many gay men off from the gay print media and print-based HIV educational campaigns waged by gay community organisations, which, as Sinnott and Todd showed, have been the most important sources of information about HIV and AIDS and about sate sex. and are also an important source of positive reinforcement for gay identity and community involvement.

In Australia, which does not have the deep racial divide which characterises the United States, issues of ethnicity and linguistic background are still important factors influencing the ability of gay men to adopt and sustain behaviour change. Most developed countries now have large populations of first or second-generation immigrants, many of them from developing countries, and many of them maintaining cultural and religious traditions which mark them off from the culture of the host country.

Gay men in these ethnic communities, who often do not identify as gay, suffer a double crisis of identity, in that they are violating their communities' accepted standards of behaviour by being gay, while being isolated from the host countries' gay community by cultural or linguistic barriers. This cuts many men off from the behaviour change messages which the gay community organisations are producing, usually in English and usually using an imagery and a vocabulary derived from the majority culture.

Alcohol and other recreational drugs have been identified as among the major villains of the HIV epidemic in the gay communities. Alcohol, it is said, lowers self-control, heightens self-delusion and makes previous decisions about safe sex harder to stick to. The fact that so many gay men find their sexual partners in places where alcohol is served make this a chronic problem. Many health educators, however, argue that the belief that alcohol makes men incapable of controlling their sexual behaviour is a myth, and a myth which serves the interests of men in many contexts. They argue that men use alcohol as an excuse to engage in sexual (and other) behaviours which they know to be socially unacceptable.

It may seem contradictory to say that gay men in relationships are at higher risk than gay men who have multiple sexual partners. There are two factors operating here. The first is that most highly sexually-active gay men have been acutely aware that they at high risk for a long time. They were the first to be targeted, and many long ago adapted to the discipline of safe sex. The sex-centered, antiromantic "culture of promiscuity" that exists around the saunas and sex clubs has served as an effective agent of behaviour change for many of these men. On the other hand, many gay men who think of themselves as relationship-centered and "not promiscuous" have been slow to perceive their own risk.

3. Lessons of the Gay Communities' Experience with Behaviour Change

It may seem a heroic leap to try to use the experiences of gay men in affluent societies to find lessons for reducing the impact of the HIV epidemic among the majority of people at risk of HIV infection in the world: men, women and children in the developing countries. But it is not an impossible task. Despite the enormous differences in circumstances and contexts, there are some underlying similarities in the experiences of the two populations which can be usefully studied.

This is particularly so when we remember that it is the sexual behaviour of men which is the fundamental behavioural problem in preventing the further spread of HIV infection in most parts of the world. The HIV epidemic in the developing countries is increasingly being understood to be a consequence of the sexual and social subordination of women in those countries. This is evidenced by a pattern of infection in which men are the vectors of infection and women the principal subjects of infection: married men who have multiple sexual partners are infecting their wives, who are prevented by economic and social restraints from protecting themselves from infection.

There are those who may feel that it is impossible to induce men to forgo sexual gratification and adopt socially responsible behaviours. The experience of behaviour change in the gay communities suggests that this is not so. The gay communities are, after all, communities of men. The gay communities offer a unique opportunity to study the sexual behaviour of men.

That the behaviour change campaigns mounted by gay community organisations have succeeded to the extent that they have in bringing about rapid and sustained change in the sexual behaviours of gay men, without resort to any kind of coercive mechanism, offers hope that changing the sexual behaviours of heterosexual men is not beyond the scope of human ingenuity.

It is difficult to judge how far the social and behavioural risk factors which have been identified as making some gay men more likely than others to engage in behaviours likely to expose them to HIV infection are applicable to other risk populations, and particularly to people in developing countries. Clearly HIV infection in heterosexual populations raises issues around gender and power imbalances between men and women which do not arise in the gay communities. It seems clear, too, that the sale of sex plays a greater role in the proliferation of HIV infection in these countries than it does in the gay communities. Nevertheless, it may be possible to draw some analogies from the research about the risk factors which have been identified among gay men.

Among the more likely candidates for social risk factors among heterosexual populations in developing countries are drug and alcohol use and relationship status. Men in all cultures use alcohol and recreational drugs of various kinds as social disinhibitors, and drinking or drug use frequently accompanies sexual activity. The extent to which alcohol abuse by heterosexual men contributes to the subsequent HIV infection of women, both sex workers and wives, is something which can be determined only by research on the spot, but it seems a fair bet, on the analogy of the experience of the gay communities, that a link will be found. If it is, it is important to remember research in the gay communities: that the link between alcohol use and unsafe sexual behaviour is not that alcohol deprives men of the ability to control their sexual behaviour, but that it gives them an excuse to behave in ways which they know would be otherwise unacceptable. The exposure of that excuse goes a long way to ending the ability of men to use alcohol in this way. Gay community HIV organisations have run campaigns stating this explicitly, such as the "Drugs and Alcohol: No Excuse" campaign of the Victorian AIDS Council.

The analogies between the transmission of HIV within gay male relationships and its transmission within marriage in developing countries is harder to develop, because of the obvious fact that a gay relationship is a voluntary and informal (in a legal sense) relationship between two men, and any power dimensions that exist within it have been largely invented by the participants, whereas a marriage is a relationship between a man and woman, contracted in law and carrying with it the legacy of centuries of accumulated tradition and assumption about gender power distribution. A marriage is usually an economic relationship as well, involving the economic dependence of the woman. Nevertheless, it may be pointed out that the belief among many gay men that participation in a monogamous relationship somehow confers immunity from HIV infection may have some parallels in heterosexual relationships. It has been pointed out that, biologically, HIV in women is a disease of fidelity, not of promiscuity, since most women who contract HIV infection sexually do so from repeated exposure to a single infected man, usually their husband, rather than from single exposures to many infected men. Behaviour change campaigns which seek to promote monogamous relationships and marital fidelity will therefore be singularly inappropriate in places where a high proportion of married men are already infected.

There are a number of lessons which may be drawn from the experiences of the gay communities in designing HIV behaviour change and prevention programmes in societies which may appear to have very little in common with those of the developed countries where most gay men live.

Information and Motivation

The first point is that the provision of information is not enough. In the early 1980s both governments and community-based organisations in the developed countries engaged in large-scale mass media and community campaigns to disseminate basic facts about HIV and AIDS and to stimulate community awareness of the disease. Some of these campaigns were restrained and confined to giving information. Others were frankly alarmist, such as the British "tombstones" campaign and the Australian "Grim Reapers" campaign. What they all had in common was their failure to bring about any significant changes in behaviour in their target populations.

Research shows that people do not change deeply-entrenched behaviour, such as sexual practices, simply on the basis of unintellectual awareness that the behaviour may be dangerous to them. A study of gay men in Los Angeles showed that those who were continuing to engage in unsafe sexual practices had exactly the same level of knowledge about HIV and safe sex as those who had adopted and maintained safe practices. The differences between the two groups were those of identity with the gay community, as discussed above. This reinforces the point that behaviour change among gay men in the developed countries has been brought about by community-based campaigns which promoted safe sex practices as a community standard of behaviour.

By contrast, populations at risk of HIV infection which have been subjected only to information-based mass media campaigns have failed to show any significant change in behaviour. An obvious example is sexually-active young heterosexuals, whose risk of HIV infection is substantial but who have failed to respond to media campaigns aimed at influencing their behaviour. There is an obvious and positive lesson here for developing countries: expensive and high profile media campaigns are ineffective in bringing about behaviour change. This is an important point for countries with limited resources and poorly developed mass media structures, and particularly those which do not have linguistic or cultural unity (such as Papua New Guinea, for example) which would find national media campaigns even more difficult.

Individuals and Communities

The second lesson is that behaviour change is not so much a process of individuals absorbing information and making rational decisions about their behaviour. It is much more a process of individuals changing their behaviour as a result of their membership of a community which is changing the standards of behaviour it expects from its members, because they identify with that community and wish to remain members of it.

The best example of this is condom use. Most gay men dislike using condoms, but have accepted that they should do so, not so much from a rational decision to use condoms because this is the best way to avoid HIV infection (although this is probably how the decision would be articulated), but because they are aware that the community of gay men to which they belong, from which they derive a sense of identity and of personal worth, and to which they wish to continue to belong, has now adopted condom use as its standard of behaviour, and condemns those who do not use them. The sanction for failure to use condoms is not so much HIV infection, a long-term and somewhat nebulous threat, especially for younger gay men who do not have personal experience of HIV, but disapproval and possible ostracism by their peers.

It follows from this that campaigns based on mobilising loyalty to and identification with specific communities offers the best hope for influencing the sexual behaviours of heterosexual men. While the gay community is a community of men who share a sexual orientation, and thus has certain unique advantages as a vehicle for influencing the sexual behaviours of its members, there is no reason why any pattern of community identification could not be adapted to the same purpose.

This is in fact precisely what has been attempted with other risk populations in the developed countries, such as female sex workers and injecting drug users. Some rudiments of community organisation and identification already existed among these populations before the advent of the epidemic. HIV organizations have sought to build on these foundations, creating a community infrastructure, and communications network to build a sense of community commitment to safe behaviours and a sense of solidarity in achieving and enforcing behaviour change in the emerging community. While the results of this strategy have been mixed, they have been at least partly successful in some places; notably in Australia, where the incidence of HIV infection among injecting drug users and female sex workers is extremely low by world standards.

Once again, of course, this is a strategy of building or, if necessary, creating communities based on an identity that relates directly to the risk behaviour involved; a community of female sex workers all share the risk behaviour of exchanging sex with men for money, and a community of injecting drug users all share the risk of behaviour of injecting drugs.

Whether it is possible to mobilise the identity of heterosexual men with other kinds of community, for example a religious community, a sporting community or a neighborhood community, to reinforce the need for changes to sexual behaviours is difficult to determine. But it is certainly possible to suggest that the mechanism of community identification and loyalty, and thus the need and desire to retain membership of the community by conforming to the expected pattern of behaviour of that community, still operates regardless of the nature of that community, and this mechanism is the mainspring of bringing about behaviour change through community-based programmes.

Greater and Lesser Evils

The third point is that behaviour change messages must give people realistic and sustainable choices. Few people welcome large-scale changes in their lives, particularly when these changes involve sacrificing behaviours which people find gratifying and which play a large role in forming their identities and sense of worth. When gay men were advised that they should abstain from sexual activity or radically reduce their number of sexual partners, most failed to respond, because these changes were too great to absorb into their lives. When the message was refined, and concentrated on the adoption of condoms for anal sex, there was a high level of acceptance, since this was a change which most gay men could accommodate without radical disruption to their lives.

The debate within gay community HIV organisations about oral sex is an instructive example of this. There have been a small number of documented cases of HIV transmission between gay men following the intake of semen during oral sex. Some gay community organisations feel that oral sex should therefore be included on the list of unsafe sexual practices which gay men should be advised to abstain from. Others have argued, however, that the risk of HIV infection through oral sex is so low, certainly many times lower than the risk of infection through unprotected anal sex, that making a recommendation against it would be counter-productive. Many men, it is argued, would look at a list of "prohibited" practices and conclude that they could not make such radical changes, and would therefore make no changes at all. It is better, in this view, to accept a continuing small risk of infection through oral sex in order to persuade the majority to abandon the really high risk activity, unprotected anal sex.

The analogy for developing countries may be that, since the really radical changes in behaviour needed to completely eliminate HIV infection cannot be achieved in the necessary time, because the intensity of community-based education needed to bring them about is too resource intensive, prevention efforts must focus on changes may be less effective in preventing HIV infection but which have a relatively low level of impact on people's lives and which thus have a greater chance of being adopted quickly.

Thus, in countries in which condoms are neither readily available, cheap nor culturally acceptable, that is, where men will not use them and women cannot compel them to do so, the best option may be to enable women, and particularly sex workers, to improve their level of genital health so that their risk of infection through unprotected vaginal intercourse is reduced to a level comparable to that of women in developed countries, where HIV infection among heterosexual women is spreading much more slowly than it is in developing countries. This strategy will buy time for a more comprehensive strategy, based perhaps on large-scale voluntary testing and partner notification, to be developed and implemented.

Horizontal and Vertical Education

The fourth point is that the source of information and education must always be as close as possible to the people who are the targets of the education campaign. Ideally, the source of the information and education should in fact belong to the population at risk of infection. This was a lesson which the gay communities in the developed countries learned only after some costly errors in the early years of the HIV epidemic. The initial educational campaigns mounted by gay community organisations were heavily media-based: they consisted of print materials such as posters and leaflets, and display advertisements in the gay print media.

As noted earlier, these campaigns were deficient in that they failed to communicate effectively with gay men who did not speak or, more commonly, read the language in which the campaign was being conducted or who lacked the literacy skills to take in the messages being put forward. But they were deficient in a more fundamental sense as well. Even though the source of these materials were gay community organisations, set up by gay activists who lived and worked in the gay community, they were still a form of vertical education: self-appointed experts were addressing messages to their communities through the impersonal medium of print. While these campaigns achieved considerable success, they failed to influence the behaviour of a large number of gay men in a sustained way.

By 1986 gay communities in some countries were evolving a more sophisticated form of HIV educations based on peer education models. While the gay activists and health professionals who worked for gay community organisations were in a sense the peers of the gay men they were seeking to educate, the techniques they were using were the same as those traditionally used by governments and other sources of authority to influence behaviour and guide opinion. Gay men, as a marginalised and in some senses oppressed group, tended to be sceptical of messages seen as deriving from sources of authority: This was particularly true of men who shared the social and behavioural characteristics discussed above which made them less likely to readily adopt appropriate behaviour changes.

The peer education strategies adopted by some gay community organizations were based on a philosophy of empowerment of individuals within the context of developing a stronger gay community. "Ordinary" gay men, that is, gay men who were not already HIV activists and were not professionally qualified were recruited to organise meetings of their friends, at which HIV and safe sex were discussed in the context of their own lives and relationships. In these small group discussions, gay men could discuss freely the difficulties and challenges of adapting to safe sex, could freely admit failures and lapses, and could offer each other support in sustaining behaviour change.

Men who "graduated" from these meetings were in turn recruited to organise more meetings, thus penetrating wider and wider strata of the gay community, and of the population of men who have sex with men but who do not identify as gay. Particular attention was paid to young men, to older men, to men from non-English-speaking backgrounds, to bisexual men, to men who injected drugs, to trans-sexuals and to male sex workers: all groups which had been identified as having particular difficulties in adapting to safe sex. More ambitious programmes were developed in some places: The "Gay Now" programme of the Victorian AIDS Council in Melbourne, Australia, organised large-scale meetings involving hundreds of gay men at which facilitators led discussions and activities both in small groups and for the whole meeting. Several thousand gay men participated in these meetings during this campaign.

While these peer education programmes were naturally uneven in their degree of sophistication and in their organisation, there is no doubt that they carried behaviour change messages to a much wider network of gay men than were being reached by more traditional behaviour change campaigns, or that these messages were being communicated more effectively in the highly personalised context of smallf group meetings than they could ever be through even the most sophisticated print campaigns.

The key to the success of gay community peer education campaigns was that behaviour change messages carry more impact when conveyed horizontally, by peers, than when they are conveyed vertically, by sources of authority to "the masses", and that individuals who are given the power to make decisions about their own lives in the context of a supportive community are far more likely to adopt and maintain appropriate behaviours than those who are spoon-fed behaviour change messages as passive and socially-isolated consumers. In this, of course, the gay communities simply rediscovered the techniques by which all knowledge was conveyed in periods before the evolution of mass communication systems.

There are models even more directly analogous, since HIV peer education campaigns have been mounted among female sex workers in some developed countries, including Australia. Their success has been less marked than that of the gay community campaigns, mainly because it is more difficult to empower female sex workers, who are usually young and economically marginalised, than it is to empower gay men, many of whom enjoy a degree of class and gender privilege. It is also much more difficult to construct a genuine community of female sex workers than it has been to construct a community of gay men. Few women positively want to be sex workers: it is harder to engender a sense of pride in being a sex worker than it is to spread a sense of pride in being a gay man. Nevertheless, HIV peer education campaigns among female sex workers have achieved some successes, and could serve as a model for campaigns among sex workers elsewhere.

4. Conclusion

In summary, there are a number of important lessons that can be drawn from the response of gay communities to the HIV epidemic. The first is that people do not change their behaviour on the basis of an intellectual awareness that the behaviour may be dangerous to them. Rather, one of the most important determinants of sustained change is membership of a community organization which actively promotes and supports such changes.

Secondly, behaviour change is less a process of individuals deciding to change than one of communities changing their standards of behaviour and values. Thirdly, behaviour change messages must give people realistic and sustainable choices from amongst which individuals and couples can choose according to their preferred sexual practices and the circumstances of their lives.

Finally, the source of information, advice and counselling should be as close as possible to the community, preferably within the community. Behaviour change messages carry more impact when delivered by friends and colleagues than by authorities. Further, having and being encouraged to exercise the power to make decisions about their own life within a supportive community is critical.

The relevance of these experiences to people at risk of HIV infection in developing countries should be obvious. The application of these lessons is independent of access to modern communication technology. Further, in countries where governments and other authority structures are either weak and ineffectual, or authoritarian ana mistrusted, it is most unlikely that government directed behaviour change campaigns will have a great impact. A strategy which has at its centre the empowerment of oppressed and marginalised individuals and the development of strong and autonomous communities will enable women and men to protect themselves against HIV infection.

24

Carrying Out HIV Sentinel Surveillance

WHO-Regional Office for South East Asia, New Delhi

1. INTRODUCTION

During the past decade, the world has seen what appeared at first to be an illness largely confined to homosexual men and drug injectors in developed countries, become a pandemic affecting millions of men, women and children on all continents. The problem predominates in sub-Saharan Africa, Asia and much of Latin America and, by the year 2000, the infection rate among women will be equal to that of men. AIDS came later to the South-East Asia Region. The first reported AIDS case was in 1984 and HIV infections in most countries were reported in 1986 or later.

In order to better characterize the nature and the magnitude of the epidemic, HIV surveillance can play a very important role. HIV surveillance studies in India, Myanmar and Thailand documented an exceptional increase in HIV infections among female commercial sex workers, injecting drug users (IDU) and other population groups. Such data are essential for advocacy as well as planning purposes. Good surveillance data can be used not only to estimate the current magnitude of the problem and make future projections of HIV/AIDS, but also to assist decision-makers in instituting appropriate and rational intervention programmes. This paper describes the steps in establishing an HIV sentinel surveillance system and the use of data so obtained for programme purposes.

2. AIDS SURVEILLANCE: PROS AND CONS

AIDS surveillance refers to the collection of data on AIDS cases. However, because of the very long latent period (average 10 years) of the disease, the incidence of AIDS provides an indirect description of the underlying and preceding HIV epidemic.

Moreover, many AIDS patients may not be correctly diagnosed or some of them may not have contact with health services/facilities. Thus, the completeness of AIDS case reporting varies widely under different settings. The data generated by this "case reporting" system may therefore not be able to help recognize the current magnitude of the problem in the country or fully understand the dynamics of HIV transmission.

Nevertheless, AIDS is a notifiable disease in most countries and the surveillance of AIDS cases and deaths at national level can give information relevant to and necessary for organizing clinical management of patients with AIDS. Notwithstanding some of the constraints mentioned above, every attempt should be made to report AIDS cases. The diagnosis of AIDS is based on clinical and laboratory evidence. WHO case definition should be used according to the available diagnostic facilities.

Voluntary HIV testing should be offered to patients with symptoms compatible with AIDS. After having provided appropriate counselling, the serum from the patient would be first tested vith one ELISA or rapid/simple assay with higher sensitivity, and reactive samples retested with a test having higher specificity and using a different assay technique (based on different antigen preparations and/or different test principles). Serum reactive in both the tests is considered HIV antibody positive. Serum that is non-reactive in the first test is considered HIV antibody negative and that which is reactive in the first test and non-reactive in the second test is also considered HIV negative.

All health institutions at primary health care level should know how to diagnose a case, and those meeting the WHO case definition should be reported to the appropriate health authority. The national AIDS progxammes in turn should report summary data to WHO using the quarterly surveillance form (Annex 1).

3. HIV SURVEILLANCE

HIV surveillance can be defined as a collection of epidemiological information of sufficient accuracy and completeness regarding the distribution and spread of HIV infection to be relevant to the planning and implementation of HIV/AIDS prevention and control programme activities. Its objectives are to:

(1) determine the geographical spread of HIV infection;

(2) monitor the trends of HIV epidemic;

(3) provide information for estimates and future projections of HIV/AIDS in a country;

(4) use such data to mobilize the national political and social

leaders as well as to generate external support for the programme; and

(5) more importantly, provide useful data for appropriate planning of health and medical care services.

Since the primary objective of surveillance is to monitor trends in HIV infection over time and place, sen-surveys need to be conducted at repeated intervals using a consistent methodology in the same population group so as to demonstrate true change, if any, in HIV prevalence. The following epidemiological aspects should be considered while designing the surveillance procedure:

(1) HIV infections are not uniformly distributed in any population. The distribution of HIV infection in the population depends on the prevalence of certain behaviours or practices associated with an increased risk of HIV infection;

(2) There are limited major modes of HIV transmission, and not everyone in the population runs the same risk of HIV infection; and

(3) HIV infections were introduced into different geographical areas and populations at different times.

Sentinel surveillance is the method of choice for obtaining data on HIV infection rates in various population groups and thereafter for monitoring trends. It is therefore recommended that all national AIDS programmes establish HIV sentinel surveillance as soon as possible.

3.1 HIV Sentinel Surveillance

Sentinel surveillance means canying out cross-sectional studies (also known as prevalence surveys) of HIV prevalence rates at regular intervals among selected groups in the population known as "sentinel groups". In other words, with sentinel surveillance trends in HIV infection are monitored over time, by group and by place. Sentinel HIV surveillance can theoretically be community-based or clinic/health facility-based; the latter is much more convenient and hence should always be preferred.

The following procedures can be used for the plaming and implementation of HIV sentinel surveillance and for analysis of the data so obtained:

Planning

(a) Selection of the Sentinel Population and Sites

The first step towards the development of a sentinel

surveillance is the selection of the sentinel population. The population can be divided by transmission pattern into higher and lower risk groups.

Some examples of groups with higher risk behaviour include:

those having sexual intercourse with multiple partners; for example, patients with sexually transmitted diseases,
those sharing inadequately sterilized needles, syringes and other skin-piercing instruments, for example, injecting drug users, where this is a problem.

An example of population groups with lower risk include pregnant women. However, it should be kept in mind that initiating surveillance in lower-risk groups may be relatively unproductive unless a critical level of HIV prevalence among those with higher-risk behaviour has been reached. Hence testing of pregnant women may not be very useful in low-prevalence countries and should, as a general rule, not be carried out if HIV prevalence in higher risk groups is below 2 per cent.

It is important to emphasize also that data from donated blood screening should also be analysed to get an indication of HIV prevalence in the lower risk population. Although not a sentinel population *per se*, such data provide valuable information to monitor blood transfusion safety. The results should however, be disaggregated, where possible, by voluntary and remunerative donations.

As far as possible, easily defined and consistently accessible groups should be selected as sentinel population. For this reason, the sites should be chosen where blood is already being drawn for some other purpose and a part of it could conveniently be separated and tested for HIV in an unlinked anonymous manner. From the programme point of view, it is preferable to select sites in such a manner that all important transmission categories in the country are covered e.g., sexual transmission, injecting drug use and blood transfusion in Thailand, India, Nepal and Myanmar, and sexual transmission and blood transfusion in all other countries. Furthermore, sites should be accessible, convenient, have sufficient numbers of patients, and have staff willing to participate in the surveillance activity. Therefore, the sites which meet these criteria include STD clinics, drug treatment centres, and antenatal clinics.

(b) Sampling

The next step during planning is to decide about the sampling methodology. For convenience, it is advisable to collect consecutive blood samples till the predetermined sample size is reached (consult (c) below for sample sizes) or, from the operational viewpoint, take all samples consecutively over the eight-week period provided the minimum sample size has been obtained.

Often patients attending a site are referred to the laboratory for blood testing and some of them opt to drop out. This leads to participation bias and therefore the drawing of blood should be arranged at the clinic site, if possible. Double counting, viz., a patient considered twice or more in the same blood collection series should be avoided. If the period of data collection is short, the possibility of double counting becomes minimum. The other method to eliminate double counting would be to include only "new" patients.

(c) Sample Sizes

The fact that HIV occurs in an epidemic form means that large differences in HIV prevalence can exist between geographical areas. As a result, the minimum sample size required for surveillance purposes should be determined for each sentinel site. The following sample sizes are considered to be appropriate for sentinel surveillance:

Patients attending STD Clinics:

250 or more over an eight-week period

Injecting drug users attending treatment clinics:

250 or more over an eight-week period.

Antenatal clinic attenders:

As the prevalence of HIV among clinic attenders is likely to be lower and change more slowly than in STD clinic attenders, a large sample size is required, e.g., 400 or more over an eight-week period. This sample size gives a greater precision, and thereby small changes in the prevalence rates can be detected.

Tuberculosis (TB) patients:

HIV surveillance in patients attending TB clinics does not give pure trend data *per se*. It does, however, give important information on HIV related disease morbidity (e.g., TB). Increased HIV prevalence in patients with tuberculosis is the effect of both increase in HIV as well as increase in TB because of HIV.

As the prevalence of HIV among tuberculosis patients is increasing in many South-East-Asian countries, a sample size of 250-300 is suggested at the initial stage. This sample size may be covered within an eightweek period. In a high priority area, surveillance should be done even if no one site can provide a sample size of >250.

(d) Frequency of Survey

As described above, sentinel surveillance should be carried out using the sample sizes given above and repeated once a year to look at HIV infection trends. Experience suggests that it is better from the programmatic viewpoint to carry out surveillance in more sites and repeat them once a year instead of fewer sites every six months. However, every possible attempt should be made to obtain good quality data. On consecutive surveys, the methodology and laboratory procedures must be similar to those used previously so that data from the various surveys could be compared to each other. If possible, in each laboratory the same technician should be made specifically responsible for running tests in order to avoid human error.

(e) Testing Methodology

The unlinked anonymous testing method must be used, where possible, as it minimizes participation bias. In this type of testing, a part of the blood sample originally collected for other purposes is used for testing for HIV. For example, at an STD clinic, when blood sample is collected for VDRL or hepatitis B virus, a part of it can be separated out and sent to the laboratory after removing all personal identifiers, namely, name, address, etc., so that the HIV test results cannot be linked with the individual. The sentinel sites should, however, be encouraged to refer the clinic attenders, when necessary, to the centres where voluntary HIV testing and counselling could be provided.

(f) HIV Testing Strategy

For HIV surveillance, WHO recommends the following testing strategy depending on the expected HIV seroprevalence in that population group:

Areas with HIV seroprevalence >10 per cent:

The serum is tested with one ELISA or rapid/simple assay. Serum that is reactive is considered HIV positive.

Areas with HIV seroprevalence <10 per cent:

The serum is first tested with one ELISA or rapid/simple assay with higher sensitivity. Any serum found reactive on the first assay is retested with a second ELISA or rapid/simple assay with higher specificity based on a different antigen preparation and/or different test principles (e.g., indirect versus competitive). Serum that is non-reactive on the first test is considered HIV antibody negative. Serum that is reactive on the first test but non-reactive on second test is also considered antibody negative.

Implementation

It may often not be possible to initiate an HIV sentinel surveillance programme simultaneously in many regions/areas of a country. The surveillance programme should initially be introduced in one or two sites, preferably in a priority area, and extended later to other areas or sites once adequate experience is gained.

After having decided on the type of population groups to test, and the sites (summary given in Annex 2), the next step is to initiate collection of blood samples, retaining minimal epidemiological data and conducting laboratory tests. In order to do so the responsible individuals at each site should be trained to carry out the following activities:

(a) Data Collecnon

While every effort should be made to unlink the HIV test result with the individual concerned, the data collection form for each serum sample should include the following information:

- # general location of the sentinel site (not the name of the clinic)
- # population group,
- # month and year of serum collection,
- # age group,
- # HIV laboratory test result.

Collection of any additional information should be carefully weighed against the fact that too much information may allow individuals to be identified. The data collection form and the laboratory result should be linked only by a unique code number.

(b) Storage and Transport of Blood Samples

At the sentinel sites, the specimen tube for HIV testing must contain a minimum of 0.5 ml of serum. These should be properly labelled and stored in the freezer compartment of the refrigerator and sent to the HIV testing laboratory in batches of not less than 50 samples. When a few samples are sent and tested, there may be a danger that a positive laboratory result could still be linked to the individual.

(c) HIV Testing

All sera collected at any one sentinel site in any one sampling period should be tested in the same laboratory at the same time, using testing strategy outlined under *HIV testing strategy.*

As described earlier, care should be taken not to test a "few" samples at a time because this may lead to potentially identifying individual(s) who might have tested positive. The intention is to make the tracing of the HIV testing results to the individual virtually impossible.

Analysis

Data collected at each HIV sentinel site and for each senitinel group at that site should be analysed and compared separately to make meaningful interpretation Primary data will be the number of sera examined for a particular group at a particular site and the proportion positive for HIV. It is advisable not to aggregate the data but try to monitor trends separately for each population group at each site. Differences in prevalence over time can be tested for significance by a chi square test, if required.

Interpretation and Use of Data

The HIV surveillance data should be interpreted to assess how rapidly HIV prevalence is increasing in different groups and areas. This helps in determining which population groups need priority attention with respect to interventions and what differences exist between sentinel sites. Also, surveillance data can be used to estimate how many people may be currently infected and how many are expected to develop AIDS in the future. The results of sentinel surveillance should be disseminated not only to those responsible for fomulating policy but also to health care providers at sentinel sites. The data should also be reported to WHO using the quarterly surveillance form (Annex 1).

3.2 Use of Other Sources of Data

Sentinel surveillance is the method of choice for assessing HIV prevalence and for monitoring trends. However, if any *ad hoc* surveys have been carried out by other researchers, these sholild be taken into account in assessing the overall picture of the HIV situation. When the data on donated blood screening are available, these should also be analysed periodically to monitor the blood transfusion safety in an area or the country.

Annex 1

WHO HIV/AIDS SURVEILLANCE REPORT

WHO AIDS Surveillance Report
(Quarterly)

I. **Country:**

Report Date	___ / ___ / ___ Day Month Year

II.

Responsible Officer	
Unit/Department	

III.

Reporting Period Ending	___ / ___ / ___ Day Month Year
Total cumulative AIDS cases	

IV. Indicate Period of Diagnosis

	Number of Cases
Cases diagnosed prior to 1987	
1987 Jan-Jun	
Jul-Dec	
1988 Jan-Jun	
Jul-Dec	
1989 Jan-Jun	
Jul-Dec	
1990 Jan-Jun	
Jul-Dec	

	Number of Cases
1991 Jan-Jun	
Jul-Dec	
1992 Jan-Jun	
Jul-Dec	
1993 Jan-Jun	
Jul-Dec	
1994 Jan-Jun	
Jul-Dec	
1995 Jan-Jun	
Jul-Dec	

V. National Definition of AIDS (check all that apply)

- ☐ CDC/WHO (1987)
- ☐ WHO Definition
- ☐ WHO Definition with HIV anitbody positiv results
- ☐ Other (Specify ___________________

Current Reporting Period:

From: / /	To: / /

VI. Age/Sex Distribution of AIDS Cases Reported during the Reporting Period

Age	Male	Female	Not Specified	Total
0 – 4				
5 – 14				
15 – 19				
20 – 29				
30 – 39				
40 – 49				
50 – 59				
60 +				
Note Specified				
Total				

VII. Risk/Transmissioin Categories

	Male	Female	Total
Adult Heterosexual Homosexual Bi-sexual Injecting Drug User Blood Transfusion/Blood Products Other Not Specified		 N.A. N.A.	
Children Perinatal Blood Transfusion/Blood Products Other Not Specified			

WHO HIV Surveillance Report
(Quarterly)

Country

Report Date	/ /
Reporting Period Ending	/ /

1. HIV Sentinel Surveillance

Sentinel Site/Region	Population Group	Number HIV Tested	Number Positive	Percent Positive	Study Methods*

Please choose one i.e. unlinked anonymous, voluntary, mandatory, compulsory

2. **HIV *Ad-hoc* Survey Results**

From: ______/ ______ Month Year	To: ______/ ______ Month Year

Survey Site	Population Group	Number Tested	Number HIV Positive	% Positive	Study Methods

3. **Screening of Donated Blood for HIV**

From: ______/ ______ Month Year	To: ______/ ______ Month Year

Region	Number Tested	Number HIV Positive*	% Positive

*On ELISA or any rapid test used.

Annex 2

SUMMARY PROCEDURES FOR HIV SENTINEL SURVEILLANCE

Procedures	Higher risk population		Lower risk population	
	Injecting drug users	Patients with STD	Pregnant women	Patients with tuberculosis
Sentinal site	Drug treatment centres	STD clinics or general clinics	Antenatal clinic	Hospital/Chest clinic or TB clinic
Sample size	250 or more	250 or more	400	250 - 400
Period of completion	8 weeks	8 weeks	8 weeks	8 weeks
Frequency of survey	Once a year	Once a year	Once a year	Once a year
Sampling	Consecutive	Consecutive	Consecutive	Consecutive
Selection criteria	New patients	New patients	Primi, 17-30 years	New patients, 15-45 years
Testing methodology	Unlinked anonymous (UA)*	UA*	UA*	UA*

*Where possible, i.e., blood is aleady collected for other purposes.

25

Women and AIDS : Agenda for Action

The Fourth World Conference on Women is talking place at a time when women are increasingly becoming infected with HIV, the virus that causes AIDS. From being almost absent from the AIDS epidemic in the 1980s, women infected with HIV now number more than seven million—with another one million women becoming infected this year. By the year 2000 over 14 million women will have been infected and four million of them will have died. Women worldwide are asking why a virus that infecs both men and women is increasingly affecting women in a disproportionate manner.

The bleak reality is that the sexual and economic subordination of women fuels the HIV/AIDS pandemic. In order to break the cycle of neglect which affects women across their life span and across generations, it is essential to undertake actions which will allow women to make informed choices and enable them to improve the quality of their lives. Women must empower themselves by networking forming alliances, and advocating for change. Top-level political commitment is needed to reduce the social vulnerability of women to HIV infection by improving their health, education, legal and economic prospetcs. Effective HIV/AIDS prevention and care efforts along with sound policies and programmes targeting women affected by HIV/AIDS need to be developed and integrated into existing national structures, particularly at the community and family level. Because such social vulnerability cannot be effectively challenged by women as individuals alone, or even as groups, building effective alliances between women and men based on mutual respect, remain the greatest challenge, but also the best hope, for the lives of tomorrow.

I. INTRODUCTION

In the space of just one decade, AIDS has turned into a pandemic affecting millions of men, women and children on all continents. WHO estimates that 4.5 million AIDS cases had occurred by late 1994 and foresees that this cumulative total will triple by the year 2000. The number of people infected with HIV—the virus that can lead to AIDS-is much greater. According to WHO's conservative estimates, as of late 1994 more than 18 million adults and over 1.5 million, infants have been infected with HIV since the start of the pandemic (Figure 25.1). By the year 2000, there will be an estimated 30-40 million infections.

To what extent has the epidemic affected women? Enormously. A decade ago women seemed to be on the periphery of the epidemic. Today they are at the centre of concern. WHO estimates that almost half of all newly infected adults are women. This means that the number of women acquiring HIV each year cannot be counted in the thousands, or even in the hundreds of thousands. In 1994, more than one million women were newly infected. Already, 7-8 million women have been infected with HIV worldwide (Figure 25.2) and this figure is rapidly growing. Estimates are that over 14 million women will have become infected with HIV by the year 2000, and about four million of them will have died.

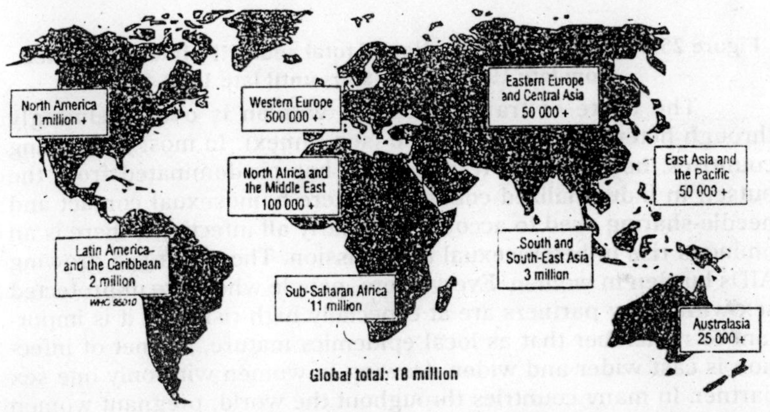

Figure 25.1. Estimated distribution of total adult HIV-infections from late 1970s/early 1980s until late 1994.

Among both men and women, the hardest-hit group is youth. WHO estimates that half of all infections to date have been in 15-24 year-olds. However, in nearly all parts of the world, the peak age of infection is lower in girls than boys. In many countries, 60 per cent of all new HIV Infections are among 15-24 year-olds, with a female to male ratio of two to one. An analysis of reported AIDS data from several African and Asian countries suggests that young women under 25 account for nearly 30 per cent of female AIDS cases and young men for approximately 15 per cent of male cases.

As infections in women rise, so do infections in the infants born to them. To date, these total about 1.5 million, of whom more than half a million have already developed AIDs. Overall, about one-third of babies born to HIV-infected mothers become infected themselves.

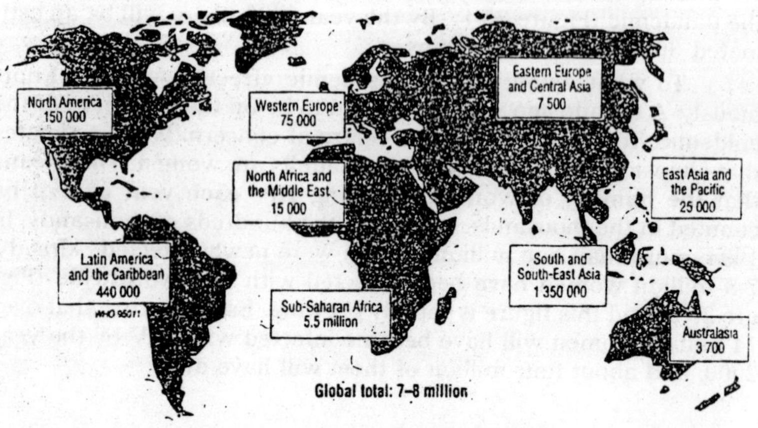

Figure 25.2. Estimated distribution of total adult HIV-infected women from late 1970s/early 1980s until late 1994

The route of transmission to women is overwhelmingly through heterosexual intercourse (see Annex). In most developing countries, heterosexual transmission has predominated from the outset. In industrialized countries, where homosexual contact and needle-sharing used to account for nearly all infections, there is an ominous rise in heterosexual transmission. The result is a growing AIDs burden in women. Everywhere, people who have unprotected sex with many partners are at especially high-risk. But it is important to remember that as local epidemics mature, the net of infection is cast wider and wider, drawing in women with only one sex partner. In many countries throughout the world, pregnant women attending antenatal clinics are showing a high prevalence of infection. Studies of women attending antenatal clinics find that many are monogamous and have been infected by their one partner—their husband.

The sexual and economic subordination of women fuels the HIV/AIDS pandemic. In order break the cycle of neglect which affects women across their life span and across generations, it is essential to undertake actions which will allow women to make informed choices and enable them to improve the quality of their lives. Given the growing dimensions of the HIV/AIDS pandemic, the need for change is literally a matter of life of death.

II. HOW HIV/AIDS IS SPREADING AMONG WOMEN?

Sexual Subordination Leads to HIV Vulnerability

In many societies, there is a significant power differential between men and women, supported by social and cultural systems that posit the control by males. Males are expected to initiate relationships, and sexual assertiveness in women is often stigmatized or punished. The gender power differential is compounded by age differences. Women typically marry or have sex with older men, who have been sexually active longer and hence are more likely to have become infected themselves. In countries with high HIV infection rates, men justify the selection of young adolescent girls, even female children, on the grounds that they are less likely to be infected with HIV/AIDS.

> **"For example, a situation like this develops. If your man comes home at 3 a.m. smelling of a perfume you don't recognize, that's the time he's going to ask for sex because he's trying to clear his conscience by making you think he hasn't alreay had it. But if he goes out drinking with the boys, he comes home and goes straight to sleep peacefully. You have to go along with what ever he asks, even if you're smelling this strange perfume, because you can't say 'no'."**

Many countries which promote monogamy and mutual fidelity, and discourage multiple casual partners as a societal norm, have also encouraged these values as a primary AIDS prevention strategy. Some societies, however, expect women to adhere strictly to this norm while tacitly condoning male deviation from it. Women are expected to have one lifetime sex partner while men are expected, or even encouraged, to have more than one partner. As a result, women are more likely to be monogamous than men and to have fewer lifetime partners. Reliance on "monogamy" or "mutual fidelity" as a principal solution can be misleading for women, as fidelity protects against HIV/AIDS only if it is completely mutual and life-long. It creates an illusion of safety for individuals who are monogamous but who cannot be certain about their partners.

In some cultures, women don't have the "permission" to talk about sex with men, or to negotiate safer sex practices. To do so many have serious repercussions, ranging from stigma to fear of violence or abandonment. Despite this, many HIV/AIDS prevention and family planning programmes have expected women to assume responsibility for the prevention of both pregnancy and sexually transmitted diseases (STDs), including HIV infection, in a context in which they have limited control over when, with whom, and how they engage in sexual activity.

Male resistance to condom use and women's inability to negotiate safer sex puts women (as well as men) at greater risk of

HIV infection. For men, the rationale for resisting the use of condoms includes concern about reduced sensitivity, ignorance about how to use the condom properly, and fear that using it will permanently interfere with fertility. In addition, within marriage or other long-term relationships, the very suggestion of condom use carries with it an indication of "infidelity" or other behaviour that could threaten the security of the relationship, making it difficult for both men and women to introduce condoms into an existing relationship.

Some countries have statutory or *de facto* restrictions based on age or gender regarding access to information about sexuality, contraception, disease prevention, condoms and lubricants, and health care. In many communities, schools and other institutions that work with adolescents are wary of providing sex education or otherwise discussing issues related to sexuality, due to social and cultural concerns about "protecting" young women from sexual experience. As a result, young women and men lack adequate information and skills to protect themselves if they are sexually active. In addition, children and adolescents, in some countries, must have a parent's permission to obtain health care services. This is a particular problem for young people who have left home or are homeless.

Women are also vulnerable to coerced sex, including rape and other sexual abuse, in and outside of the family, and forced sex work. Any non-consensual penetrative sex can carry an increased risk of transmission of HIV and other STDs, particularly as men who rape are not likely to use condoms. Moreover, even when sex is non-consensual, women are often stigmatized and blamed, causing them to be ostracized from family and support networks. The problems associated with rape and other forms of violence against women are often intensified in war situations, in which occupying or invading armies, systematically rape women as part of a strategy to intimidate the local population.

In all countries there are customs related to women's sexual activity. Some have become deadly.

Economic Subordination Leads to HIV Vulnerability

In virtually every society, women face discrimination in education, employment, and social status, resulting in economic vulnerability to HIV/AIDS. This includes, for example:

discrimination that girls face in both educational institutions and the family; for example, girls who are encouraged to take different subjects from those taken by boys have less access to financial and other family resources,

and are often withdrawn from school to assume domestic responsibilities;

occupational segregation of women into low-paying clerical and service jobs, unequal pay and fewer promotions (vis-a-vis men), fewer workplace benefits and concentration of women in the informal sector;

lack of access to technical assistance, training and credit; for example, in agricultural sector development, policies have traditionally provided funds and technical training to men involved in cash crop farming and not to women, who have been more likely to be engaged in subsistence farming.

Households headed by women are much more likely to be financially poor than those in which there is a working resident male. Women's economic dependence on male partners in order to avoid poverty for themselves and their children makes it difficult for women to negotiate safer sex practices to protect themselves from infection.

Some national laws reinforce women's economic dependence on men. Laws that restrict property ownership and inheritance to men, and in some cases limit women's ability to enter into independent contracts or obtain credit under their own names, impede women's ability to control income and property, and reinforce their economic dependence on male relatives. This dependence makes it difficult for them to refuse sexual practices that put them at risk of STDs and HIV infection. Laws regarding marriage, divorce, and child custody can impede women's ability to leave relationships in which they or their children are physically or sexually abused, or exposed to the risk of HIV infection.

Worldwide, many women rely on prostitution, or sex work, for economic survival. The proportion and the number of women who do so, in both developed and developing countries, is often directly related to the economy and the level of unemployment. In many parts of the world, prostitution is illegal and underground, which means that prostitutes my have to work without adequate control over the conditins of the sex work transaction.

"A woman in Asia put in a nutshell the dilemma faced by so many women like herself across the world: "AIDS might make me sick one day," she said. "But if I don't work my family would not eat and we would all be sick anyway".

Migration as a result of war, famine, political oppressin or poverty, can increase a women's vulnerability to HIV infection if she is isolated from community structures, and does not speak or read the local language. Furthermore, women who are migrant workers, refugees or returnees are often more vulnerable than other women to some kind of sexual barter, (e.g., to obtain entry or residence permits, in exchange for transport, or to obtain or hold onto jobs), receiving financial support from men with whom they have sex, or engaging in formal prostitution. Similarly, when men migrate to urban centres, leaving wives and girlfriends at home, they may have other partners in cities.

There is often a lack of social and financial support to help women with HIV infection plan for the care of their surviving, and often healthy, children. This lack of support increases the emotional and psychological stress among women who understand that they are going to die while their children are still young. In some countries, as the number of children orphaned as a result of the epidemic has increased, some women have assumed responsibility for these children, taking them into their homes, often without any financial or other support, and often with inadequate space, food, or other supplies.

Female Biological Vulnerability to HIV

AIDS is essentially a sexually transmitted disease (STD), which like some other such diseases can also be spread through blood and blood products, and from an infected women to her unborn or newborn child. Women are biologically more vulnerable then men to HIV infection and other STDs. Studies in many countries have found that male-to-female transmission of HIV appears to be 2-4 times as efficient as female-to-male transmission. Postulated as the major factors responsible for differential transmission are the larger mucosal surface areas exposed to virus in women and the greater viral inoculum present in semen compared with vaginal secretions. Male-to-female transmission of some STDs is at least 15 per cent more efficient than female-to-male transmission. Young girls are particularly vulnerable. Their immature cervix and relatively low vaginal mucus production presents less of a barrier to HIV, making them biologically more vulnerable to infection than older premenopausal women.

Other data suggest that STDs— especially those, such as chancroid and syphilis, which cause ulcerative lesions—greatly facilitate both the acquisition and transmission of HIV. However, women with STDs are often asymptomatic and fail to recognize any infections. As a result, women are more vulnerable to HIV infection because they are more likely to have untreated STDs. Often their vulnerability to STDs is the result of their partners' behaviour rather than their own. This increases the likelihood that they will not recognize lowgrade infections. At the same time, women tend to avoid STD clinics for fear of being recognized and stigmatized. Women who do seek medical services often choose to go to primary health, family planning, and material and child health clinics for their care. Unfortunately, such facilities are often less well equipped to diagnose and treat STDs or may be unsympathetic or judgmental towards women with STDs.

Finally, women are disproportionately the receipients of blood transfusions and other blood products (e.g., for anaemia or childbirht complications). In the absence of adequate blood screening, women's vulnerability to blood-borne HIV transmission increases.

Impact of HIV/AIDS on Women

Because women are sexually, economically and biologically vulnerable to HIV/AIDS, they are often stigmatized and blamed for "causing" HIV/AIDS and other STDs. Women are frequently identified as "reservoirs of infection" or as "vectors for transmission" to their male partners and their offspring. This inaccurate view is iactually harmful in a number of ways: it fails to focus on men's equal responsibility to prevent HIV/AIDs; it prevents programmes from developing services which meet the needs of women; and it underlies some research and intervention strategies which have been designed more to protect men from women than to enable women to protect themselves.

> *"All the gender issues we had never tackled came up at once", says Theresa Kaijage, a founding member of the Tanzanian AIDS Service Organization called WAMATA. "Initially we ignored them or thought they were irrelevant. We thought it was Eurocentric to tackle them in Africa. We thought our African culture was different and dealt with things in a different way. All the agendas that we had ignored- legal, educational and health problems, inequitable gender relations—suddenly we are dealing with these multiple issues, which people have not learned to analyze in a way that promotes equal sharing of both resources and power at all levels. In order to deal with AIDS, we have had to confront these."*

Many people assume that if a woman has HIV infection, she has had multiple partners or engaged in prostitution and that such behaviour marks her as a "bad woman". As a result of this social stigma associated with HIV infection, women known or thought to be infected have been dismissed from their jobs or not hired, evicted from their homes, abandoned by their husbands or other long-term partners, and denied the custody of their children. In addition, women perceived to be at risk of HIV infection have been denied health insurance, and health care personnel have refused to treat women they thought were or might be infected.

Some countries have implemented mandatory testing schemes targeting women. Women who test positive or who are suspected of being infected suffer from increased discrimination, random and institutional violence, arrest, incarceration, and deportation. Most often such testing is without the women's informed consent, and without appropriate pretest and post-test counselling.

Most societies rely on women to be voluntary caregivers for their families, as well as occupational caregivers for the community. Older women may be expected to assume a major caregiving responsibility at the same time that adolescent daughters may be kept out of school to care for younger children or other family members who are ill. The expectation that women will provide most of the care for people with HIV infection and AIDS results in high stress, especially if such care must be provided in addition to other work, including paid work outside of the home and family-centred work, such as subsistence farming. Such stress is compounded when the women become ill themselves, often with no one to care for them.

If the vulnerability of women to HIV infection is to be reduced, both men and women must work to counter gender discrimination and the subordination of women. Policy makers, community leaders and other people in positions of power must recognize the connection between women's economic and social status and their vulnerability to HIV infection. Men and women need to reassess the way they see themselves and each other, the way they relate as husband and wife, partners, lovers, brothers and sisters, parent and child, coleagues and friends.

The inequality between men and women fuels the spread of HIV/AIDS. Unless the interaction between HIV infection, cultural values and the rights and needs of women is reconized, the fundamental change required to stem this pandemic is unattainable. While women require urgent consideration in the response to the epidemic, interventions must mobilize all sectors of society, including, and in particular, men.

It is important therefore, to develop complementary and interlined strategies for action, incorporating a gender analysis of the socio-economic and cultural causes and effects of the pandemic. Specific activities are listed below.

> *"To enable women to protect themselves there are three issues at stake : improving the social and economic status of women: providing a method over which they have sufficient control: or getting more men to adopt safer sex. This is not an academic exercise in setting priorities, but a question of-life. and death for many women".*
>
> *Dr. Eka Esu Williams, Nigeria*

Reducing the Vulnerability of Women to HIV/AIDS

Preventing HIV Infection Among Women

Support the development of HIV/AIDS prevention interventions that provide the necessary messages, skills, and support services to men and women, including marginalized or hard-to-reach groups, such as migrants, the wives and non-marital partners of migrat.ing men, women and men in prison, and adolescent girls and boys both in and out of school:

increase girls' access to education including access to scholarships and other financial assistance;
support programmes that target both men and women with informed messages about the importance of using condoms to protect both partners from HIV and other STD, and about their mutual responsibility to engage in safer sex practices;
support sex and HIV/AIDS education for young people (male and female) in school and out of school to iricrease their understanding and skills in human sexuality;
support the development of sound HIV/AIDS work-place polices and effective workplace educations programmes;
remove obstacles to women's ability to earn money and engage in productive labour'by supporting' child care services, equal pay for equal work,employment training programmes, as well as small business and agricultural-development programmes;
ensure a safe blood supply through blood donations from low risk,' voluntary, non-renumerated blood donors'and test all blood for HIV.
reduce unecessary blood transfusions by improving women's nutrition, preventing anaemia, treating infections, preventing the loss of blood due to complications in pregnancy, and using blood substitutes wherever possible;

Reduce the incidence and prevalence of STDs among women by increasing their access to and utilization of appropriate STD services:

develop appropriate educational programmes that target both men and women concerning the increased risk of acquiring HIV infection in the presence of an STD;
fund activities that educate women how to prevent and recognize signs and symptoms of STDs and to seek appropriate health care services;
provide high quality condoms through effective social

marketing programmes and promote the use and distribution of lubricants and other agents that reduce the likelihood of microscopic vaginal lesions associated with sexual intercourse;

improve the provision of STD diagnostic and treatment services for women, regardless of age or marital status;

Support research to better understand women's biological vulnerability to HIV, and the impact of contraceptives and other means of fertility regulation, and of pregnancy, on HIV infection and disease progression;

advocate that biomedical scientists and. private industry give top priority to developing a vaginalvirucide or microbicide active against—HIV and other STDs.

Reducing tbe Impact of HIV/AIDS on Women

Reduce the stigmatization and discrimination of women regarding HIV infection:

encourage countries where mandatory testing or routine HIV screening programmes exist to replace them with voluntary, confidential testing supported 'by counselling services;

support programmes that work with families and communities of women with HIV/AIDS in order to reduce the likelihood that women will be ostracized due to their HIV status;

plan and implement HIV/AIDS prevention interven-tions with sex workers, and support self-help and advocacy organizations for sex workers;

review the impact of laws and regulations relating to prostitution on working conditions as well as on the ability of HIV/AIDS and STD prevention activities to operate effectively.

Caring for Women with HIV/AIDS

Increase the availability of support services for HIV positive women who want help with reproductive decision-making and for women with children who need help with planning for their care:

ensure that women have access to voluntary, safe and affordable contraceptive measures;

support programmes—to assist women with HiV/AIDS . in family planning decisions and planning for their surviving families;

ensure that HIV-positive women are not pressured or forced to be sterilized, and that pregnant women with HIV infection are not pressured or forced to terminate pregnancies.

Ensure that women do not carry the entire burden of care for people with HIV/AIDS:

encourage men and women to share in the caregiving role, and support interventions that provide training for women and men in basic health care procedures;

support community-based institutions that can provide professional alternatives to home care and respite care for primary caregivers;

encourage families to keep their daughters in school, and discourage them from relying on adolescent girls for caregiving responsibilities,

support programmes and interventions to assist women and men who provide foster care to children orphaned as a result of HIV/AIDS and other diseases.

IV. CONCLUSION

The sexual and economic subordination of women continues to fuel the HIV/AIDs pandemic. Women are increasingly becoming infected with HIV and at a significantly younger age than men. At the same time, proportionately more girls and young women are becoming infected in their teens and early twenties than women in any other age group. Today, the stakes are higher than ever. The ways in which we respond to the pandemic now will influence the ways in which women participate and contribute in the twenty-first century.

26

Female Genitile Health and Risk of HIV Transmission

Dr. Regina Mc Namara
Assistant Professor of Clinical Public Health Centre for Population and Family Health, Columbia University, New York City.

INTRODUCTION

This paper is concerned with preservation of the intact surface of the female genital tract as a defense against heterosexual transmission of HIV. If the vaginal epithelial mucosa, the female's normal barrier against infection, is not intact when the male deposits infectious semen, susceptibility to HIV transmission may be significantly increased. STIs are one source of damage to that barrier and their association with HIV transmission is well-documented. (See e.g. Wasserheit, 1990; WHO, 1990.) Other causes of genital trauma and infection in both women and men that may open a pathway to HIV infection have been given little attention. For women, cultural conditions and inadequate health services compound the disadvantages of sexual and social inequality, increase their vulnerability to infection and limit their resources for treatment.

This discussion of genital infection and trauma is intended to convey the widespread nature of the problem and its roots in the social and economic context of the lives of women in developing countries. Barriers to diagnosis and treatment of genital conditions are often specific to women varying in different cultures but with common themes: lack of information; differential access to health care; violation of norms of personal modesty; and ignorance or denigration of women's needs. These barriers can be lowered with education, economic opportunities, better and more available health services and preventive methods that women can control themselves. To accomplish this, the health and well-being of women must be prominent on national and international research and aid agendas.

GENITAL INFECTION AND TRAUMA

In—the following discussion it is understood that: intact vaginal epithelial mucosa alone may not be sufficient protection against HIV transmission during intercourse; the use of condoms is important even in the absence of a sexually transmitted infection or other genital condition; and the study of HIV continues and current knowledge indicates that genital health can decrease, but not eliminate, susceptibility to infection.

Sexually Transmitted Infection

Genital ulcers caused by syphilis, chancroid and herpes are believed to facilitate penetration of HIV through disruption of epithelial mucosa or through the increased local concentration of lymphocytes which are target cells for HIV. A World Health Organization (WHO) expert committee meeting in 1989 concurred that it is biologically plausible for all STD pathogens that cause genital ulcers or inflammation to be a factor in increased infectiousness or susceptibility to HIV (WHO, 1989). Other sexually transmitted infections, such as gonorrheal, chlamydial and trichomonal infections, may also enhance susceptibility (Oxtoby and Gayle, 1990). Trichomoniasis may be a far greater risk than genital ulcer disease because of its extensive prevalence in many parts of the developing world (Wasserheit, 1990).

The term sexually transmitted infection extends the list of traditional venereal diseases (gonorrhea, syphilis, chancroid, lymphogranuloma venereum and granuloma inguinale) to cover more than 20 organisms and syndromes, including chlamydia, genital herpes, and human papillomovirus infections. The major primary manifestations of sexually transmitted infections throughout the world include urethritis in men, cervicitis and vaginitis in women and genital ulcers, genital warts and enteric infections in both men and women. With infections of the lower reproductive tract, women can experience abnormal vaginal discharge, a burning feeling with urination, abnormal vaginal bleeding and genital pain or itching.

The prevalence of sexually transmitted infections, and thus the patterns of disease, vary greatly among and within world regions and within countries. In western countries, at present, the Herpes Simplex Virus (HSV) is the most common cause of Genital Ulcer Disease (GUD); in many developing countries, syphilis and chancroid appear to be the most common causes (Hatcher *et al.*, 1989). Infection rates are approximate since facilities for testing and treatment are scarce in developing countries, private physicians in developed countries frequently do not report their patients' sexually transmitted infections, population-based studies are rare and much of the research is subject to biases inherent in studies of selected groups (e.g., commercial sex workers, STD clinic patients, prenatal and family planning clients).

Although a female is more likely than a male to be infected from a single act of intercourse with a partner who has a sexually transmitted infection (Hatcher et al., 1989), women are seriously undercounted in sexually transmitted infection data in all countries, in part because their conditions are often asymptomatic, but also because services they can or will use are not available. Clinical diagnosis or screening for infection is rarely incorporated into services offered at family planning antenatal or maternal and child health (MCH) clinics. Sexually transmitted infection clinics, when they are available, are usually not acceptable to women. Consequently, estimates of the gender distribution of the incidence of sexually transmitted infections cannot be made with any confidence.

Wasserheit (1989), in an international review of female reproductive tract infections, found greater prevalence reported in African-studies than those conducted among Asian or Latin American populations. The median of the rates of gonorrhea was 10 per cent in the studies in African countries; 1 per cent in Asian countries and 6 per cent in Latin America. Median rates of trichomoniasis were 19 per cent, 11 per cent and 12 per cent for African, Asian and Latin American studies, respectively (Dixon-Mueller and Wasserheit,-1991).

Although a female is more likely than a male to be infected from a single act of intercourse with a partner who has a sexually transmitted infection, women are seriously undercounted in sexually transmitted infection data in all countries, in part because their conditions are often asymptomatic, but also because services they can or will use are not available.

Since the major immediate causes of infertility in women are probably gonorrhea, chlamydia and other reproductive tract infections, infertility serves as an indirect measure of sexually transmitted infection prevalence. Untreated, these infections lead to pelvic inflammatory disease, which leads to tubal inflammation, damage or distortion, which leads in turn to inability to conceive or to spontaneous abortion (Sherris and Fox, 1985). The measure of female infertility used in most population studies is childlessness at the end of the reproductive years. However, this incorrectly assigns all childlessness to female rather than male infertility, and misses infertility that follows first or later births. The indices vary widely, from as low as 1.0 to 1.5 per cent in Korea and Thailand to as high as 13 per cent in urban areas of Colombia and 23 per cent in one rural area of New Guinea (Belsey, 1980).

In sub-Saharan Africa, the highest levels of childlessness have been found for the most part in three zones: southwestern Sudan and northwestern Zaire; Cameroon and Gabon; and southeastern Angola and northeastern Zambia. These areas, and regions in Burkina Faso and Uganda, have reported infertility levels of over 21 to 40 per cent. In adjacent areas, levels of childlessness are still well above 3 per cent which is considered a normal fertility benchmark. (Frank, 1983). A large multicenter study conducted by the WHO found tubal occlusion, often resulting from sexually transmitted infection, as a cause of infertility in 11 per cent of infertile women from developed countries, 16 per cent from non-African developing countries, and 49 per cent from African countries (cited in Hatcher et al., 1989). Differences in the prevalence of sexually transmitted infections, or in access to treatment, may well explain differences in infertility rates.

Genital Trauma

Sexually transmitted infections are a major but not the sole source of damage to the female genital tract. Additional sources of infection or trauma that could damage the epithelial barrier include female genital mutilation, childbearing, insertion of objects into the vagina and trauma during sexual intercourse. Maintaining cleanliness of the genital area under the harsh conditions of nomadic life, drought or life-long water scarcity requires heroic measures. Infections probably caused by inadequate cleansing—of cloths used to absorb menstrual blood are also reported (Wasserheit et al., 1989).

Female genital mutilation is a plausible cofactor for HIV transmission which has not been adequately studied. Of the three types of operations performed on young girls, the gravest is infibulation, also called pharaonic circumcision. The clitoris, labia minor and parts of the labia major are removed and the two sides of the vulva are fastened together, leaving a small opening for urination and menstruation. Consequences of infibulation, such as inflammation of the genital area, partial closure of the vaginal orifice, abnormal anatomy or friable scar tissue are conditions that, according to the WHO, may increase susceptibility to HIV (WHO/GPA, 1990). Long-term consequences of infibulation are chronic urinary retention, urinary tract infections, incomplete healing and excessive scar tissue (or keloids) which can cause vaginal obstruction. Childbirth (when the infibulated section is cut open for passage of the infant) can be severely traumatic with consequences as grave as rupture of the vagina. Complications caused by these female genital operations are not reported with any regularity, in part because of the reluctance of the women to expose their genitals for medical examination (Gordon, 1991).

In northern Sudan, according to preliminary reports from the demographic and health survey, 82 per cent of married women had undergone pharaonic circumcision. A additional 15 per cent of the married women underwent Sunna circumcision, the "mildest form in which the tip of the clitoris is removed or an intermediate type of excision when the whole clitoris and often adjacent parts including the labia minor are removed (Ahmed and Kheir, 1990). The intermediate and Sunna forms are practiced more widely in subSaharan Africa and the Middle East than is the pharaonic (which is reported mainly in southern Egypt, Ethiopia, Somalia, Djibouti and in other Red Sea coastal areas). Current estimates of the total number of African women who have undergone some form of circumcision or infibulation approach 100 million (Women's International Network, n.d.).

The Safe Motherhood Initiative launched in Nairobi in 1987 brought to the fore of international discussion the problems of maternal mortality in developing countries. Research and interventions have focused on the risk of death yet, during each delivery, women confront the risk of damage to the genital tract. Tears or incisions during childbirth, with potential for infection, are common traumas of childbirth and massive infections can result from induced or spontaneous abortions. Very young women are especially vulnerable to risks associated with delivery (especially when childhood nutrition has been poor, infections are frequent and growth is stunted). Childbirth at very young ages is not a rare event. In Mauritania, for example, 15 per cent of girls have given birth by age 15; in Bangladesh, 21 per cent have had at least one child by age 15 (United Nations, 1991:59).

When the pelvis is immature or underdeveloped, cephalopelvic distortion and prolonged obstructed labour can cause damage as severe as vesico-vaginal fistula (VVF). With VVF, there is an opening between the urinary bladder and the vagina and the afflicted women continuously leak urine, wetting their clothes and excoriating their mutilated vulvae and vaginas. Reports on VVF from Egypt, Ghana, India, Kenya, Nigeria, Pakistan, South Africa, Sudan, and Turkey indicate obstetric causes for 80 to 100 per cent of the cases identified (Tahzib, 1989). In one Nigerian hospital, 30 per cent of those suffering from VYF were under age 15; 59 per cent were under age 18 (Ampofo, et al., 1990). The number of women with VVF is not known; many are believed to be suffering quietly out of sight, shunned as pariahs by family and community and without protection.

Other causes of genital trauma abound and include such traditional practices as the 'gishiri' or 'salt cut' in Nigeria which involves incision of part of the interior vaginal wall by a traditional birth attendant, traditional healer or occasionally by the woman herself. The purpose is to cure a variety of vaginal conditions and infertility (Adebajo, 1989).

Herbs, traditional preparations and foreign objects inserted into the vagina can cause inflammation, abrasions and infections, and so increase risk of HIV transmission. Practices may be intended to increase the male partner's pleasure during intercourse. Among pregnant women studied at a hospital clinic in Malawi, 12 per cent reported using one or more of the following to tighten the vagina: herbs, aluminum hydroxide, cloth or stones (silica gel, potassium permanganate or pumicelike stone). Not surprisingly, stones were found to have an irritating and erosive effect on vaginal mucosa and the data reported suggest that they may facilitate entry of HIV (Dallabetta et al., 1990).

Globally, women are known to insert objects into the vagina as medication, for contraception or to induce abortion. The array of items used for these purposes in Mexico for example, includes herbs, pills, soap and lime (Shedlin and Hollerback, 1981). A more complex process is described in Nigeria:

> To prepare [the abortifacient], leaves and seeds from certain local trees (ejirin seeds and itu leaves) are ground and the juice from another tree (epin) added to form a paste. The paste is then made into small balls and dried. As they become dry, more juice is added two or three times. The balls are inserted into the vagina and, according to our informants. they have the effect of destroying the foetus (Adebajo, 1989:14).

A cross-cultural study of indigenous fertility regulation conducted in seven countries illustrates the diversity of potentially damaging objects (Newman, 1985). In Afghanistan, women reported intravaginal insertion of wooden spoons or sticks treated with copper sulphate to cause heavy bleeding and abortion (Hunte, 1985). Egyptian women use aspirin, lemon juice, black pepper and plant stems (Sukkary Stolba, 1985). In other countries, bamboo leaves. grass. the midrib of the coconut palm, water pumped under hiah pressure, hangers, knitting needles and umbrellas are used as abortifacients (Ngin. 1985; Low and Newman, 1985).

Genital conditions conducive to HIV transmission may also result from sexual intercourse especially in the absence of foreplay when the unlubricated surface is irritated by penile penetration. Among older women, atrophic vaginitis may cause mucosal tears during sexual intercourse (Peterman. 1990). The contraceptive sponge may absorb vaginal secretions excessively and cause dryness (Hatcher *et al.,* 1989), and drying out the vagina before intercourse to increase penile friction has been reported in Zambia (S.K. Hira, cited in Feldman, 1990).

Damage to the female genitalia and increased susceptibility to HIV infection can result from rape or other modes of violent assertion of sexual supremacy by men. This is a risk factor, especially for sex workers who have repeated encounters with drunk and violent clients. In a Harare, Zimbabwe study, half the sex workers interviewed said that their most recent client was drunk (Wilson et al., 1989). An additional genital hazard comes with the use of condoms for frequent acts of intercourse in a short time period. According to recent reports from focus groups with sex workers in Thailand, the customer with a condom takes a longer time to ejaculate, the lubricant wears off, and friction and irritation follow (Sittitrai et al., 1989).

DIAGNOSIS AND TREATMENT: THE OBSTACLES

Recognizing the major role played by the integrity of the female and male genitalia in reducing heterosexual transmission of HIV can be an important contribution to global prevention efforts, but diagnosis and treatment are possible only when women and men can present themselves to someone with the skills and means to identify correctly the conditions and supply appropriate medications .

Utilization of Health Services

Little is known about what use women in developing countries make--of health services for themselves. They are usually questioned only about their use of services that are related to reproduction or to their children's health. The most recent, comprehensive source of information on use of services related to pregnancy is the demographic and health surveys conducted in the 1980s in 29 developing countries. They indicate that many of the women interviewed had at least one visit to a trained midwife or physician at some time during pregnancy, but far fewer delivered with trained assistance. Table 26.1 shows socio-economic and geographic differentials within countries, as well as between countries, in prenatal visits and delivery assistance in Egypt, Ghana, Guatemala, Mali and Thailand.

> *The obstacles many women face in access to health care are caused by poverty, lack of education, inferior position in society, and inadequate health systems, among others. The result is that, if a woman does not have prenatal care, or if her one or two visits do not include an internal examination, she may pass through her entire life and bear her children, yet never have an internal examination.*

TABLE 26.1: PERCENTAGE OF WOMEN WITH PRENATAL VISITS AND TRAINED ASSISTANCE AT DELIVERY, IN SELECTED COUNTRIES, BY RESIDENCE AND EDUCATION

	EGYPT %	GHANA %	GUATEMALA %	MALI %	THAILAND %
Residence					
Urban					
Prenatal	69	94	58	70	95
Delivery	57	70	60	77	96
Rural					
Prenatal	42	78	26	19	73
Delivery	70	26	13	26	46
Education					
None					
Prenatal	42	72	18	27	49
Delivery	20	26	13	26	46
Primary					
Prenatal	55	—	40	—	79
Delivery	34	—	34	—	59
Complete primary					
Middle					
Prenatal	65	92	64	—	79
Delivery	49	55	64	—	59
Secondary					
Prenatal	81	97	86	95	97
Delivery	78	79	87	98	95

* Educational levels for Thailand: 0-3, 4-7. 8+

Sources: Demographic and Health Surveyes: Egypt. Ghana, Guatemala. Mali and Thailand.

In Egypt, 42 per cent of rural women receive some prenatal care from a physician or trained nurse or midwife; yet only 19 per cent deliver with trained assistance. Seventy-eight per cent of rural women in Ghana have at least one prenatal visit; only 29 per cent have trained assistance at childbirth. In rural Guatemala and Mali, fewer than 20 per cent have trained help at delivery and percentages with prenatal care are scarcely greater. In all countries, urban women are more likely than rural women to use these services.

Strong upward trends in utilization of trained assistance are seen as women ' s educational levels rise from no education to secondary school education. In Guatemala, for example, prenatal care increased from 18 to 86 per cent, in Mali from 27 per cent to

95 per cent in Mali (Chayovan, 1988; Sayed, 1989; Ghana, 1989; Guatemala, 1989; Traore, 1989).

Distance from home to the health facility, lack of transportation and lack of funds undoubtedly explain some of the births not attended by trained personnel, yet the differential between source of care for prenatal visits and deliveries also suggests that deliberate choices are being made. The value given to a natural and familiar setting and the spiritual and material support for the cosmological conceptions of the patient offered by traditional birth attendants strongly influence a decision to give birth in the home community (Twumasi, 1987). These factors weigh heavily against the lack of privacy in a health facility, the use of unfamiliar positions during childbirth, shame at crying out before others and the indignity of exposure (Auerbach, 1982; Rehan, 1984; Schuler et al., 1985; Beeson et al., 1987; Kerns, 1989).

The statistics on utilization do not take into account the quality of care (training and skills of the provider or shortages such as supplies or equipment, including specula and gloves for internal examinations). In a typical prenatal examination, the woman is weighed, blood pressure is taken, the abdomen may be palpated, urine may be tested and sometimes blood may be drawn for testing. The woman may be asked about vaginal discharge, itchiness or other symptoms, but a pelvic examination is not always performed if it is not indicated by her history or condition. Even a woman using a modern family planning method, unless it is an intrauterine device (IUD) or tubectomy, might not be examined internally.

Women often are not aware they have vaginitis and cervicitis, which are the most common syndromes in lower tract infections (Hatcher et al., 1989; Wasserheit, 1989). It is estimated that 10 to 50 per cent of women with trichomoniasis, 25 to 30 per cent with gonococcal cervicitis and probably over 50 per cent of women with chlamydial cervicitis or bacterial vaginosis experience no symptoms (Wasserheit et al., 1989 citing Holmes et al., 1984). Such symptoms as vaginal discharge may be taken to be a fairly normal condition, not requiring medical attention (Orubuloye et al., 1990). The discharge and even a substantial degree of discomfort are often ignored (McFalls and McFalls, 1984).

Access to Health Services

Differences in access to health care between men and women, as widely reported, are acute with regard to conditions affecting sexual organs. A man with symptoms might go for STI treatment, at least at an advanced stage; his wife is more likely to remain untreated. This is not always because women are unaware of what is happening-to their bodies but because their bodies are devalued and are not seen as requiring care. Preferential health care for male children —is documented— in Asia, principally in Bangladesh and India, and in the Middle East (Cook, 1987). This apparently leaves its cultural mark on the adult female.

In the rural areas throughout developing countries, women doctors are rare; in the Moslem culture especially, women are not allowed to be examined by a male doctor. Distances to health facilities can be very great, and women lack autonomy and money. They are often not released from household and child-care duties to go to a clinic during office hours or to wait at hospitals or dispensaries. Travel outside their immediate community may be forbidden (Kloos, 1987) or inhibited by lack of education and the confidence needed to deal with the official systems. More efficient means of transportation — such as bicycles, motorbikes, horses and donkeys — may be for use only by males (Stock. 1983).

Where they are confined to purdah, as in Hausa society, a woman must obtain the permission of her husband before leaving the home compound. Many men are reluctant to allow their wives to make long, unescorted journeys for health care, particularly if the husband perceives the wife's illness to be non-threatening and amenable to traditional treatment (Stock, 1983).

Men are often the intermediaries between women and health services and assessment of the severity of a condition and the choice of an appropriate source of treatment, if any, may be made by the husband or by senior male members of the family. In Zaire, sufferers retain decisionmaking rights only if they are adult, capable of walking and travelling, financially able to pay for care and, usually, male (Janzen, 1978).

The obstacles many women face in access to health care are caused by poverty, lack of education, inferior position in society, and inadequate health systems, among others. The result is that, if a woman does not have prenatal care, or if her one or two visits do not include an internal examination, she may pass through her entire life and bear her children, yet never have an internal examination.

Personal Modesty

Even if symptoms are recognized, and even if services are available, obstacles remain. For women, a strong deterrent is reluctance to undergo a pelvic examination. This was emphatically demonstrated by a survey on female genital operations in the Sudan. Ninety-five per cent of the sample population, 3,210 women, were interviewed, but only 12 of the women were willing to be examined (Gordon, 1991). Some of the women may have wished to conceal the evidence that they had undergone mutilation; the majority were more likely to be expressing a strong sense of personal modesty.

Reluctance to expose the genitals is not unique to women in developing countries. In the United States, for instance, fear of a pelvic examination was cited by 25 per cent of adolescents queried as to their reason for— not coming sooner to a family planning clinic (Zabin and Clark, 1981). As Scrimshaw states emphatically: "Any woman from just about any culture who has ever had a pelvic examination knows how undignified and embarrassing it feels" (1973: 10).

Embarrassment or shame has particular force in some cultures, as is evidenced by the unpopularity of contraceptive methods that require genital exposure and contact. Injection, for example, has been recommended for women in India so that they might avoid both the mortifying experience of exposure to medical scrutiny and the need to handle their genitals when using a method (Marshall, 1973). Embarrassment with genital exposure associated with IUD insertion is reported from Indonesia where the Islamic religion plays a major role in choice of contraceptive method. Many Moslems object to the intimate physical contact between IUD providers and their clients, despite recent rulings from high Moslem councils conditionally endorsing IUD use (Molyneux et al., 1990).

Modesty as a value central to the image of womanhood is notable in the care taken to cover the genitals of females even in infancy, as in Latin America, while male children are free to expose their genitals until they approach puberty. Douches and coitusdependent contraceptive methods which violate standards of modesty are rarely used by women in Colombia (Browner, 1985) and never among the Aguarunas in Peru, who interpret any viewing or manipulation of female sexual organs as erotic (Berlin, 1985). Some Mayan women in Guatemala do not remove their skirts even for childbirth (Beck, 1991). Mexican women asked to name the parts of their bodies could find no word for the vagina except "la parte" (the part), and that was uttered with manifest embarrassment (Shedlin, 1982).

The depth and force of modesty is exemplified by the pregnancy and childbirth practices of rural Hausa/Fulani women in the northern region of Nigeria. Muslim women in purdah do not openly admit to their pregnancies. They often labour alone in their compound (with other women keeping within hearing distance in case assistance is required). The traditional birth attendant (TBA) is called in after the child is born to cut the cord and look after the mother and baby (Sokoto Maternal Health Project, 1990).

Fear and stigma surround problems relating to the sexual organs and women suffer in silence. In India, inhibitions about drawing attention to the body can be so great that even female health workers must rely upon verbal accounts of the symptoms of women who will not subject themselves to a physical examination (Ramasubbam, 1990).

Feelings of "verguenza", or shame, and their influence on attendance at family planning clinics, were examined by Scrimshaw in detail (1973). Many of the women interviewed in Guayaquil, Ecuador, who never undressed completely before their husbands, were forced to expose themselves to male doctors at the clinic without even a drape over their legs during the pelvic exam. With a drape, at least, the woman cannot see the doctor and has some illusion of privacy.

Moroccan women report feeling inhuman when they are ordered to take off their pants and sit in a drafty hall where people walk by while they are waiting to see the service provider for family planning (Mernissi, 1975). This study, the Scrimshaw work also from the 1970s and a much earlier study by Stycos in Puerto Rico (1955) gave serious scientific attention to a subject that is still acutely and universally felt by women, still a grave problem and still for the most part ignored.

> *. . . when men are infected, their wives are suspected of infidelity; when women are infected, they are assumed to have strayed...*

Sexual Inequality and Stigma

Restrictions on travel, fear of pelvic examination and violation of the sense of personal privacy are formidable barriers in themselves, without the added stigma of a sexually-related infection. An association of STIs and promiscuity, references to sexually transmitted infections as the woman's disease in popular parlance in some languages and common use of the term reservoirs of infection to describe prostitutes place the onus solely on the female, regardless of the male's multiple relationships. Research in Zaire found that when men are infected, their wives are suspected of infidelity; when women are infected, they are assumed to have strayed (Schoepf, cited in Bledsoe, 1989:11). The image of women as the source of disease is reinforced by the media and public health announcements, as in the Zambian advertisement: —Avoid AIDS. Take Time to Know Her (Bledsoe, 1989:11).

Counseling women about prevention and the need for treatment of their partners may presume incorrectly that they are free to discuss sex and condom use without jeopardy. Discussion of this emotionally charged topic is rare in many cultures. A survey of spousal communication in Asian countries, for example, found that close to one third of the women interviewed in the Philippines never talked to their husbands about sexual matters, nor did 47 per cent in Singapore or 53 per cent in Iran (UNESCAP, 1974). In sub-Saharan Africa, sexual activities are rarely discussed either between spouses or between the generations (Caldwell et al., 1989). In Latin American culture, communication between men and women (or parents and children) regarding sex is not the norm (Worth and Rodriguez, 1987; Santos Ortiz, 1990). In a study of decision-making on the use of family planning in Mexico, 35 per cent of the survey sample had never discussed the subject of birth control with their spouse (Folch-Lyon, 1981). In focus groups, women expressed the difficulties they experienced in any discussion of sexual relations with their husbands. Castro de Alvarez (1990) observed that cultural norms in their patriarchal society dictate that Latin American women appear naive about sexual matters and that a woman knowledgeable about and prepared for a sexual encounter is considered loose. It is thus very difficult to realize the necessary conditions for promoting condom use and persuading a partner to be treated for a sexually transmitted infection. They are: relative sexual equality between men and women; the possibility that other sex partners can be acknowledged; and options other than motherhood to define self-identity or self esteem (Worth, 1989).

When there is no communication about sex, and when women fear that their relationships will be jeopardized by asking for safe sex practices, promotion of condom use among women is likely to fail.

When there is no communication about sex, and when women fear that their relanonships will be jeopardized by asking for safe sex practices, promotion of condom use among women is likely tofail. The anger at being made to feel responsible for men's sexual behaviour expressed by women in a New York City study probably has near universal application. Women claimed men decide what is going to happen sexually and that if the staff wanted men to wear condoms, they would have to talk to them, not to women (Worth, 1989). Prevention strategies that place the onus on women ignore the subordinate position of the many who are economically and emotionally dependent on their male sexual partners. For these women, negotiation, even perhaps discussion, is not an option (Maldonado, 1991).

Among the socio-cultural and psychological constraints to overcome in promoting condom use in Zaire are strong beliefs and feelings about the contribution of semen to women' s health and the importance of reproduction (Schoepf et. al, 1988). The decision to use a condom is a decision not to reproduce as well as not become infected. The general use of condoms may. therefore, be in direct conflict with the desire of women to fulfill their reproductive roles and with the expectations of their partners and families that they do so. It is also a decision that must be made for each act of intercourse. Women must repeatedly address the issue of sexual decision-making and sexual control, and each time this is done they are emotionally, sexually, physically and economically vulnerable (Worth, 1989).

SUMMARY AND RECOMMENDATIONS

The causes of damage to the epithelial barrier that allows vaginal transmission of HIV are numerous: sexually transmitted infections insertion of objects into the vagina, trauma during sexual intercourse and genital mutilation practices, among others. Obstacles to prevention. diagnosis and treatment are also numerous. Most are embedded in the cultural and economic context of women's lives and can be overcome only with concerted effort at the level of both local communities and the national health systems. These issues must be given priority in national and international research and aid agendas.

Recommendations in this section are given with the caution that a change in women' s knowledge. and behaviour is necessary but women alone do not carry the responsibility for prevention of HIV transmission. Men, in their political and economic positions of power as well as in their sexual partnerships, are responsible for change, as it is women's subordination -lack of control over their bodies and their lives — that is the primary HIV risk factor (Hamblin and Reid, 1991; Carovano, 1990).

Community Level

On the level of the local community, the starting point for education of women and men is the message that women's health is important for reasons other than childbearing. Knowledge about their bodies ability to speak of sexual organs and processes without shame, hygienic practices (especially as regards menstruation) and signs and symptoms of genital-urinary problems must be communicated through social networks in the community. By whatever means, women must be helped to talk of these things together in their own-idiom, without embarrassment, and to help each other devise strategies for raising these issues with men. Men must be helped to be at ease speaking of their own and women's sexuality, with each other and with women, candidly and not crudely. Role models must come forth who in their knowledge of and attitudes toward women can redefine the masculine image.

> *Women's groups are a near universal resource and women can use them to learn to speak of their bodies, sexuality and genital health in their own way, according to their own customs.*

Knowledge about sexuality and reproductive biology is transmitted by older experienced women, in many societies, especially where social separation of sexes emphasizes communication between women rather than between partners (Newman, 1985). The local setting may suggest other rules for discussion of sexually-related matters, as in Tunisia where women never speak of family planning with their daughters or with anyone of a different age group (Huston, 1978). Women's groups are a near universal resource and women can use them to learn to speak of their bodies, sexuality and genital health in their own way, according to their own customs.

Preferences for local, familiar and predictable midwifery services for childbirth suggest that traditional midwives can play an important role in developing awareness of threats to genital health and the ability to recognize symptoms of STIs and in providing advice on resources for treatment. Training TBAs for safe delivery and health education is a fairly widespread practice. Although the trainers usually discourage midwives from performing internal examinations, in order to avoid infections, and their curricula do not usually cover sexually transmitted infections and other genital conditions, midwives can be trained to ask about symptoms, to advise and, when linked to a health service system, to refer women for diagnosis and treatment.

Research on traditional medicine rarely examines conditions other than pregnancy that motivate women to seek care. However, evidence generally supports the view that traditional practice is popular and addresses a broad range of women' s conditions. Traditional medicine co-exists with modern medical practice, and it is not uncommon for consultations with both systems to occur serially or concurrently (Janzen, 1978; Cosminsky and Scrimshaw, 1980; Heggenhougen, 1980; Green and Makhubu, 1984; Cleland and van Ginneken, 1988; Good, 1988; Ingstad, 1990).

In Malaysia for example two traditional systems (Ayurvedic and Chinese) and the local Malay folk medical system, accepted as parts of general Malaysian culture and society, are linked to the official health system and used widely as additions or alternatives to modern medical practices (Heggenhougen, 1980). A Guatemalan plantation population can have simultaneous access to folk curers (curanderos), herbalists, midwives, spiritists, shamans, injectionists, pharmacists, private physicians, public and private clinics and hospitals and home remedies (Cosminsky and Scrimshaw, 1980). Good (1988) estimates that most African rural areas have at least one part-time traditional healer for every 200 to 300 persons; in the towns, there is one healer for every 400 to 800 persons. In Swaziland. at least 85 per cent of the population is believed to make use of the services of traditional healers (Green and

Makhubu, 1984). Many of these opinion leaders and therapists are female. While the role of traditional healers in communicating information on genital health and its protection is not universal, they are an ubiquitous and influential resource.

Health Systems

Strengthening health service systems for prevention and treatment of genital infections and other conditions must be a major national and international priority that should go beyond traditional categories of service. The narrow focus of public health programmes concerned with women is apparent in their labeling as maternal and child health services. The rationale for this lies in the belief that improving women's health is an important precondition to child health. A recent variation on this reasoning focuses on the woman as a potential transmitter of HIV to her infant and as a caregiver to people with HIV infection and related illness and orphaned children.

Health systems reflect this limited view of women's lives and potential and the pervasive gender inequalities which deny women control over their own bodies. Expansion of the concept of women's health to encompass the breadth of their activities and concerns is an immediate public health responsibility. Grants for study and research, support for networks of organizations, forums, training, policy analysis, advocacy and new and improved programmes are all required to bring attention to the restrictions on the health services women are now offered. These health services are restrictive both because they are difficult of access in many areas and because they respond only to a narrow range of women's health needs.

Prenatal services provide a good opportunity for health care workers to counsel women on protection of the genital tract and to diagnose and treat genital-urinary tract infections. Training of clinical personnel to be alert to adverse genital conditions is necessary; equally necessary are respect for the patients' sense of inappropriate or shameful exposure and care to ensure privacy to the maximum degree possible. Screens constructed from local materials, drapes made from local cloths—to shield exposed areas, minimum time without full clothing—these are in themselves indications of concern for feelings as well as relatively simple measures to make services more acceptable to women. Increasing the supply of female medical personnel on all levels is essential. In the prevailing absence of educational opportunities for women from the earliest grades through university degrees, more women must be given scholarships.

Much of the work needed does not require advanced training and extensive employment. In-service training of local women in health centres and in the community can reduce barriers while extending the availability of services. Primary health care and family planning services have amply demonstrated the value of recruiting and training paramedical personnel from the local population. If there is genuine community participation, especially of women's organizations, in facility and service planning, then needs, perceptions, problems and expectations can be freely expressed, respected and addressed.

Family planning providers can lead the formal sector in exploring how health services can reduce the institutional obstacles women encounter. Their programmes could provide services for diagnosis and treatment of genital lesions, inflammations and infections, and could be the only available source of health care for sexually active women, especially poor women. Functions that would be relatively easy to integrate into family planning services, given appropriate training and supplies and a commitment to genital as well as reproductive health are as follows: substituting modern contraceptives for objects damaging to the vagina (which will also diminish their use as abortifacients); educating women and men about risks; and diagnosing, treating and counseling sex partners.

The scarcity of resources for health care in developing countries is glaringly evident. There is a shortage of laboratories and supplies for diagnosis, as well as medication for treatment of STIs. In the shorter term, rapid expansion of laboratory testing is not feasible. However, it is possible to develop and subsidize distribution of supplies for inexpensive, relatively simple diagnostic techniques using cervical swabs, vaginal KOH odor and dipstick assessment of vaginal pH, as demonstrated in a study of reproductive tract infections in Bangladesh (Wasserheit, et al., 1989). As appropriate tests are developed, the health systems must undergo the changes necessary to put them to use.

Research and Aid Agendas

Priorities for research and development assistance are not easily set for a topic so seldom examined in its personal and social complexity. It is urgent that technological advances be made to develop and provide inexpensive diagnostic tests for women in developing countries. Female providers in traditional and modern sectors must be trained to educate, diagnose and treat. Their work should be evaluated through operations research.

The dilemma, or paradox, of condom use as the main strategy to prevent women from contracting HIV stems, of course, from the fact that it is a strategy for men. Since it can not be used when the male is dominant and resistant, alternative means of mechanical or chemical barrier protection must be found quickly, they must be distributed widely at little or no cost and they must have appeal to women.

> *A vaginal virucide which would offer protection against transmission without preventing conception is vital for women who desire children and who need to have them in societies where their status and economic security depend upon procreation.*

Spermicides and diaphragms shift the focus of control over prevention to the woman, a preference demonstrated by women who were given the choice in studies in Cameroon and Ghana (Spieler, 1990) and Rwanda (Allen et.al., 1988). Barriers that depend on the woman alone may be less effective than condoms, yet more effective in the long run if they are consistently and widely used and the condom is not (Stein, 1990). Laboratory and clinical studies indicate that vaginal spermicidal contraceptives which place a chemical barrier between infected fluids and vulnerable mucous membranes offer women considerable protection against STIs (see North, 1990, for a literature review), although use with a condom is more certain. Nonoxynol-9 (N-9), the most widely used spermicide, has been tested as an HIV virucide and laboratory findings suggest that it offers some protection. However, it has not been determined whether spermicides alone, without any mechanical barriers, protect against HIV infection (Cates and Stone, in press). Problems encountered in interpreting results of clinical studies have stemmed from a research focus on special populations (e.g. prostitutes with rates of sexual activity far exceeding the general population) and confounding factors such as use of N-9 with a vaginal sponge, which could itself cause microlesions or irritation from high concentrations of N-9 (Gollub. 1991). Female condoms (e.g., pouches made of polyurethane or latex) are being tested although they are not now in a form that is likely to have wide acceptability.

A vaginal virucide which Would offer protection against transmission without preventing conception is vital for women who desire children and who need to have them in societies where their status and economic security depend upon procreation (Stein, 1990). A promising avenue for the research is the possibility that concentrations of N-9 lower than recommended as a spermicide may be effective as a virucide (Stein and Gollub, 1991). The urgency of the need to investigate this and other virucides and the necessity for rapid development of a method women can use to protect themselves cannot be overstated.

The literature on the possible association of female mutilation with HIV transmission is sparse and speculative. Infections of the mutilated area, trauma caused by sexual intercourse, and blood transfusions necessitated by excessive bleeding at childbirth are plausible reasons. The universality of the practice in some African regions suggests that there may be a group of women at risk of infection of appalling dimensions as the epidemic expands geographically. A vigorous investigation of the relationship between female mutilation and HIV transmission must be undertaken.

Societal Transformations

> *Collectively, women are developing strategies to stand up to the official systems, to change men 's behaviour and to realize the strength of unity for survival. They must be assisted with information, with legal aid, with health services and with opportunities for education and economic independence. A woman 's lack of control over the resources for her own physical and mentul health and well-being is a violation of human rights that constitutes a direct threat to her life.*

The place of women in society is a primary cause of exposure to risk of HIV infection and a primary barrier to use of health services. Some of the consequences of this role of women are: little or no information; restrictions on movement outside the local community; fear of strange environments that are often with justification perceived as hostile; and the role of the men as mediators between women and the health system. The changes that must be made in the legal, economic and cultural spheres over the long term are immense and must be made largely by those who are favoured by the present inequities.

Yet over the short term there are collective actions women can take in their local communities. Women working together are learning to develop strategies for communication with their sexual partners about HIV, sexually transmitted infections, use of condoms and other sexual behaviours, finding as well the courage and determination to face opposition. Collectively, women are developing strategies to stand up to the official systems, to change men's behaviour and to realize the strength of unity for survival. They must be assisted with information, with legal aid, with health services and with opportunities for education and economic independence. A woman's lack of control over the resources for her own physical and mental health and wellbeing is a violation of human rights that constitutes a direct threat to her life.

REFERENCES

Adebajo, Christine Olufunke (1989). "Traditional practices that are harmful to health." Paper presented at a meeting of the Inter African Consultative Expert Group on the Possible Link between Traditional Practices and the Transmission of HIV. Addis Ababa, Ethiopia. 911 May.

Ahmed, Samira Amin and E. Haj Hamad M. Kheir (1990). "Sudanese sexual behaviour in the context of socio-cultural norms and the transmission of HIV." Paper presented at the IUSSP Seminar on Anthropological Studies Relevant to the Sexual Transmission of HIV. Sonderborg, Denmark, 19-22 November.

Allan, Susan et al., (1988). "Acceptability of condoms and spermicides in a population based sample of urban Rwandan women." IV International Conference on AIDS. Stockholm, Sweden, 12-16 June. Book 1, 1989:349, Abstract 5137.

Ampofo, E. Kofi et. al., (1990). "Risk factors of vesico-vaginal fistula in Maiduguri, Nigeria: a case control study." *Tropical Doctor*, July. pp. 138-139.

Auerbach, Liesa S. (1982). "Childbirth in Tunisia: implications of a decision-making model.' *Social Science and Medicine* 16. pp .1499- 1506.

Beck, Diane et al ., (1991) . American College of Nurse-Midwives. Personal Communication. May .

Beeson, Diane et al., (1987). "Client-provider transactions in family planning clinics." In *Organizing for Effective Family Planning Programmes,* edited by Robert J. Lapham and George B. Simmons. Washington, D.C. National Academy Press, pp.435-456.

Belsey, Mark A. (1980). "Infertility: etiology and natural history." *In Workshop on the diagnosis and treatment of infertility,* Nairobi, Kenya, 21-22 February 1979, edited by P.J. Rowe and S.R. Raharinosy-Ramarozaka. Bath, England. Pitman Press, pp.11-42.

Berlin, Elois Ann (1985). "Aspects of fertility regulation among the Aguaruna Jivaro of Peru. In *Women's medicine: a cross-cultural study of indigenous fertility regulation,* edited by Lucile F . Newman . New Brunswick, N .J . Rutgers University Press, pp .125- 146.

Bledsoe, Caroline (1989). "The cultural meaning of AIDS and condoms for stable heterosexual relations in Africa recent evidence from the local print media." Paper presented at the IUSSP Seminar on Population Policy in Sub-saharan Africa: Drawing on International Experience, Kinshasa. 27 February - March 2.

Browner, C.H. (1985). "Traditional techniques for diagnosis, treatment and control of pregnancy in Cali, Colombia." In *Women's medicine: A cross-Cultural study of indigenous fertility regulation*, edited by Lucile F. Newman. New Brunswick, N.J. Rutgers University Press, pp. 99-123.

Caldwell, John C., Pat Caldwell, and Pat Quiggin (1989). "The social context of AIDS in sub-Saharan Africa." *Population and Development Review* 15(2) pp.185-234.

Carovano, Kathryn (1990). "More than mothers and whores: redefining the AIDS prevention needs of women." *International Journal of Health Services* 21(1)pp.131-142.

Castro de alvarez, Virginia (1990). "AIDS prevention programme for Puerto Rican women." *Puerto Rican Health Science Journal 9*(1)pp.37-41.

Cates, Jr., Willard and Katherine M. Stone (1992). "Reproductive Tract Infections and Contraceptive Use. Safely." In *Reproductive Tract Infections in the Third World: National and International Policy Implications*, edited by A. Germaine, K. Holmes, P. Piot, J. Wasserheit. New York. Plenum Press, in press.

Chayovan, Napaporn, Peerasit Kamnuansilpa, and John Knodel (1988). Thailand Demographic and Health Survey 1987. Bangkok. Institute of Population Studies, Chulalongkorn University and Demographic and Health Surveys, Institute for Resource Development/Westinghouse. May

Cleland, John G. and Jerome K. Van Ginneken (1988). "Maternal education and child survival in developing countries: the search for pathways of influence." *Social Science and Medicine* 27(12)pp.1357-1368.

Cook, Robert (1987) . " Current knowledge and future trends in maternal and child health in the Middle East." *Journal of Tropical Pediatrics,* 3 (Suppl. 4) pp. 3-10.

Cosminsky, Sheila and Mary Scrimshaw (1980). "Medical pluralism on a Guatemalan plantation." *Social Science and Medicine,* 14B, November, pp. 267-278.

Dallabetta, Gina et al.. (1990). "Vaginal tightening agents as risk factors for acquisition of HIV." VI International Conference on AIDS, San Francisco California, 20-24 June 1990. Vol .1, p. 268, Abstract No. TH .C. 574.

Dixon-Mueller, Ruth and Judith Wasserheit (1991). *The Culture of Silence: Reproductive Tract Infections Among Women in the Third World.* New York. International Women' s Health Coalition.

Feldman, Douglas A. (1990). "Sexual practices in traditional Africa: planning for culturally appropriate HIV-related interventions." Unpublished. p.19 pages.

Folch-Lyon, Evelyn, Luis de la Macorra, and S. Bruce Schearer (1981). "Focus group and survey research on family planning in Mexico." *Studies in Family Planning* 12(12) pp. 409-432.

Frank, Odile (1983). *Infertility in sub-Saharan Africa.* Center for Policy Studies Working Papers, No. 97, June. New York, The Population Council.

Ghana Statistical Service and Institute for Resource Developmenti Macro Systerns, Inc., (1989). *Ghana Demographic and Health Survey 1988.* Columbia, Maryland. Ghana Statistical Service and Institute for Resource Development/Macro Systems, Inc., September.

Gollub, Erica (1991) . School of Public Health. Columbia University and HIV Center for Clinical and Behavioural Studies, New York State Psychiatric Institute. Personal communication, June.

Good, Charles (1988). "Traditional healers and AIDS management." In *AIDS in Africa: the social and policy impact,* edited by Norman Miller and Richard C. Rockwell. Lewiston, NY, Edwin Mellen (published in association with the African-Caribbean Institute and the National Council for International Health), pp.87-95.

Gordon, Daniel (1991). "Female circumcision and genital operations in Egypt and the Sudan: a dilemma for medical anthropology." *Medical Anthropology Quarterly* 5(1) pp. 3-23.

Green, Edward C. and Lydia Makhubu (1984). "Traditional healers in Swaziland: toward improved co-operation between the traditional and modern health sectors." Social Science and Medicine 18(12)pp.1071-1079.

Guatemala Ministerio de Salud Publica y Asistencia Social (1989). *Encuesta nacional de salud materno infantil 1987.* Columbia. Maryland. Instituto de Nutricion de Centro America y Panama and Institute for Resource Development/Westinghouse, May.

Hamblin, Julie and Elizabeth Reid (1991). "Women, the HIV epidemic and human rights: a tragic imperative." Paper prepared for the International Workshop on "AIDS: A Question of Rights and Humanity, International Court of Justice, The Hague, May.

Hatcher, Robert A. et al., (1989). *Contraceptive Technology: International Edition.* Atlanta. GA., Printed Matter, Inc.

Heggenhougen, H K. (1980). "Bomohs. doctors and sinsehs—medical pluralism in Malaysia." *Social Science and Medicine* 14B, pp. 235-244.

Holmes, Kino K. et al. (eds), (1984). *Sexually transmitted diseases.* New York. McGraw Hill.

Hunte, Pamela A. (1985). " Indigenous methods of fertility regulation in Afghanistan." In *Women's Medicine: a Cross-Cultural Study of Indigenous Fertility Regulation,* edited by Lucile F. Newman, New Brunswick. N.J., Rutgers University Press, pp.43-75.

Huston, Perdita (1978). *Message from the village.* New York, The Epoch B. Foundation.

Ingstad, Benedicte (1990). " The cultural construction of AIDS and its consequences for prevention in Botswana." *Medical Anthropology Quarterly* 4(1) pp. 28-40.

Janzen, John M. (1978). *The Quest for Therapy: Medical Pluralism in Lower Zaire.* Berkeley, University of California Press.

Kerns, Virginia (1989). *Women and the Ancestors: Black Carib Kinship and Ritual.* Urbana and Chicago, University of Illinois Press.

Kloos, Helmut et al., (1987). "Illness and health behavior in Addis Ababa and rural central Ethiopia. " *Social Science and Medicine* 25(9) pp.1003-1019.

Low, Setha M. and Bruce C. Newman (1985). "Indigenous fertility regulating methods in Costa Rica." In *Women's Medicine: A Cross-Cultural Stud} of Indigenous Fertility Regulation,* edited by Lucile F. Newman. New Brunswic};, N.J., Rutgers University Press, pp.147-160.

Maldonado—Nugyekuba (1991). "Latinas and HIV/AIDS." *SIECUS Report* December 1990/January 1991. pp .11-15.

Marshall, John (1973). "Fertility regulating methods: cultural acceptability for potential adopters." In *Fertility control methods: strategies for introduction,* edited by G.W. Duncan et al. New York, Academic Press, pp. 125-132.

Mcfalls, Joseph A. and Marguerite Harvey McFalls (1984). *Disease and Fertility* New York, Academic Press.

Mernissi, Fatima (1975). "Obstacles to family planning practice in urban Morocco." *Studies in Family Planning* 6(12) . pp .418-425.

Molyneaux, John W. et al., (1990). "Correlates of contraceptive method choice in Indonesia. Population studies in Sri Lanka and Indonesia based on the 1987 Sri Lankan Demographic and Health Survey and the 1987 National Indonesian Contraceptive Prevalence Survey. The Population Council and Demographic and Health Surveys, Institute for Resource Development, Demographic and Health Surveys Further Analysis Series, No. 2, March.

Newman, Lucille F. (1985). "Context variables in fertility regulation." *In Women's Medicine. a Cross-Cultural Study of Indigenous Fertility Regulation,* edited by Lucile F. Newman. New Brunswick, N. J., Rutgers University Press, pp.179-191.

Ngin, Chor-Swang (1985). "Indigenous fertility regulating methods among two Chinese communities in Malaysia." In *Women's medicine: a cross-cultural study of indigenous fertility regulation,* edited by Lucile F. Newman. New Brunswick, N.J., Rutgers University Press. pp. 25-41.

North, Barbara B. (1990). "Effectiveness of vaginal contraceptives in prevention of sexually transmitted diseases." In *Heterosexual transmission of AIDS,* edited by Nancy J. Alexander et al. New York, Wiley-Liss, pp.273-290.

Orubuloye, I.O., John C. Caldwell and Pat Caldwell (1990). "Sexual networking and the risk of AIDS in southwest Nigeria." Paper delivered at the IUSSP Seminar on Anthropological Studies Relevant to the Sexual Transmission of HIV. Sonderborg, Demnar;. 19-22 November.

Oxtoby, Margaret J. and Helene D. Gayle (1990). "AIDS in women and children." *Outlook* 8(4)pp .2-6.

Peterman, Thomas A. (1990). "Facilitators of HIV transmission during sexual contact." In *Heterosexual transmission of AIDS,* edited by Nancy J. Alexander et al. New York, Wiley-Liss, pp. 55-68.

Ramasubban, Radhika (1990). "Sexual behaviour and conditions of health care: potential risks for HIV transmission in India." Paper prepared for the IUSSP Seminar on Anthropological Studies Relevant to HIV Transmission, Sonderborg, 19-22 November.

Rehan. Nagma (1984). "Knowledge, attitude and practice of family planning in Hausa women *Social Science and Medicine* 18 (10) pp. 839-844.

Reid, Elizabeth. Women, HIV and Development. Paper presented to the Conference on the implications of AIDS for Mothers and Children, Paris, 27-30 November 1989.

Reid, Elizabeth. "Young Women and the HIV Epidemic". *Development,* (Journal of the Society of International Development), No. 1, 1990, p. 16.

Santos-Ortiz, Maria del Carmen (1990). "Sexualidad femenina antes y despues del SIDA." *Puerto Rican Health Science Journal* 9(1)pp.33-35.

Sayed, Hussein A. et al., (1989). *Egypt Demographic and Health Survey 1988.* Cairo, Egypt, National Population Council and Institute for Resource Development/Macro Systems Inc., October.

Schoepe, Brooke Grundfest (1988) . ' AIDS and society in Central Africa: a view from Zaire. " in *AIDS in Africa: The Social and Policy* Impact, edited by Norman Miller and Richard C. Rockwell. Lewiston, NY, Edwin Mellen (published in association with the African-Caribbean Institute and the National Council for International Health), pp. 211-235.

Scheler, S. et al., (1985). "Barriers to Effective Family Planning in Nepal." Studies in Family Planning, 6(5) pp.) 260-270.

Scrims Law, Susan, C. (1973). *Lo de Nosotras: Pudor and Family Planning Clinics in a Latin American City.* New York. International Institute for the Study of Human Reproduction. January.

Shedlin. Michele G. (1982). *Anthropolog and Family Planning: Culturally Appropriate Interventions in a Maxican Community.* Ph.D. Dissertation, Columbia University.

Shedlin Michele, G. and Paula Hollerbach (1981). "Modern and traditional fertility regulation in a Mexican community: the process of decision making." *Studies in Family Planning* 12(6/7) June. July, pp. 278-296.

SHERRIS. Jacqueline D. and Gordon Fox (1983). "Infertility and sexually transmited disease: a public health challenge." *Population Reports*. Series L, No. 4, July (reprinted July 1985).

Sittitrai, Weerasit, Rapeepan Sujaritraksa, and Anchalee Wisuttimak (1989). "AIDS education materials for Thai commercial sex workers; preliminary report." Center for AIDS Research and Education. Science Division, Thai Red Cross Society, January.

Soko to Meternal Health Project (1990). "Report of planning activities." Usmanu Danfodiyo University Sokoto. and Ministry of Health Sokoto, Report of maternal health project for prevention of maternal mortality June.

Spieler. Jeffrey M. (1990). "Summary discussion" (remarks of Dr. Lamptey). In *Heterosexual transmission of AIDS* edited by Nancy J. Alexander et al. New York, Wiley-Liss. pp.419-426.

Stein, Zena A. (1990). "HIN prevention: the need for methods women can use." *American Journal of Public Health* 80. pp.460-462.

———and Erica Gollub (1991). Testimony submitted to the National Commission on AIDS. Denver. Colorade. 5 June.

Stock. Robert (1983) Distance and utilization of health facilities in rural Niveria." *Social Science and Medicine* 1 7(9) pp.563-570.

Stycos, J.M. (1955). "Birth control clinics in crowded Puerto Rico." In *Health, Culture and Community*. edited by Benjamin D. Paul. New York, Russell Sage Foundation, pp.189, 210.

Sukkary-Stolba, Soheir (1985). "Indigenous fertility regulating methods in two Egyptian villages." In *Women's Medicine: a Cross-Cultural Study of Indigenous Fertility Regulation,* edited by Lucile F. Newman. New Brunswick, N.J., Rutgers University Press, pp.78-97.

Tahzib, Farhanq (1989). "An initiative on vesicovaginal fistula." *Lancet* June 10, pp. l316, 1317.

Traore, Baba, Mamadou Donate, and Cynthia Stanton (1989). *Enquete demographique et de sante au Mali 1987.* Columbia, Maryland: Centre d'Etudes et de Recherches sur la Population pour le Developement, Institut du Sahel and Institute for Resource Development/Westinghouse, January.

Twumasi, P.A. (1987). "Traditional Birth Attendant Review Programme in Ghana." Commissioned by Ghana Ministry of Health. October.

United Nations (1991). *The World's Women 1970-1990: Trends and Statistics.* New York United Nations Publications, Sales No. E.90.XV11.3.

United Nations Economic and Social Comission for Asia and the Pacific (UNESCAP) (1974). "Husband-wife communication and practice of family planning." *Asia Population Studies Series. Bangkok.* 16, pp .26-27.

Wasserheit, Judith N. (1989). "The significance and scope of reproductive tract infections among third world women." *International Journal of Gynecology and Obstetrics* Suppl. 3 pp.145-168.

———(1990) . " Reproductive Tract Infections . "In *Special Challenges in Third World Women's Health.* Presentations at the 117th Annual Meeting of the American Public Health Association, Chicago, October 1989. New York, International Women's Health Coalition, March, pp. l-15.

———et al., (1989). "Reproductive tract infections in a family planning population in rural Bangladesh." *Studies in Family Planning* 20(2)pp.69-80.

Wilson, D.P., C.S. Lavelle, and C. Mutero (1989). "Sex workers, client sex behaviour and condom use in Harare, Zimbabwe." *AIDS Care* 1(3) pp. 269-280.

Women's International Network (n.d.). "Women and health summary facts: genital and sexual mutilation of females (1)." *News.* Lexington, Maine.

World Health Organization (WHO) (1989). "WHO consensus statement: sexually transmitted diseases as a risk factor for HIV transmission." *Journal of Sex Research* 26(2) pp. 272-275.

———(1990). Consensus statement from the consultation on global strategies for co-ordination of AIDS and STD control programmes, Geneva, World Health Organization, WHO/INF/90.2.

World Health Organization/Global Programme on AIDS (WHO/GPA) (1990). *AIDS Prevention: Guidelines for MCH/FP Programme Managers. II. AIDS and Maternal and Child Health.* Geneva, World Health Organization, May, WHO/MCH/GPA/90.2.

Worth, Dooley (1989). "Sexual decision-making and AIDS: why condom promotion among vulnerable women is likely to fail." *Studies in Family Planning* 20(6)pp.297-307.

———and Ruth Rodriguez (1987). "Latina Women and AIDS." *SIECUS Report* January-February. pp.5-7.

Zabin, Laurie Schwab and Samuel D. Clark Jr. (1981). "Why the delay: a study of teenage family planning clinic patients." *Family Planning Perspectives* 13(5) September/October, pp.205-217.

27

Sharing the Challenge of the HIV Epidemic

Ms. Elizabeth Reid
UNDP, New York

Conceptual Complexity

There are two important characteristics of the HIV epidemic which need to be acknowledged and understood, by national leaders in particular, for they will affect and determine the nature of the response to the epidemic in the Asian and Pacific region.

Firstly, the epidemic is at one and the same time both a crisis and an endemic condition. It is a crisis because the speed of spread of this virus can be so awesome. Infection rates can, and have even in this region, increased from two per cent to 25 per cent in adult populations in less than four years. There is no reason to assume that this is not happening in this region. Before people are even aware that they are surrounded by infected family and friends, their communities have been deeply penetrated. This fact alone should be sufficient for the epidemic to be viewed as a calamity, albeit too often invisible in its early stages, as much in need of an immediate response as the invasion of one country by another. For war nowadays rarely has the toll in human lives that this virus is causing and will cause.

That it is an endemic condition may best be simply illustrated by the fact that even if in an affected country there were to be no further cases of infection as from today, the pain and trauma of the deaths of those already infected will continue for the next twenty years and the social and economic repercussions of their deaths will continue on for decades and generations after that. We know that nowhere in the world is the spread abating or even slowing down. Each day of continuing spread adds to the ramifications and duration of its devastating impact.

Both dimensions, the epidemic as crisis and the epidemic as

endemic, need to be recognized. leach has its own appropriate responses.

Secondly, the epidemic manifests itself both as a specific problem but also as a pervasive one. Its specificity is revealed in its associated morbidity and mortality, in increasing numbers of people, mostly healthy, productive young women and men, getting sick and dying. The response of the first decade of the epidemic addressed this quality of the epidemic. It focused on the epidemic as a health crisis and on its ramifications for health service delivery.

However, the repercussions of these deaths will permeate and affect every facet of human life and national development, more so in countries where men and women are infected in more or less the same numbers. The causes and the consequences of the spread of the virus embrace poverty and wealth, disempowerment and influence, wellbeing and disease, deprivation and development, trust and bad faith; the very way we are as human beings.

Both of these dimensions of the epidemic, its particularity and its ubiquity, must also be recognized. Each of these too has its own appropriate responses.

Thus this epidemic is conceptually complex: at once a crisis and an endemic condition; at once a specific issue and a permeating one.

Programme Imperatives

These two characteristics of the HIV epidemic impose a set of imperatives upon us:

the imperative of an effective response;
the imperative of a sustainable response; and
the imperative of a co-ordinated response.

The prerequisite of an effective response is a common understanding of the nature of the epidemic, which takes into account the above two characteristics, and a shared vision of the way forward. This we do not yet have. This should not surprise us for the epidemic is a new and complex phenomenon for which there is no likeness in living memory, not one drawn from war, not from disease, not from natural disasters nor from man-made ones.

This is not to say that we are blindly groping. We are doing what we know needs to be done while we search for new and more effective ways to respond. The more we share a vision of an effective way forward, the more co-ordination and the building of partnerships will naturally follow.

The second imperative is that of a sustainable response. The commitment and contributions of affected individuals and communities have yet to be recognized or valued but they are extensive.

They lie at the heart of a sustainable response to this epidemic but in most cases they need to be supplemented by further human and financial resources. The closeness of these individuals and communities to the problems and needs created by the epidemic generally ensures that their responses are appropriate. Similarly, governments are increasingly beginning to allocate national resources to the epidemic although in most cases they still have to be persuaded that it affects all aspects of societal development both now and in the future.

The required human and financial resources must be available for effective responses. However, these responses must also be ranked in order of effectiveness since resources, whether of individuals, communities, nations or of external support agencies, will continue to be limited and will themselves be reduced by the epidemic.

Thus priority must be given to strengthening national capacity to ensure that these resources, and that of the external support agencies, are used in the most effective manner. There is not time and there are not sufficient resources for illconceived, inappropriate or ineffective responses. The selection must be ruthless for the demand on resources, both human and financial, will continue and increase inexorably for decades. Communities and governments must have the ability to monitor, assess and evaluate their interventions and to modify, redesign and expand them.

Where the response to the epidemic is effective and sustainable, hope is brought into being that the desolation and distress of this epidemic can be eased, a hope that can turn back the tides of fatalism and despair

The third imperative. that ot a co-ordinated response, means that we must build the partnerships required to ensure that the search for effective and sustainable policies and interventions is an ongoing process and that duplication is minimized. Such partnerships are needed among the community groups responding to the epidemic, between such groups and government, among government ministries, between the public and the private sectors, among external support agencies, especially within the UN system, and between donors and countries.

The Challenges to be Shared

Before we elaborate further on the partnerships required by this epidemic, we need to identify the challenges facing the Asian and Pacific region that we are being called upon to share.

I want to identify just three such challenges;

the challenge of making the invisible visible;

the challenge of creating an ethic of compassion; and
the challenge of placing people and their communities at the centre of the response to the epidemic.

The first challenge to make the invisible visible, is a clear imperative in this region. We must find the means to belter understand and make known the speed and the surreptitious patterns of spread of the virus. Surveillance systems tell us where the virus has been but we need predictive systems that map out for us where it is likely to go. Understanding the factors which determine this will enable us to put faces to the figures, to see ourselves in its path or in its wake.

But more than just numbers and silhouettes of those affected need to be made visible. Those living within the epidemic, those at the forefront of change, must create a new language that makes more visible the new realities of life in the post-HIV era.

This is already happening in two important aspects of the epidemic. Firstly, we are beginning to develop a language of optimism: affirmations of the possibility of behaviour change, of the centrality of compassion and concern, of care and commitment. Secondly, we are developing a language of process rather than of interventions, of people as responsible actors rather than manipulable objects. It is a language of empowerment, of participation, of listening and talking, of counselling of deciding together.

However, there is still a silence, an inarticulateness, about the dark side of the epidemic: the doubt, the trembling, the uncertainty, the distancing, the denial, the fear. We do not yet have a language that reflects the reality of living with the knowledge that one is infected or that someone one loves dearly is infected: the constant companion of mortality, the sadness, the tentativeness of desire, the longing for love, the stripping raw of self by death after death after death of partners, of children, of childhood friends, of companions.

There is another silence around a central reality of this epidemic: that it evokes a wilderness of emotional and psychological states with whose very existence we are uncomfortable, for which our vocabulary is too limited and which we are reluctant to acknowledge and express. These include hatred, anger, shame, guilt, humiliation, grief, indignity. There is a deep unease which permeates families and societies about using a language of sexuality, of mortality and of vulnerability.

Even those emotional states we value and which are central to our belief that the epidemic can be overcome, we hesitate to publicly acknowledge and express. We lack a familiarity of usage of words such as care, compassion, happiness, humility and wonder.

For that which is invisible about this epidemic to be made

visible we must spin this language, weave it into our lives and grow strong in the courage to use it.

The second challenge we face is to create an ethic of compassion. Let me begin by delineating what this is not. Compassion is not pity, which strips one of dignity and individuality. Compassion cannot be expressed in authoritarian relationships structurally based on inequalities of power: doctor and patient, men and women, parent and child, caste and class. For this reason an ethics of compassion will threaten conventions of distancing and objectivity, norms of control and domination, prerogatives of position and wealth.

An ethic of compassion will value concern over ambition, connectedness over individualism closeness over control mercy over judgment. An ethic of compassion will require the presence of men who pay attention to daily life.

An ethic of compassion is not a matter of appeasing hunger, of providing shelter, of resolving conflict. These are as compatible with charity or pragmatism as with compassion. Rather it involves seeing ourselves as one with others, our lives essentially intertwined with their lives.

An ethic of compassion will bring a particular focus to our work. It will add a sense of urgency to keeping people uninfected. It will place high importance on keeping those affected by the epidemic, the infected, those who love and care for them and those who survive them, within our families, workplace and communities.

Keeping those infected alive for as long as possible will be not only an economic imperative but also a human imperative for even when sick and dying, those infected can nurture their children, touching them smiling, talking, keeping them company and can pass on to them their own skills for economic survival, be they farming, brewing, fishing, street selling, cobbling weaving, repairing or whatever.

Helping those infected to die with dignity through, for example, the treatment of opportunistic infections or the provision of shelter and assistance, will reduce the psychological trauma of the children left behind. Their memories will be of the person they loved not of their unseemly condition.

The third challenge is that of placing people and their communities at the centre of the response to the epidemic.

Again this can be defined by contrast. It means that primary focus will not be placed on technologies (condoms, test kits, etc.) or on interventions (education campaigns, STD services, for example) but on the initiation of processes whereby both individuals and communities can change and through which agents of change are created. The technologies and interventions will become the handmaidens of, not the masters of, change, there to be called upon as required.

Placing people at the centre of the response to the epidemic will enable that response to reflect and build upon the complex nature of people's daily lives and to address their needs in a cohesive manner. It will begin the process of breaking down a compartmentalized development approach to essentially interlinked conditions: poverty, disempowerment, disease, subordination, illiteracy, land ownership, to mention a few, and HIV infection. It recognizes and accepts that little is simple in the face of this epidemic

An approach that values and builds on the vagaries of human life and human nature will lead to realistic and therefore sustainable responses. It will provide the basis for the hope. the belief, that we are not powerless in the face of this pathogen and that we will indeed overcome the epidemic and its consequences.

The most striking feature about this epidemic is that individuals and communities have been mobilized and empowered by it. People are speaking out; community groups are coming into existence. We see this already in this region. This conference has honoured Dominic de Souza. There are many other courageous men and women like him in our communities, speaking out, working with others. However, in a non-supportive environment, too often the impact of such individual initiatives wanes over time as people move on or die or groups lose their initial momentum.

The Partnerships to be Built

The energy, vision and commitment of these agents of change needs to be transformed into an active force for change, a force which can transcend the particular and permeate communities and nations. For this to happen, four social contracts or partnerships must be built.

The first partnership must be a new social contract between men and women.

The HIV epidemic and its impact will only be overcome if men and women begin to forge true partnerships of mutual respect and trust and of equitable sharing of the burdens of sadness, pain, care and support created by the epidemic. Men and women must seek to establish the kind of honest communication about sexuality and sexual behaviour needed to prevent the transmission of HIV in their partnerships. They must work to restructure the sexual relationships in which they take part.

Women alone cannot stop this epidemic nor care for its sick and its survivors. Women alone cannot bear the burden of its psychological, social and economic impact. Nor should this be expected of them. To do so would be to build in the certainty of failure. Not because of any failing in women, but because sexuality, love and coping are essentially shared experiences.

Changes in individual relationships between men and women will occur only in the context of the emergence of a new social contract, not one simply governing men's or women's behaviour, but one which changes what it is to be a man or a women. The social contract must encompass the way we nurture and raise our children. the way society constructs its gender archetypes. It must further allow for community explorations of the appropriateness of accepted community values and standards of behaviour. Such a social contract must be supported and reaffirmed by laws, policy budgetary priorities and programme design and delivery.

The family in all its diverse forms thus becomes the basic nexus of change. For although individual men and women can decide on ways to protect themselves from infection, the likelihood of this happening and being sustained resides in factors which long precede adulthood and sexual activity. They have their origin in how people are brought up in family life, whether that be an extended or nuclear family or another environment.

It is in the family context, from birth, that personalities are formed gender identity is created. moral values are instilled. In particular it is in families that boys are brought up to be boys and girls, girls, with their attendant sexual and social identities, attitudes and behaviours. We know that self respect, self confidence, respect for others and an ability to talk about personal and intimate matters are all characteristics which help people to remain uninfected.

Thus it is within family contexts that the basic prevention.strategies must be put into place. Love and nurturing must be given to both boys and girls so that they may grow into independent, confident human beings, able to form respectful and non-violent relationships, whatever their sexual orientation may be. Parental-child discourse must be developed on bodily care and sexuality and strengthened on community norms and moral values, especially with regard to respect for self and others. We must change the ways that girls and boys are raised so that as adults they will be less likely to put themselves and others at risk of infection This will require significant changes in the social construction of masculinity and femininity.

These gender paradigms must be reconstructed in particular ways. The new paradigms should lead to the greater valuing of compassion, concern for others and love of family in men and, for women, in a simple recognition of their value and worth. It is hard to reconcile the oft claimed valuing of women, even as mothers, with the widespread acceptance of female infanticide or the mortality rates associated with pregnancy and childbirth, as high as one woman in 21 in some parts of the world: 1 million women per year. New patterns for the sharing of the responsibilities and joys of women's lives must emerge.

But families individually do not determine cultural meanings, social customs or community values. They inherit, accept, respect and instil them. Thus, for families to change, communities and societies must also change. The new social contract will therefore require a radical reassessment by societies of the very way men and women see themselves and each other, of the way they relate as husband and wife, lovers, brothers and sisters, parent and child, as partners, colleagues and friends.

The second partnership must be a social contract between the affected and the not yet directly affected.

The infected and those close to them are amongst the most powerful agents of change in the world today. They can give us glimpses of how we can peacefully co-exist with the virus, of how we can become empowered through the trauma and the tragedy of the epidemic. Within the desolation of this epidemic, they give us snatches of laughter and happiness. They can help us explore and better understand the nature of intimacy, desire and sexuality in the age of the virus.

But these insights of the affected will not be shared, this gift will remain ungiven, if, in the sharing, the affected are stripped of their self esteem and dignity, subjected to humiliation and discrimination, left alone in a hostile limelight without support and companionship.

These insights, these glimpses of the world within the epidemic. must be shared if our response is to be grounded in human experience, if this experience and knowledge is to shape and reshape theory and practice.

The stories of the affected provide access to lives which are subtle and various, which present the experience of living within the epidemic in the complex, interrelated way life usually asserts itself. The stories bring to light different perspectives, different points of view and so make the understanding of how to live with the epidemic accessible across class, gender, educational and lifestyle barriers.

Women are more aware of the dynamics of gender in their daily lives. Thus how gender affects the epidemic emerges more clearly in their stories. Life situations such as being infected or caring for someone infected can be understood only if gender roles and interrelationships are taken into account. Women' s stories both present and interpret the dynamics of power between women and men and the relationship between the individual and society. They provide glimpses into men's lives as well as into women's lives and relate individual agency to social and economic structures.

Stories, however, do not capture systems of relationships which affect individuals but whose locus is beyond the individual and her or his realm of vision. The relationships between poverty and infection status may form a critical part of the story but the relationships between structural adjustment programmes, for example, poverty and the tragedy of being infected may not. Hence, stories need to be complemented by system level analyses. A full understanding of the nature and impact of the epidemic requires both kinds of analysis .

This partnership between the affected and their communities is critical. It is an acknowledgement within the community that the epidemic concerns the community as a whole and not just certain individuals perceived or assumed to be at risk. The absence of this social contact favours discrimination, marginalization, denial and infection. The Them/Us mentality which dominates in the absence of this partnership has, sadly, too often characterized perceptions of and responses to the epidemic. There is no other in the shadow of the epidemic. We are all there.

This second partnership or social contract, once in place, will enable the creation of a supportive milieu that encourages the affected to speak out. tell their stories, reflect on their lives and hopes and help us all to live peacefully with this epidemic.

The third social contract must be between communities and government.

The responses we have seen occurring within affected communities provide us with the hope that the epidemic can be overcome, and the insights into how this can come about. These responses are universal. Wherever the virus has spread, communities have responded, to provide care and support, to stop further infection, to assure the rights of the affected to minister to spiritual, emotional and physical needs.

But individuals, families and communities cannot carry this epidemic alone. There must be a social contract, a partnership, between governments and affected communities. Governments must provide an enabling environment that will evoke, nourish and sustain these responses. This enabling environment must include national policies that acknowledge the centrality of community responses, a body of legal and human rights laws that respect the principles of non-discrimination and respect for the rights and dignity of affected individuals, mechanisms for interaction between government and communities, and assistance, as required, for programme design, delivery and financing by communities.

The need for additional resources for this epidemic is frequently mentioned. Whilst it is clear that external resources are needed, it is important to stress that the initial financial resources mobilized to respond to this epidemic are invariably those of individuals, families and communities. As yet, these remain unrecognized and unquantified. We must name these contributions and quantify them for, sadly. this is the way that most people recognize and establish the value of such actions.

These resources—peoples' volunteered time, the food, means and insights they share, the transport provided, the labour contributed, the funds raised—lie at the heart of a sustainable response.

Yes, the resources must be supplemented. They are not without end. They themselves are depleted by the epidemic. They are not, always or usually. sufficient. Communities know what additional resources, human or financial, they need for sustenance and growth. They need to be empowered to be able to define their external support requirements, select them, manage them and account for them in appropriate ways whether these resources come from national or international sources.

Mutual trust and respect is a sine qua non for a social contract between communities and their government. This may not be easy for either but it must come about.

The fourth partnership must be a global contract.

As the epidemic deepens, its devastating potential impact on all aspects of human life and national development is becoming better understood. Certain nations may be brought towards the threshold of destitution. Will the world wait until this stage is reached in some countries? When will there be a global response? Will the world community provide the resources for investment in the education, health and social welfare of people and in the technological development required to enable these nations to continue to function? Will there be global social safety nets to allow nations rendered poor by this epidemic. and the poor within nations, to survive?

The working of global trade agreements and markets have increased the disparities between rich and poor nations and rich and poor individuals. At the national level, many governments try to offset such tendencies by redistributing income through systems of progressive income tax and by supplementing this with social safety nets to prevent people from falling into poverty and absolute destitution. No such systems exist at present at the global level.

The closest the world comes to a global safety net is the current system of development assistance. However, this system is fatally flawed, not only in the way it is programmed, but in the inadequacy of its extent, and because its allocation is unrelated to levels of poverty. Less than 7 per cent of global aid is spent on human priority concerns of basic education, primary health care, family planning, safe drinking water and nutritional programmes. Only a quarter of overseas aid flow is earmarked for the ten countries containing three-fourths of the world's absolute poor. In fact, India, Pakistan and Bangladesh contain nearly one-half of the world's poor but get only one-tenth of total aid.

Twice as much development assistance per capita is given to high military spenders among the developing world as to more moderate military spenders. The international financial institutions, like the World Bank and the IMF, are now taking more money out of the developing world than they are putting in, adding to the reverse transfer of around $50 billion per year to the commercial banks.

If overseas aid is to be able to serve as a social safety net for the world's poor, it will have to be based on principles requiring that aid should be directed to priority concerns for human survival and human development.

These four social contracts or partnerships are essential to an effective sustainable response to this epidemic. They will be difficult to forge and will not come about without the commitment and courage of our leaders and friends. There is an ever increasing urgency to embark upon the endeavour to build them.

The Way

At the heart of this epidemic, either there can be violence and fragmentation or there can be stillness. In the hearts of those yet personally untouched by it, it is the same. It is the same in the hearts of those affected.

For all of us, knowing how to live with HIV can bring a certain stillness to the centre of our lives. It can still the violence and the fragmentation the fear and the denial. It is this stillness which creates the possibility of living.

We need to reach out to each other, as one human being to another. There can be no Them and Us if this epidemic is to be overcome. We are all seeking to pass from untruth to truth, from darkness to light, from vulnerability to ease.

There is a special truth and light, a special love and laughter, which can be given to us by those who are courageous enough to tell their stories. We must learn to share in their sadness and hope, their tears and laughter. We must partake of their dignity and courage.

That we have gathered here at this Congress bears witness to the tact that we are pilgrims, engaged upon a voyage of understanding.

This voyage will require from each of us truth, compassion, faith wisdom, respect for others and courage.

It will be a voyage of understanding what is, of understanding reality, not of asserting what we would like to be the case, what we would prefer to believe.

It will be a voyage of sharing, the sharing of a sense of mystery, of a burden of sadness, of the pain of care, of the laughter of life.

It will be a voyage to change for each of us, for none of us are untouched by this epidemic.

It will be a voyage of the heart and the mind to communities of concern and commitment.

It will be a voyage through pain, through the dark side of the epidemic, with hope.

28

Responding to the Challenge of HIV and AIDS

The UNDP Regional Projeet for Asia and the Pacifie Region will have completed its initial phase by the end of December 1992, leading to a new four-year Project in 1993. The response to the Project, initially enthusiastic but guarded, indicates that the socio-economic implications of the HIV epidemic have already moved closer to the centre of policy-making concern. Organizational and bureaucratic barriers have begun to crumble, leading to dynamic partnerships across operational sectors.

The challenge now is to build on the increased level of awareness. New initiatives are coming forward from NGOs and business sector allies; government departments and policy institutes. New strategies are emerging for improving HIV awareness, communicating information and advice, counselling those affected, combating prejudice, and promoting behavioural change. New service delivery approaches, such as some just starting in the hotel and transport sectors, need to be monitored for application elsewhere. The human rights lobby is starting to defend people with HIV from discrimination and privacy invasion. This mushrooming volume of activity needs encouragement and concrete support.

Consciousness-Raising Among Decision-Makers

There is still much to be done in changing the policy climate towards HIV. AIDS as a subject exerts a powerful fascination. Unfortunately, even hightly educated and relatively well-informed people tend to believe that AIDS is confined to special groups and that HIV must—and can—be kept at bay by isolation of people known to be infected. Familiarization with a less alarmist, more positive approach so that it becomes embedded in policy-making attitudes cannot be achieved overnight. Many politicians, government officials, academics, NGO leaders, and captains of industry and commerce, still need to be introduced to HIV as a social and economic phenomenon. The existing concern of others needs reinforcement if it is to be translated into action.

The UNDP country and regional workshops have provided all opportunity to identify researchers keen to make a contribution to the analysis of the epidemic participants from a variety of disciplines have become resource persons for further workshops, or for the preparation of new components in AIDS country plans. A regional network is developing or socio-economic expertise in the field of HIV and AIDS related studies. Data and authoritative analysis is not only vital *perse*, but of great importance in providing the evidence needed to persuade the sceptical that HIV and AIDS are, indeed, a threat in their own country and will reach their own social milieu; and that something can be done to reduce this threat both by health professionals and others.

Country workshops and regional consultations are primarily aimed at consiousness and knowledge building, they also have an advocacy function. When individuals participate, for example, in discussions on education about HIV in the workplace, they are also confronting—often for the first time in their professional capacity - the need to take the personal, social and economic consequences of the epidemic seriously. The intent is to create a snowball effect of HIV concern, which will be taken forward during the new project phase.

Support to Community-Based Initiatives

UNDP's guiding principles for policy development in the field of HIV and AIDS emphasize the importance of enhancing the capacity of community-based organizations (CBOs). As a result of the presence of AIDS in Asia, new CBOs have emerged spontaneously to address various aspects of the epidemic. Other NGOs, mostly those concerned with health, but also some concerned with urban community development, or with human rights, have added concerned about HIV to their existing agendas.

The role of the NGO sector vis a vis the HIV epidemic is very special. Whether interest.-, creed-, or profession-based, NGOs exist to address preoccupations shared by a specific group of human beings. They are driven therefore, by human motivation and experience; not by the constructs familiar to professional planners and policy-makers.

Those that are community-based are, by definition, close to their constituencies. The connection between HIV infection and intimate behaviour make this a difficult subject to address at a personal level—where all behavioural change takes place. To bring about such change requires eliciting people's confidence and empathy, which is especially difficult among those engaging in behaviour which is 'not respectable' or illegal. Helping people to avoid H1V infection will require a process of building alliances with organizations and authority figures people trust. These are most likely to be found in the NGO and CBO community.

The UNDP Regional Project therefore playes a strong emphasis on these groups. It. keeps abreast of new developments, initiates contacts, and networks between organizations enabling them to learn from each other's experiences. Organizations that have sprung up in response to HIV and AIDS have high motivation but little experience, and need organizational and management skills. In the ease of existing NGOs, the challenge is to find common ground with their own agendas so that they can be persuaded to undertake HIV-related initiatives among their own membership or clients. UNDP has already held a number of formal and informal consultations for NGOs.

The inspirational role of NGOs is also an important tool for HIV prevention. Case histories, both of HIV-related human predicament, and of effective nurturing or preventive strategies, can have a profound effect on the caring human conscience and are important in dispelling prejudice and rallying resources. The impact not only on the public at large, but on decision-makers, of people's courage in the face of AIDS has had a major effect on the overall campaign, world-wide and in their own societies. During the next four years, the Regional Project will offer support to up to six innovative community-based pilot projects. These will be fully documented with a view to cross-fertilization of information and the stimulation of similar approaches, where suitable, in other environments.

A promising area of partnership for NGOs is with the business sector. A recent regional consultation organized by UNDP brought together NGOs and CBOs with representatives of the hotel, advertising, retail, and pharmaceutical industries and Chambers of Cormmerce of India and Thailand. This was the first ever occasion on which the business and NGO communities have met together in a structured context to discuss how they can work together on AIDS related projects.

The need to shed preconceptions and find common ground between corporate and NGO agendas as a pre-requisite of joint action was the theme underlying the consultation proceedings. The business perspective is that NGOs are unprofessional and have little to offer; the NGO perspective, that companies' objectives are barely compatible with social concern and they can best be seen as an occasional source of funds. NGOs need to learn how to target their approaches by analyzing the corporate culture, offering services appropriate to the employer and employee setting, and building up personal contacts.

Hua Hin Consultation to promote NGO/business sector partnerships for AIDS prevention, June 1992

The objectives of the Consultation were to increase awareness of successful NGO/business partnerships in programmes relating to HIV and AIDS; to share guidelines for establishing such partnerships; and to identify and develop the skills required to make such partnerships work. Among the topics addressed at the meeting were the following:

Characteristics of Partnerships: the Business Perspective (Bill Timmerman, Saatchi & Saatchi, Singapore)

Characteristics of Partnerships: the NGO Perspective (Teresita Bagasao, Kabalikat, Philippines)

Partnerships: Lessons Learned (Royal Garden Resorts/ Population Development Association, Thailand)

HIV: Social Security and Insurance Schemes (Nikom Chandravithun, Thamasart University, Thailand)

HIV and Workplace Personnel Policies (Lee Dilokvidhyavat, Chulalongkorn University, Thailand)

Seeking Business Sector Support: Presentation Techniques (Margie Maciolek, Northwest Airlines, Thailand)

HIV: Labour Law and Other Legal Issues (Vitit Muntarbhorn, Chulalongkorn University, Thailand)

Marketing NGO Services to Business (James Reinnoldt, Northwest Airlines, Thailand).

Among the outcomes of the consultation was a new sense among the representatives of the commercial world that NGOs can provide a useful technical resource for workplace initiatives; and that there is a need to develop policies and prepare management for coping with HIV, as well as to educate staff concerning all aspects of HIV infection. Progress was also made towards developing strategies across the NGO-business divide. Although there is no quick-fix method of partnership development fruitful relationships are practicable if NGOs develop the skills and confidence to form them.

Action for AIDS Prevention

'I'he UNDP Regional Project will maintain as a primary focus the need to prevent further HIV transmission. At present, the only sure guard against the spread of HIV is the observation, throughout society, of a strict personal sexual code. (Drug users will also need to use sterile needles for drug-injection.) For people to adopt such behaviours, they have to be both properly informed and motivated. This requires an open discussion on sexual mores.

In most, societies of the region the topic of sexuality is not openly discussed, even between husbands and wives, parents and children. However, the challenge of AIDS has brought a realization that as long as sexual behaviour remains a taboo subject, correct information about how to avoid HIV will remain locked away. In this context, the work of many NGOs in breaking down communications barriers needs to be encouraged and emulated.

Compounding the dangers inherent in the silence surrounding sexual affairs are certain cultural practices which increase the vulnerability of the entire population. These include the assignment to sex workers of the task of initiating male children into sexual activity; and the dedication of certain women to a state of sexual servitude, often under the guise of traditional marriage, and their subsequent sale or abandonment. to the commercial sex market.. Both the silence surrounding sex, and the practices in question, have to be sensitively addressed. In this context, further research is required, and the work of NGOs concerned with women's and children's rights needs to be supported.

Particular audiences - the young, workers in occupations which take them far from home, those in the entertainment industry have to be targeted and reached persuasively. All media need to be used in advertising; television; group and individual counseling through NGO's, religious congregations, and personnel net departments. More attention will in future be paid by UNDP to the role of the communications media in reporting HIV and AIDS. Most people derive their notions about AIDS and HIV from newspapers and television. Ghoulish and sensational reports, particularly where they depict AIDS as a disease of the socially outcast have contritbuted to many misconceptions. Failure to emphasize that the means of transmission are limited, and that casual infection is impossible, arouses unnecessary fears. UNDP hopes in time to build an informed network of journalists concerned about AIDS issues.

Working to Change the Legal Climate

UNDP has begun t.o work with lawyers, policy-makers, and human rights activists in the region to create an ethical and legal environment which support rather than discriminates against people living with HIV. While the detention of HIV-positive individuals is an extreme case of the negative use of the law, there are other examples of discriminatory legal practice. Hospitals and laboratories have been required to report the names of all those testing HIV -positive, often leading to leaks of confidentiality and social rejection. Regulations which expose people to loss of jobs, household eviction, and victimization in ways that seem infinitely less endurable in the present than the prospect of sickness and death in the future support the process of denial, HIV's deadliest ally.

The repressive use of the law, by driving HIV underground, also obstructs the process of charting the epidemic. Where it restricts the advertisement of condoms or of safe sex messages, it inhibits action for prevention. Since the law reflects moral judgments made by society at large, it is important that it be used to provide a supportive policy framework. Policy-makers must be encouraged to use the law to prohibit discrimination and support the rights of people with HIV to privacy and aceess to services. The decriminalization of some activities, such as homosexuality and prostitution, may help the building of bridges to socially outcast groups in order to gain their co-operation in HIV prevention.

The law can also be used indirectly to lessen the vulnerability of certain groups exposed to HIV infection. Improvements in the status of women would enable them to protect their sexual health and their rights of inheritance to property; also to give them better access to decent, reasonably paid, jobs. In some countries, a review of the marriage code and the family code, particularly elements which do not afford sufficient protection to girls from early marriage, easy abandonment, and sexual exploitation, is needed in response to the threat which AIDS presents to women and family life.

UNDP is setting up an HIV legal network in the region to raise awareness about the need to integrate considerations about the law into HIV and AIDS policy, and to promote appropriate legal responses. This network will include policy-makers, lawyers, people living with HIV, and community-based organizations. The first step in this process is a Regional Consultation to be held in late 1992.

In Conclusion

The presence of AIDS in a country characterized by a poor standard of human development can set off a downward spiral of damage to hard-won gains in health and living standards. Existing social and economic deprivation produces an environment in which the spread of HIV occurs; and, in turn, the HIV epidemic intensifies deprivation among families already operating within perilously overstretched margins. Because AIDS cuts down people in the prime of life, the ramifications of HIV infection demand a special response from bodies at local, national, and regional levels, in the government, commercial, and non-governmental sectors.

THE HIV/AIDS EPIDEMIC AND ITS CONSEQUENCES

Phase I Spread of the virus	Phase II Illness and death	Phase III Survivors	Phase IV Social and economic impact	Phase V Long-term potential impact
		DISCRIPTION		
Initial spread is hidden but increasing numbers of people becoming infected	Spread of virus continues and infected people increasingly become ill and die.	Children, spouses elderly and others left without support	Depletion of the labour force and military; adverse impact on productive and social sectors, families, communities.	Possibility of social and political unrest, destitution, social disintegration, devastation of aspiration and economies
		POLICY CONTEXT		
Behaviour change: * Education * Prevention * Legislation Other preventive measures Surveillance	Attitudinal Change: * Living positively * Fear * Discrimination Confidentiality Income maintenance and housing Social and psychological support Home care and services Treatment Employment and education Legal rights Community management	Maintain in community Immediate assistance programmes Counselling and social support Education and health Income-generation Legal protection	Monitoring systems Sectoral strategies Personnel policies Education, training policies Strengthening of health/ social sectors Planning methodologies	Minimizing potential impact on individuals, communities and nations.

Countries of the Asian and Pacific Region will have to make the following critical choies:

The type of prevention policies adopted and the extent of resources directed to the epidemic in its early stages.
The extent to which community responses are integrated into and complemented by the governmental response.
The extent to which governments assist the infected, their families and carers, to remain an integral part of their Communities.
Whether, and at what stage, governments, the private sector and others begin to plan to minimize adverse social and economic impacts.

Upon the choices made will depend the degree of crisis posed by HIV and AIDS to human and economic development in Asia and the Pacific.

29

Facing the Challenges of HIV/AIDS/STDs: A Gender-based Response

1. Why Gender and HIV/AIDS/STDs?

> *"One of the most striking features of the response to the HIV epidemic to date is how few of the policies and programmes we have developed relate to women's life situations. The daily lives of women and the complex network of relationships and structures which shape them are well known to women and well documented. Despite this, our theories, research agendas, policies and programmes have not been grounded in and informed by these experiences."*
>
> Elizabeth Reid[1]

As the HIV/AIDS epidemic and sexually transmitted diseases (STDs) continue to advance worldwide, we are learning ever more about how they affect individuals, households, families, communities, organizations and nations The individual loss has been enormous, particularly in those countries and regions affected early on. AIDS is increasingly recognized in developing countries as a serious concern for socio-economic development as a whole. Its impact is seen in family and community structures and relationships and in sectors as varied as education, employment, health care, social welfare, agriculture and the judiciary.

Economic consequences are already apparent. In highly affected countries, the business sector is experiencing increased absenteeism as employees fall ill, care for the sick or attend funerals. Loss of experienced and skilled workers in the formal and informal sectors may lead to lower productivity, savings and investments. In subsistence and small-scale agriculture, loss of labour may result in changes in farming patterns and food shortages.

Strategies to prevent the spread of HIV have focused on the promotion of condom use, reduction of numbers of sexual partners and treatment of STDs[2]. Many of these responses, however, have failed to address social, economic and power relations between women and men, among men and among women. These relationships, together with physiological differences, determine to a great extent women's and men's risk of infection, their ability to protect themselves effectively and their respective share of the burdens of the epidemic:

— Women are physiologically more vulnerable to HIV infection than men. Young women are especially at risk and AIDS death rates are highest in women their 20s.

— Stereotypes related to HIV/AIDS and STDs and their association with marginalized groups (e.g., sex workers) contribute to blaming women for the spread of HIV. Fear of stigmatization inhibits people from taking preventive measures and leads women and men to assess their own risks inadequately. Moreover, many ideas and expectations regarding male and female (sexual) behaviour neither encourage men to act responsibly and protect themselves and their partners from infection nor stimulate women to challenge notions of female inferiority and social structures which keep them vulnerable.

— Low social status and economic dependence prevent many women and young people (e.g., street-children) from controlling their own risk With little negotiating power, they are often unable to insist on safer sex; disproportionately poor, they may have little choice other than to barter sex for survival.

— As society's traditional care-givers, women carry the main psychosocial and physical burdens of AIDS care. Yet they have the least control over and access to the resources they need to cope effectively; few men share domestic responsibilities and family care with their partners.

Although the necessity of focusing on women's needs has been highlighted time and again, especially since 1990 when the theme of World AIDS Day was "Women and HIV/AIDS", women continue to bear the brunt of the epidemic and to be highly vulnerable to infection. Reducing their—and men's—risk of infection demands gender-based responses that focus on how the different social expectations, roles, status and economic power of men and women affect and are affected by the epidemic. This involves analysis of gender stereotypes, redefinition of male and female relationships and roles, promotion of cultural beliefs and values supporting mutually responsible behaviour and exploration of ways to reduce inequalities between women and men. A supportive environment can be created thereby, enabling women and men to undertake prevention and cope better with the epidemic.

Women and men both have much to gain from increased gender sensitivity in general development policy, planning and programmes and particularly by national AIDS/STD programmes, AIDS service organizations and related services. At all levels a gender-based focus on problems and solutions is urgently needed.

A gender-based response to HIV/AIDS and STDs focuses on how different social expectations, roles, status and economic power of men and women affect and are affected by the epidemic.

It analyses gender stereotypes and explores ways to reduce inequalities between women and men so that a supportive environment can be created, enabling both to undertake prevention and cope better with the epidemic.

This publication aims to provide policy-makers, planners and programme implementers with information and ideas to help them incorporate a gender-based approach to HIV/AIDS and STDs into their policies and programmes. It highlights the nature and scale of the epidemic, explores the concepts of gender and a gender-based approach and the ways HIV/AIDS and STDs affect and are affected by gender. Suggestions are made for approaches and strategies to address some of the problems.

It is hoped that the analysis, information, ideas and examples will help stimulate many more gender-sensitive initiatives to help us cope with HIV/AIDS and STDs more successfully.

2. How Extensive are HIV/AIDS and STDs?

At the end of I994, a cumulative total of I,025,073 AIDS cases (adults and children) worldwide had been reported to WHO. The actual number of AIDS cases is unknown because of under diagnosis, incomplete reporting and reporting delays. However, an estimated 4.5 million AIDS cases have occurred in adults and children since the beginning of the epidemic (Figure. 29.1).

An estimated I8 million adults (I3-I5 million alive) and 1.5 million children have been infected with HIV. Of the adults, 7-8 million are women (most of childbearing age, Figure 29.2). WHO forecasts that, by the year 2000, 30-40 million HIV infections will have occurred, 90 per cent in developing countries. Moreover, an estimated 5 million children under I0 years of age will be orphaned, losing one or both parents.

The proportion of women with HIV and AIDS has increased dramatically. By I994, women represented 40 per cent of all new AIDS cases; up to 50 per cent of all new HIV infections were in women, mainly those aged 15-24 years.* Female vulnerability has

---

* *All figures are based on WHO reports unless otherwise indicated.*

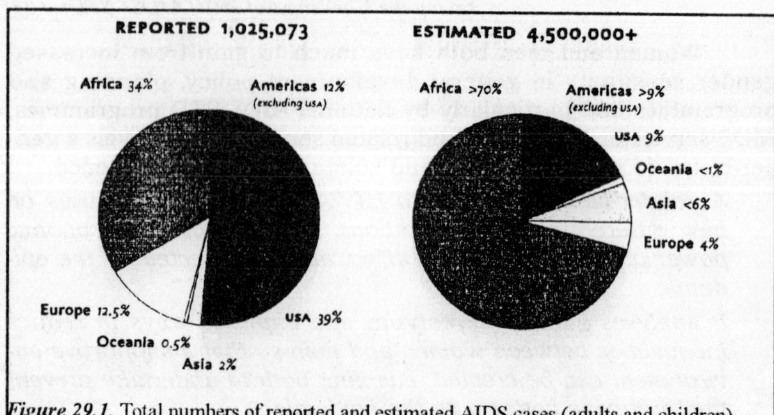

Figure 29.1. Total numbers of reported and estimated AIDS cases (adults and children) from the late 1970s/early 1980s until late 1994 ***(Source: WHO/GPA)***

become increasingly clear in Africa and Asia. By the year 2000, an estimated I4 million women will have been infected with HIV and about 4 million will have died of AIDS.

HIV is transmitted predominantly through sexual intercourse (70-80 per cent of infections). Mother-to-child transmission and needle-sharing by drug users each account for 5-I0 per cent of all HIV infections, while needlestick accidents among health workers account for less than 0.01 per cent of resorted cases.

Higher proportions of young women than young men acquire HIV infection through sex. Their exposure to the virus at an earlier age, coupled with physiological factors, increases their risk. In countries with high HIV prevalence, the greatest numbers of reported AIDS cases occur among women aged I5-34 years and men aged 25-44 years (Figure 29.3).

HIV infection due to blood transfusion is more common in women than men.Women more often have blood transfusions because of anaemia and complications during pregnancy and childbirth. Perinatal transmission occurs during pregnancy, delivery or breast-feeding. The chance that a child of a seropositive woman will also be infected with HIV-I is 33 per cent overall, with transmission reported to be as high as 48 per cent in some developing countries. [3]

Regional Patterns

In regions where initially more men than women were infected, there is now a marked increase in infections transmitted through heterosexual intercourse. In Europe, 15.4 per cent of new infections in adults in I993 were due to heterosexual transmission. In France, heterosexual transmission increased from I9 per cent in

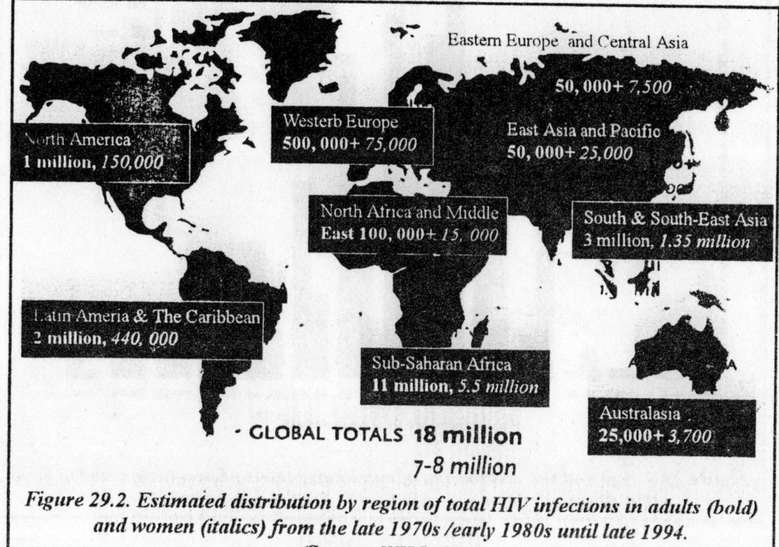

Figure 29.2. Estimated distribution by region of total HIV infections in adults (bold) and women (italics) from the late 1970s /early 1980s until late 1994. (Source: WHO/GPA)

I991 to almost 25 per cent in I993. In I993 in the USA, AIDS cases in women were almost Is per cent higher than in I992; in nine major cities AIDS has become the leading cause of death among women of childbearing age.

In sub-Saharan Africa, HIV has been transmitted predominantly through heterosexual intercourse since the beginning of the epidemic. More than half of newly infected adults are female (11-12 women for every 10 men). The annual number of infections is still increasing. In Francistown, Botswana, for example, HIV prevalence in pregnant women rose from 8 per cent in 1991 to about 35 per cent by I993. In some countries, e.g., Cote d'Ivoire, Zaire and Uganda, AIDS has become the leading cause of adult death[4].

Seroprevalence rates in North Africa and the Middle East appear relatively low but are increasing. In Djibouti, for example, HIV prevalence has reached I4 per cent among men attending STD clinics and 4 per cent among women seeking antenatal care.

In Latin America and the Caribbean region, a shift from transmission through primarily homosexual intercourse to bisexual and heterosexual transmission as well as injecting drug use has taken place since the early I980. In Brazil, one woman was infected with HIV for I00 men in I 984; by I 994 this was one woman for four men.

Half of the newly infected adults in Asia are women. In a border town in Shan State, Myanmar, 6-I0 per cent of women registered at public maternal and child health centres were already seropositive in early I995 [5].

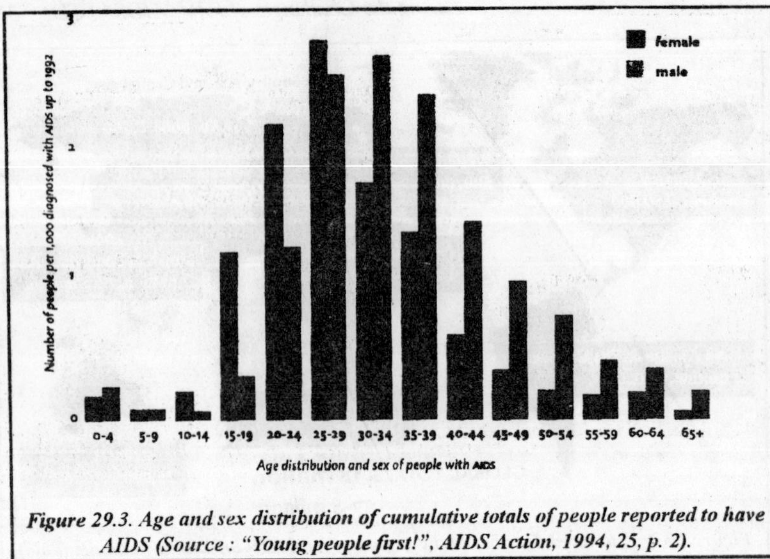

Figure 29.3. Age and sex distribution of cumulative totals of people reported to have AIDS (Source : "Young people first!", AIDS Action, 1994, 25, p. 2).

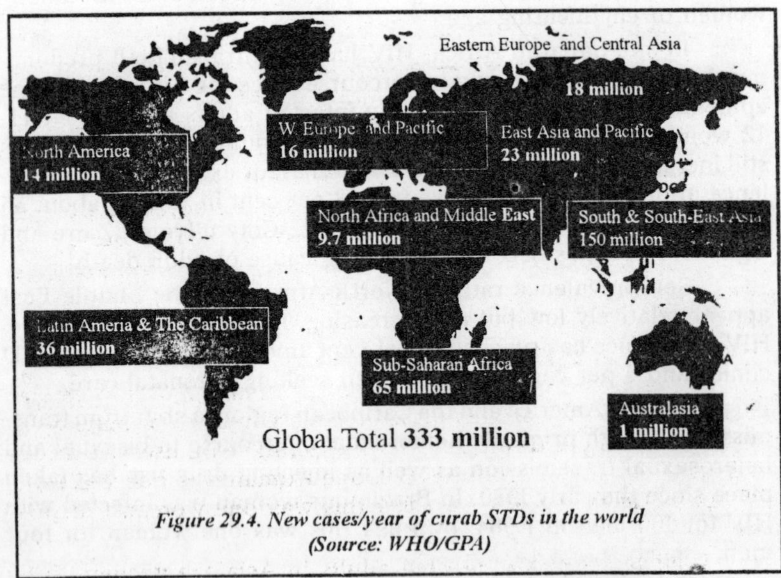

Figure 29.4. New cases/year of curab STDs in the world (Source: WHO/GPA)

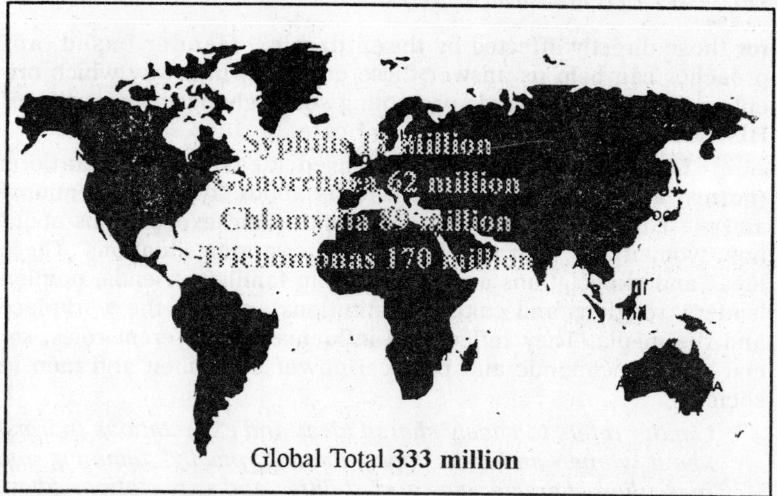

Figure 29.5. Estimated new cases/year of treatable syphilis, gonorrhoea, chlamydia and trichomonas
(Source: WHO/GPA)

Sexually Transmitted Diseases

STD rates remain high in much of the world. Each year about 330 million new cases of STDs occur, of which more than 90 per cent are in developing countries (Figures. 29.4-29.5). Overall infection rates for STDs are higher in women than men. Ulcerative STDs, including syphilis and chancroid, and STDs causing inflammation, such as gonorrhoea and chlamydial infection, facilitate transmission of HIV in both women and men. Women, however, are disproportionately affected. As with HIV, women often acquire STDs at an earlier age than men. Gonorrhoea and syphilis are asymptomatic in 50-80 per cent of women against less than I0 per cent of men. In women, they often go untreated, especially in countries with inadequate STD programmes. The secondary health consequences of STDs are more serious for women as they may contribute to infertility, ectopic pregnancy, cervical cancer, premature delivery, stillbirth, low birth weight and neonatal infections. Ectopic pregnancy, cervical cancer and sepsis following pelvic inflammatory disease can be fatal.

3. What Does a Gender-based Response Involve?

What changes are needed to create an environment enabling women and men to protect themselves and each other? How can they collaborate equally in providing adequate care and support for those directly affected by the epidemic? Gender-based approaches can help us answer these questions in a way which orients programmes towards promoting social changes supportive of HIV/AIDS and STD prevention and care.

Gender refers to widely shared ideas and expectations (norms) about women and men: ideas about "typically" feminine and masculine *characteristics* and abilities and expectations about how women and men should behave in various situations. These ideas and expectations are learned from families, friends, opinion leaders, religious and cultural institutions, schools, the workplace and the media. They reflect and influence the different roles, social status, economic and political power of women and men in society.

> *Gender refers to widely shared ideas and expectations (norms) about women and men: ideas about "typically" feminine and masculine characteristcs and abilities and expectations about how women and men should behave in various situations. These ideas and expectations are learned from families, friends, opinion leaders, religious and cultural institutions, schools, the workplace and the media. They reflect and influence the different roles, social status, economic and political power of women and men in society.*

Status and power affect the individual's risk of infection and communities' abilities to cope with the epidemic. The low status and power of women and young people lead to their subordination and restrict their possibilities of taking control of their lives in relation to HIV/AIDS and STDs. Societal pressures also make it difficult for men to change their behaviours in this regard. Their sexual behaviour may be influenced by their relations with other men and women (e.g., fathers, sons, mothers, sisters, peers)[6].

Below, three examples show how gender is related to norms affecting HIV/AIDS and STD prevention and care. The examples are simplified. In-depth gender analysis would also consider other differences that interact with gender to create situations of dominance and subordination, such as age, class, ethnicity and religion[7].

Norms Concerning Parenthood

In most societies, women's primary role in life is to bear and nurture children. Although responsible fatherhood may be promoted, nen's main duty is seen to be earning a living and dealing with the broader society on behalf of the family.

Such norms have two broad implications in relation to HIV/AIDS and STDs. First, a false division is made between "reproductive" (women's) and "productive" (men's) roles[8]. The expectation that women must care for the children is extended to all household members needing support, e.g., the elderly, those who are ill with HIV/AIDS and/or orphaned children. Men are not usually expected to undertake care roles.

This supposed division does not correspond entirely to reality, however. Almost universally, women have always undertaken productive as well as reproductive work; it has simply been unpaid, unrewarded materially and unrecognized. In many African countries, for example, zell over half of the agricultural work is undertaken by women (68 per cent in Central African Republic and the Congo, 70 per cent in Gambia). Yet women do not gain equal access to educational opportunities or the paid labour market, both of which may contribute to social and economic indepenence and more self-assurance.

A second consequence is that childless women are not viewed as "fully adult" or may be considered deviant. Their social status is often low. If their childlessness is due to infertility, they may not know this or refuse to accept the diagnosis and try repeatedly (even with a variety of partners) to become pregnant. This of course implies that they have unprotected sex, thereby increasing their risk of exposure to HIV/STDs.

Moreover, when childless women express their opinions about community measures needed for HIV/STD prevention and care, their suggestions may not be fully respected or accepted by other community members. The voices of women who are mothers may also be given less credibility, because they are expected to confine themselves to household matters.

Sample statements reflecting the idea that women lure men into sex:

"Women should wear purdah [head-to-toe covering] to ensure that innocent men do not get unnecessarily excited by women's bodies and are not unconsciously forced into becoming rapists. If women do not want to fall prey to such men, they should take the necessary precautions instead of forever blaming men" (comment by a member of Malaysia's parliament during debates on the reform of rape laws[9].

"The child was sexually aggressive" (reason given by a Canadian judge for suspending the sentence of a man who had sexually assaulted a 3-year-old girl [9]).

"The female condom will increase immorality among women and single mothers. It is worse than the male condom, giving women the opportunity to do what they want. We are going to preach against these condoms-the church cannot condone their use"

(Parish priest in Kenya[10]).

Norms Concerning Sexuality

Among the numerous norms related to sex, many societies share ideas that women seduce men into having sex and that because male sexual needs are so strong, men cannot resist this. Such notions make men appear to be governed by their instincts, unable to control their behaviour and victims of female power. As a result, men are not expected to behave responsibly, while women's sexuality and behaviour are controlled. For example, in many countries, girls who become pregnant must leave school, while boys who father children can continue their education with no requirement to contribute to child care. To protect men from themselves, social rules may also deprive women of the freedom to move about freely and lead to situations in which women, instead of their attackers, are blamed for sexual abuse.

These ideas form an obstacle to HIV/STD prevention because they absolve men from taking responsibility for they sexual behaviour. They may also prevent women from taking measures to protect themselves. For example, women may be reluctant to buy and carry condoms because they will be accused of wanting to "entice" men into having sex. Women may be reluctant to report abuse because they fear this will affect their position in society: if it becomes known that a young girl has been sexually abused (the result, of a tial in some countries she will have difficulty marrying because both women and men see her as "spoiled".

Norms Concerning Power in Relationships

In many societies, men are expected to control women in all aspects of relationships. This involves desicion-making on when and whom a a girl/women will marry, when and how she will have sexual relations, when and how many children she will have, household expenditures, etc.

This type of male power is supported by tradition and social norms. Women learn, for example, that their first loyalty must be to their kin and families, causing them to act in ways that reinforce rather than challenge female subordination. Oftén, female family members enforce community norms saying, for instance, male relatives must assume authority over widows. In addition, men may impose their will on women, even resorting to violence to do so. Coupled with economic dependence on men, ideas and expectations concerning so-called "proper' male and female roles make it difficult or impossible far women to demand that men share responsibility for preventing sexual and perinatal transmission of HIV/STDs.

Gender analysis and gender-based programmes can help

women and men redefine their relationships in a mutually beneficial way. As women move into traditionally "male domains", men can be encouraged to begin sharing responsibilities in the "female domain". Some women already exert considerable power, if often in subtle ways. Their existing strengths should be recognized and their self-confidence and social skills expanded. Men can be helped to see how their privileged position and social roles orient them more towards relationships involving authority and competition and, perhaps, conflict than Collaboration. As the dynamics of male-female relationships change, communities will be able to benefit from the potential of all their members to minimize the impact of HIV/ AIDS and STDs.

— "Right now I'm pregnant. It was an accident, I was planning to go to the clinic but my husband took away my card. He wanted more children so I became pregnant" (woman in Kenya [11]).

— " I told my husband that it was better to use condoms, the doctor said so. The doctor had also given me some to use at home. My husband became very angry and asked who gave me permission to bring those condoms home" (woman in Kenya [12]).

4. Why do HIV / AIDS/ STDs affect Women more?

Women's vulnerability to HIV/AIDS and STDs is partly determined by physiological factors. It further reflects their wider social, sexual and economic vulnerability. The central issue is inequality. Economic need, lack of job opportunities, poor access to education and training and cultural expectations of female submissiveness and male dominance combine to prevent women from actively making choices and decisions about their lives, particularly with regard to limiting sexual risks and protecting their and their families' health. For the same reasons, men are led to deny risk and avoid responsibility, not only for their partners but for themselves. For both sexes this situation needs to change.

Physiological Vulnerability

Women and Men

Researchers estimate that women's risk of HIV infection from unprotected sex is at least twice that of men. Semen, which has high concentrations of virus, remains in the vaginal canal a relatively long time. Women are more exposed through the extensive surface area of mucous membrane in the vagina and on the cervix through which the virus may pass. In men, the equivalent area is smaller, mainly the entrance to the urethra in a circumcised man plus, in an uncircumcised man, the delicate skin under the foreskin. Circumcision in males (not in females!) appears to have some protective value against STDs, including HIV. Men and women's risk of HIV escalates manyfold if STDs are present [13].

Young Women

Young women are at even greater risk than mature women (except for menopausal women in whom thinning of the vaginal mucosa increases susceptibility to infection). A teenager's vagina is not as well lined with protective cells as that of a mature woman. Her cervix may be more easily eroded, potentially enhancing risk of HIV infection. She also faces potential bleeding at first intercourse through tearing of the hymen. In cultures where sex with very young girls is condoned, sexual intercourse is especially likely to cause trauma. In some countries, girls as young as 12 may be married to men three times their age. In addition, girls aged 17 years or younger who have unprotected sex are at increased risk of developing cervical cancer. Sexually active young women may easily contract herpes simplex and human papilcomavirus infections.

All these factors make young women especially vulnerable at a time when their negotiating and economic power is last making them easier targets for sexual coercion and exploitation. This situation is worsened when more men, especially in high HIV-prevalence areas, seek out ever younger female partners in the belief that they are least likely to be infected. This is the most risky pattern of sexual partnership, as a group more likely to have HIV already (older men) transmits the virus to a group with low levels of infection (young girls).

Sexually Transmitted Diseases

Who estimates that about 330 million cases of treatable STDs exist worldwide at any time yet women may have these infections without realizing it some 50-80 per cent of STDs in women are asymptomatic or gounnoticed because they are internal. Women are much less likely than men to seek timely treatment for STDs for this reason. Stigma attached to STDs, especially for women, inaccessibility of clinics, lack of money and too many other responsibilities further prevent them from getting treatment. Negative attitudes of health workers towards women presenting with STDs may be another major deterrent to their seeking treatment or even contraceptive advice. This is true of teenage girls in South Africa, for example[14].

***Shyamala, India:** "From one end of the room, partitioned by a curtain, a voice, loud and haranguing, came through the silence. It was unmistakably the doctor's. 'Spread your legs!.......Tell me, where is it paining? Now tell me properly! Is it or isn't it paining? How are we supposed to understand anything if you won't talk? OK. Now you can go'...Suddenly the nurse's voice boomed: 'Everybody go and pass urine and come back! I quickly followed three other women towards the single toilet...Back in the waiting room, some men had appeared. Two seemed to have come with their wives and two others .....powere hospital orderlies. I noticed their eyes stray towards the gap in the curtain"[15].*

Culture Practices

Certain cultural practices may exacerbate women's physiological risk of HIV infection, especially when HIV is widespread in the population. Many women actively support these practices because they enhance their social status and security with their partners. Examples:

— In some parts of the world, women use herbal and other agents in the vagina to cause dryness, heat and tightness. This practice is carried out because people believe men prefer "dry sex" (in which women feel like virgins) and because they think that female secretions are unclean. The substances used can cause inflammation and erosion of the vaginal mucosa, making it easier far HIV to enter.

— Excessive rubbing of the genitals during foreplay and intercourse, or "rough sex", can lead to sores in the mucous membrane.

— Anal intercourse carries higher risks of HIV transmission because of frequent lesions. Although H is often associated with homosexual contacts, heterosexual couples practise it to preserve virginity, to protect against pregnancy, far (usually male) sexual pleasure and in a search for sexual variety.

— Female genital mutilation (circumcision) is practised in various Countries. Infibulation fin which the labia minora and majora are cut away and the vulva is sewn shut leaving a pinhole opening for urination and menstruation) leads to extensive tearing and bleeding when sexual intercourse is attempted. it may also cause couples to practise riskier anal sex instead. The procedure itself could be risky if unsterilized instruments are used for several patients in succession. Less extreme circumcision, like removal of the clitoris hood, carries little risk during sex, but the procedure itself is potentially risky. Bleeding aver circumcision may lead to the need for blood transfusions with unscreened, possibly contaminated, blood.

Gender-Related Vulnerability and Obstacles to Prevention and Coping

Male Sexual Priority

Commonly, though not universally, male sexual needs are acknowledged to a greater extent than female needs. This may be reflected in the very terminology describing male sexual desire, genitals and partnerships compared with female equivalents. Many cultures use words to describe male sexual desire, genitals and partnerships compared with female equivalents. Many cultures use words to describe male sexuality in a positive way and female sexuality in a more negative and judgemental way. Many women and men define sex largely according to what they believe gives men pleasure, particularly penetration. Often women do not explore, let alone assert, their own preferences, because this is considered inappropriate.

"Everything is centred around the pleasure of the man," says a Zimbabwean women at a market. She sells herbs which, when put in the vagina, cause dryness and tightness. "So if these substances are harmful or even if discomfort is caused, it doesn't matter to the woman. She's doing what she thinks he wants. This is how we have been conditioned" [16].

The dominance of male needs and denial of female needs impedes open discussion between the sexes and limits people's chances of achieving mutually satisfying, respectful and safe forms of sexual behaviour. To curb HIV transmission, both partners should be able to express their worries about infection and use protective measures such as condoms out of respect and affection rather than as a sign of mistrust.

Sex within marriage,in particular, needs to be a source of mutual pleasure and bonding, rather than only a duty and a condition for procreation. However, it is within marriage or with regular partners that wonnen may have most difficult negotiating safer sex, such as condom use as this implies lack of trust and infidelity. But it is essential that they be able to do so, as most HIV-inicted women have been infected by their husband/regular partner.

Economic Vulner ability and Sexual Services

For women and men struggling with daily, concern about a disease that may kill[10] years hence is a luxury they can ill afford..Women's economic dependence makes them vulnerable and, for many, training and employment opportunities are few. If selling sex enables them to survive today, long term concerns remain out of focus. A Ghanaian woman engaged in sex work in Abidjan, Cote d'lvoire, commented, "I need to feed and clothe my children now. How can I worry about something that may not affect me for many years?"[17]

A ready market for sexual services exists almost worldwide and is a significant factor promoting the HIV epidemic. In some countries, it is reportedly the norm for young men's first sexual experiences to be with sex workers. Demand for sexual services is fuelled by cultural attitudes condoning or even encouraging male sexual freedom while repressing female sexuality. Migration, with its associated disruption of family life, partly promotes the demand for and supply of sexual services. Members of the armed forces away from home, displaced populations and affluent sex tourists from Europe, Japan, the Middle East, North America and the Pacific region further contribute to demand.

VULNERABILITY TO SEXUAL EXPLOITATION

Nhlungwane, ***South Africa:*** *"A woman may go to look for employment all day and fail. On her way back home she might meet a man who wants to have sex with her. she will accept any amount of money in exchange for sex in order to purchase meals for herself and her children. She could get AIDS from that person".* [8]

In Asia, daughters may be sold by the family to the sex industry because they need the income.

In Fiji, 8 out of 70 domestic workers reported that they are sexually abused by their employers. Female industrial workers are paid a pittance; some are also sexually abused by supervisors and employers. Because of these problems and increasing poverty, more of the women (often deserted wives) are engaging in sex work. As one sex worker said: "Why put up withyour boss demanding sex and receiving $ 30 a week when you can get more a day by selling your body?" [19].

At the same time, the boundaries of sex work are often blurred: payment and intimacy may range from a brief anonymous sex act for a specified fee through a gradation of casual and commercial interactions. In many societies, not only those with marked gender inequality, men entertain women or provide them with desired goods in return for sexual access on a one-off, short- or long-term basis. Sex may be demanded or bartered in the workplace to gain a job, promotion or trade permit. This is not usually considered sex work but is nonetheless related to economic need. Unfortunately, sex in these situations is often unsafe.

Control Over Sexual Relations within and out side Marriage

Marriage may be viewed as a social and economic commitment between individuals and families. Sexual access, procreation, childrearing and other services are universal to social expectations of marriage; romantic love and affection are not. Because of this, as well as lower social status and economic dependence, married women may be unable to challenge their husbands' extra-marital affairs or insist on condom use for themselves even when they know they are at risk. One philosophy professor used the Bible to justify this, arguing that women vowed to follow their husbands "in sickness and in health". in his view, this absolved husbands of the need to protect their wives; it did not apply the other way round.

Double standards—different sets of sexual rules for women and men—also may hold for other informal long- and short-term relationships. Various societal institutions may promote fidelity, on the one hand, yet also transmit the message that women should not question male unfaithfulness. Thus, heavy deep pressure may make it difficult for boys to resist experimenting with multiple premarital partners, while girls are expected to remain virgins until marriage or at least to remain faithful to one partner.

Havinei, Zimbabwe: [My husband] told me he'd been going with all sorts of women. He said that he couldn't see a woman passing by without falling in love with her. . . He always told me that I was lucky to be his wife. He said the ladies that he'd fallen in love with could fit into four or five buses, but he never took any of them as his wife. He told me to pray to God to say thanks for the husband that I'd been given" [20],

Richard, Uganda: "After dropping out of school at age 17, I made friends with four boys who were prominent. We had quite a lot in common, only they engaged themselves in business and sexual life. We used to have evening walks from place to place, especially where there was entertainment and drinking. At such places, these boys could meet rnore than one sexual partner. They tried their best to persuade rne to do what they were doing, by sending me different girls so that we could exchange a word or two relating to sexual activity. I usually had fears and shyness. I didn't know how to start: what could she think of me and what could she say afterwards? How would I engage in actual physical intercourse?

After all their pressures, the group was not happy with me at

all. They felt that I didn't belong and started tc tease me with a lot of embarrassing questions and statements like: 'You will suffer from backache because of not releasing the semen. Richard, you seem to be impotent - were you castrated?' To sum it up, they deserted me on those grounds". [21],

A further potential source of risk is polygamy, usually meaning multiple wives rather than multiple husbands. If no partner has sex outside the group, this can be a safe system but if any one is infected, all may be at risk.

To curb the epidemic, marriage should be squarely acknowledged as a major risk factor for women in many societies. The simplistic message of lifelong monogamy is a poor one if one partner already has HIV infection and will not use condoms. It has been observed that some men who learn or fear they have HIV infection marry to ensure someone will care for them when they become sick [22].

Violence Against Women

Violence against women, especially rape, is a risk factor that is inadequately recognized or addressed. In South Africa, an estimated 370,000 women are raped every year; in the United States, the Department of Justice reports that a woman is raped every six minutes[23]. Ironically, marital violence is more tolerated by society than violence outside marriage, to the extent that rape within marriage is not a recognized offence in many parts of the world. The woman's word is usually given less credit than that of the rapist. It is also traumatic and difficult for women to report rape and secure a conviction; the extreme is reached in some Islamic countries where a male witness to the rape is required.

Young girls who may be raped by a male relative or who are married off as children are especially vulnerable to HIV/STD *infection. At a maternity hospital in Lima, Peru, 90 per cent of the young' mothers aged 12-16 years had been raped by their (step)fathers or another close family member. In Jamaka, 40 per cent of pregnant girls between 11 and 15 years of age reported that their first intercourse was forced". Meanwhile, in India, nearly 16 per cent of 133 middle and upper-class postgraduate students said they hadbeen sexually abused before the age of 12 years* [21].

Violence against women is sometimes socially condoned. Many would argue that widely distributed films and television portrayals of women as sex objects and victims of abuse reinforce the acceptability of violence against them. In some countries ritualized violence, including rape, is condoned in certain circumstances.

In Papua New Guinea, various factors in tribal life combine to place women in situations of HIV/STD infection risk. Customs encourage strong male bonding mechanisms that are played out during frequent group sex events. Many men participate in having sex with one woman and several other men. Even though this is often against the woman's will, it is not considered rape in the legal sense or condemned [24].

In the worst situations, physical and sexual violence against women are commonplace. Wars and armed conflicts, generally accompanied by widespread rape, now have the added risk of spreading HIV and STDs. The physical trauma of violent sex, often multiple rape, makes transmission particularly likely. Indeed, any coerced sex increases the likelihood of micro-lesions in the vaginal mucosae which may then be entry points for HIV.

Blame and Rejection

Despite the realities of infection patterns, gender stereotypes allow women to be blamed for spreading HIV/STDs. Men are often reported to be infected by sex workers or casual girlfriends, who may be castigated by men and women alike, while less blame tends to fall on men than women who have multiple partners. Indeed, in some African and Asian cultures, it is believed that men must regularly release semen to avoid ill hearth.

Married women in Palembang, Indonesia, who knew little about AIDS, associated it with "loose women" rather than believing themselves to be at risk. They believed that AIDS was contracted through "sexual contact with the lower class of commercial sex workers" and that the high class had usually been protected from STDs. They also said that AIDS comes from "promiscuous women and multiple partners" [25].

Although for both sexes alcohol consumption reduces a sense of responsibility and leads to risk taking, women are more likely to be criticized for this. Male drunkenness is widely tolerated, men being excused for giving way to "natural urges".

Men in some societies may boast about STDs because these show they are "real men" who have sexual relations. For a boy growing up this may be part of his initiation into manhood. But for a woman the story is different; she is more likely to be looked down on as loose or unclean. In much of southern Africa, for example, STDs are derogatorily termed "women's disease" and men blame women for their infections. A doctor's wife in Australia with pelvic inflammatory disease was told by her health worker that she should be ashamed of herself: "someone in your position coming in with a problem like this"[26].

If HIV infection is discovered first in a wife, perhaps because she is the first tested when a baby falls sick, she is readily blamed. Her husband may refuse to be tested or, if found positive, accuse her of infidelity to cover his own behaviour. She may equally be blamed by other relatives, regardless of whose infection was discovered first.

At the same time, the denial of women's sexuality and the social assumption that they must be "pure" make it hard for women to acknowledge any other sexual experiences they may have had even before marriage. To do so is to court divorce or blame, even from female relatives. This blocks women from assessing their own risk and discussing risk behaviours and situations with their partners. Women living with HIV (perhaps more so than men) are even expected to become sexually inactive.

BLAME AND REJECTION

Sylvia, The Netherlands: *"I only dared tell my two sisters after a year. One thought I might be imagining it because I still looked healthy, didn't I? My other sister felt it was my fault. If I had lived well, with a complete family [including a husband], it wouldn't have happened to me. . . My ex-partner told others, too.. . Because people gossiped about me, the vice police started following me; they had heard I was whoring around and infecting everyone. Of course, they couldn't prove that"* [27].

Reina, The Netherlands: *"When a person is infected with HIV, that does not mean that sex disappears from her or his life, even though some people think those living with HIV/AIDS should never have sex again. Of course, none us of living with the virus wants to pass it on to others. . . we want to have sex for the same reasons you do: because we like it, to express love, to gain consolation or security. In that, we are like everyone else"* [28].

Blame can also lead to institutionalized human rights violations, e.g., the compulsory screening of sex workers. Women carrying condoms may be charged by police as sex workers; thus even when they act to safeguard themselves, this may backfire.

Lack of Information

Many women have poor understanding of their own bodies, mechanisms of HIV/STD transmission and their level of risk in unprotected sex. Many men also lack adequate information about their own bodies and tend to have even less information about women's bodies and needs.

Addressing these gaps in information and understanding is difficult because many poor men, and even more women, have low level of education and literacy and have lime access to printed information on HIV/AIDS and STDs. Men are more often able to gain information from radio and television. Consequently women hear about HIV/STDs later and not infequently have little or incomplete information about transmission. This may prevent them from assessing adequately their own risks. A female merchant in Senegal commented: "I don't need condoms because I am not a prostitutes have a husband and children. It is rare that during my travels I fall to the advances of a man. When I do, it is with someone I trust. I only choose to have sexual relations with men who are clean and visibly healthy, polite, and capable of respecting me. These men know me, trust me and know that they don't need to use condoms with me."[29]

Communication

Poor communication between parents and children and between partners about relationships, male and female sexual needs and responsibilities exacerbates risk..Youth as well as adult can be taught to discuss sex-related issues (health, needs, relationship; ideally, this should become an accepted norm.

Communicating can be hard

Somchai, Thailand: "I want someone to talk to, but it is very difficult to open up. I cannot talk to my wife about this. she does not have much to say about it and rarely exchanges conversation with me. I don't really know how she feels or what she really thinks. She is a very good wife but we cannot be friends[30].

Woman, South Pacific: "I was aware my husband was having casual sex when not with me, but I was too ashamed to ask him to take precautions. I kept telling myself, next time. My advice to young mothers is, 'Don't ever wait for next time.' Now I have big regrets. I'm so lucky that I didn't have any more children after I was infected"[31].

Family Stress

Women's traditional family roles are arduous. Rural women in many pans of the world are primarily responsible for subsistence agriculture and, in rural and urban areas, informal sector activities. Women usually undertake most household tasks, go through pregnancy, childbirth and lactation, and rear children. Large numbers of women are in fact household heads but lack sufficient authority, money and material resources, family and formal support to provide adequately for their children and themselves. AIDs-related stigmatization and the extra care burdens brought on by the disease worsen existing gender inequalities, increasing women's vulnerability and exploitation.

In an African country, when Janet's husband learned that she had HIV infection, he threw her out with their two small children. Janet's father had died of AIDS and her mother was sick but trying to look after Janet's seven younger siblings. The logical outcome was for Janet to return to her parents' home and help. Her mother has since died, leaving Janet to care for all nine children. None are in school, all are malnourished. They live in one room, a corner of which is partitioned off and rented out to provide a small income. This, and what the older girls can earn from selling sex, keeps the family alive. No help has been forthcoming from Janet's husband nor from other relatives on either side.

The impact of AIDS on the family may be devastating, with both parents and sometimes one or more children becoming ill and dying. Girls may be withdrawn from school to look after their families, thus increasing their economic and social vulnerability when they grow up. The elderly also take up an increasing care burden when they themselves may be frail.

"A nurse: "In many countries in Africa families admit they have had to disrupt the schooling of the girl children; first, because they need another pair of hands to help them in caring for the sick, and second, because the family resources are reduced and the little funds available go into meeting the basic survival needs of the family.... They seem to see this as one big disadvantage of the home-care programme activities".[32]

AIDS makes decision-making about child-bearing, abortion and breast-feeding much more difficult. Available services may or may not provide helpful advice or be sensitive to the stress women face around these and other sexual health issues. In fact, women and couples may face humiliation and misinformation in the very centres and at the hands of the so-called professionals supposed to help them.

Pung, Thailand: "It all happened with my first pregnancy when I had a blood test. The nurse asked me some questions and finally told me I was infected with the HIV virus.. . I brought my husband in for testing and he tested HIV-positive. . . I remember crying when both of us sat in front of the nurse. She asked us what we wanted to do with our unborn child. She suggested aborting the child and added that it would be free of charge. If I agreed to do so, I was also required to have a hysterectomy.

I talked to my husband and we both agreed to have an ultrasound to see if our child was healthy. The technician said the child was healthy and strong. Then she looked at my HIV status and suddenly replied: 'No, no you cannot keep the child'; her voice was so threatening. 'You must abort the child', she insisted.

My husband said it is probably better to abort the child, letting go now was better than losing it when the child grew and became as lovely as our dreams. I was not sure myself but was in a state of shock. I asked the nurse if I could have a sterilization that was reversible. She looked at me with surprise and asked if I still had hope for a cure. On the form there was only a hysterectomy so she wrote that I wished not to have a permanent sterilization operation.

I had my child aborted, with a special deal: abortion with sterilization — free of charge. But I still don't know what kind of sterilization I got. I am not sure if it is a reversible or permanent sterilization. I have no way of knowing what has been done to my own body"[33].

Home Care

In areas where the epidemic is already severe, particularly sub-Saharan Africa, hospitals cannot cope and much patient nursing is done at home Numerous home-care programmes have been developed by church and community groups or as hospital outreach programmes. AIns service organizations provide counselling, material and practical help, spiritual support nursing care and advice. Excellent work is performed by dedicated staff, yet coverage remains low, often under 10 per cent. Visits from support teams may be on a fixed and infrequent schedule, and cost-effectiveness and sustainability remain serious concerns. The extra burden inevitably falls on the family, in particular on women.

In other regions, such as Latin America, the Middle East and Asia, some hospitals, clinics and social services do not provide care because staff are still afraid to accept people with HIV/AIDS. Stigmatization and discrimination may also prevent families and community members from providing support.

The growing orientation towards home care may, in fact, worsen women's situation, particularly as men are often the first to become sick. The wife may have to nurse her husband while her own health deteriorates, but the main expenditures are for his care. There may be no appropriate care-givers to nurse her through her sickness. Rather than an excessive focus on home care, developing a continuum of care between hospitat clinic, local hospice and other community care is preferable, a strategy supported by WHO. This enables health workers at the local clinics, community health workers and neighbours to help when appropriate and when requested by the family.

ASPANE, in Mexico, helped Yolanda, 26 years old. She lived in a "house" of carton near garbage dump in a Mexico City suburb with her 3-year-old son and 5-year-old daughter. When her partner died of AIDS and her neighbours discovered that Yolanda was also HIV-positive, they tried to drive her away. Yolanda sought refuge with her mother-in-law, but her daughter was sexually abused by a brother-in-law in that household. In desperation, Yolanda turned for help to a charitable organisation for abandoned children. After proving that her children were HIV-negative, so that the organization would accept them, the Department of Social Welfare helped Yolanda to transfer custody of the children legally to the organization. They went there when she died.

Men need to be motivated to assume stronger care roles in the family, both for the sick and in general around child care. Health and welfare concerns cannot remain women's preserve. If this can be achieved, husbands may be less likely to desert women who are found to have HIV and will write wills or other wise provide for their families when they themselves are dying.

Legal and Human Rights

At present, women's rights in many countries are curtailed. They may have little right to land, to inherit property, even to keep their own children when their husbands die. AIDS throws these problems into stark relief because more women are being widowed at a young age and will themselves face an early death. Safeguarding their children's future may be a desperate worry for these women, yet they may lack the means to provide for them without extended family support. In some countries, women am traditionally inherited by the deceased husband's brother. Their economic and social survival may depend on their acquiescence.

On the other hand, after the death of, husband, women around the world may be disinherited by the husband's relatives, particularly if they blame the woman for his death.

At another level, marries women's confidentiality may be broken with relative impunity leading to violence or desertion if their husbands blame them for infection. Meanwhile, women may not be informed of their partners' HIV status. The right of partner notification versus strict confidentiality is being debated in many countries and different policies are being developed. For women the outcome is particularly crucial as infection often enters the family through the husband. Uninfected wives could, in theory, protect themselves but only if access to information is accompanied by the economic, social and legal means to take preventive action.

VIOLATIONS OF HUMAN RIGHTS

ASPANE in Mexico helps Rosa, who contracted HIV from her bisexual husband. He abandoned her and their four children when he learned that she, too, was HIV-positive. Rosa's in-laws blamed her for the HIV infection and consequently refused to offer her any help or information about her husband, who went into hiding for fear of being made legally responsible for child support.

Deborah in Uganda lost her husband to AIDS and is herself very sick. Her brother-in-law tried from the very beginning to inherit her, but she categorically refused so as not to infect him and his wife. He repeatedly told her he does not care that she has AIDS and is willing to take the risk of becoming infected. He harassed her for almost a year; when she held firm and refused, he cut off all financial support to her and he four children. Once she refused him, she was ostracized by the entire family and cannot rely on them for anything, even moral support. Now, he is trying to claim the land that his brother left jointly to them[34].

The rights of women living with HIV to bear children or seek an abortion are hotly debated. A British woman living with HIV was angered and upset by accusations that her choice to have a baby was selfish as the child risked infection or, if it lived, would certainly be orphaned fairly young[35]. In many developing countries a woman's status is highly dependent on motherhood; much more than in Britain it may be of great importance to an HIV-positive woman to have a child.

The issue of sex work also raises difficult legal and ethical problems. While soliciting remains illegal in most countries, sex workers remain vulnerable to abuse, are difficult to reach with HIV/STD prevention and support programmed and face increased stigma. Yet arrangements for sex work may involve minors, abduction and coercion; these aspects of the trade must be stopped. AIDS is giving rise to increased public outrage about these human rights violations.

"When life became difficult in her native village of Melamchi in the Nepali hills, Geeta moved to Kathmandu where she worked as a housemaid. When her cousin promised her a better job in a carpet factory in India, she jumped at the opportunity: 'I didn't realise that I was sold to a Nepali brothel keeper in India until the lady told me to engage in business. . . I wept and wept. I was shocked to be sold by my own relative. I went mad. They admitted me into a mental hospital. After a year, I was ultimately forced into prostitution. I never liked it—that was not what I had wanted. But you can't fight against luck and fate.'

Geeta was sent home with 200 Indian rupees (US$ 6.50) for her transport after she tested HIV-positive. Back in Melamchi, she found her mother had died and her father refused to take her back. Determined to begin a new life, she rented a liquor shop with her savings. The shop was successful until her HIV status became known in the village-then business collapsed and she was forced to close down". [36]

Another neglected area is the rights of homosexual women and men to social acceptance, child care, marriage and inheritance. Lesbian relationships are a preferred lifestyle for some women and generally carry a low risk of HIV infection. However, societal intolerance precludes many women from exploring this option even if they would like to. Male gay relationship are more common in some societies, but their very existence may be denied or condemned, leading gay men to marry and engage in bisexual contacts even if they prefer only to have sex with men. "Talk to any African government about homosexual issues and the spread of AIDS, and they simply tell you that homosexual activities only go on in the Western world," said Obi Zikora, president of Gentlement Alliance, in Nigeria [37]. "The stigma attached to homosexuality frightens away many who should be examined from going to doctors."

As with sex workers, legal rights for homosexuals and lesbians need to be strengthened and societal intolerance challenged if they are to cope better with HIV and AIDS and not be driven underground.

Structural Patterns

Economic policies widening the gap between rich and poor countries and rich and poor people within nations exacerbate the conditions for HIV/STD transmission. For example, economic structural adjustment programmes may have a negative impact on rural and urban poverty, national debt and trade relations. These policies hamper countries' capacity to provide social, educational and medical support to affected families and communities, especially if food subsidies are cut and social, welfare and health expenditures are reduced.

The epidemic has hardest the developing world and the poor inner cities of industrialized countries, which are least able to cope. Furthermore, poverty increasingly has a female face: UNDP estimates that 70 per cent of the world's poor are women. As prevention efforts are stepped up, communities' abilities to cope must also be strengthened. Only through improving coping capacity will fear and stigma around AIDS be reduced, allowing prevention strategies to really work.

Within this framework, empowering women and reducing gender inequalities are critical. The structural basis of gender inequality must be challenged by promoting personal attitude and behaviour change. Women must gain access to the education, training and employment they need to achieve sexual relations on equal terms and to control their risk of HIV/STDS. Cultural expectations that exonerate men from taking responsibility for health and welfare concerns must be transformed, along with the structural conditions of work, housing, migration, etc., that prevent this from becoming a reality.

Woman, Zimbabwe: "My husband passed away from AIDS when he was 35; he was ill for six months. He used to work as a general labourer in a big firm and only came home at weekends. We had eight children, but the last two both died. This leaves me with six children to feed. It is very hard. The two eldest have had to leave school to try and earn money, but I am trying to keep the youngest four in school.

In the early stages of my husband's illness we could cope. It became difficult when he lost his job. We had to spend a lot of his savings on special food for him, and he lost his medical aid cover. I grow maize and try to make money selling crochet work, but it is not sufficient. I cannot get a proper job —in these days it is even more difficult as a woman because it is men who are expected to work.

My husband's workplace helped with the funeral and will pay me a small pension for four years. But he had not worked there long so the amount is low. My husband's brother is supposed to take care of us. He knows our problems but did not help at all during my husband's illness nor after his death. Now he wants to marry me, but I think it is in order to take my husband's estate, not to help us. I am lucky because my husband left a letter instructing that his property was to remain with us and that I should not marry his brother in the traditional way. Fortunately, the headman and the other village elders support this decision because they know that this brother did not help us when my husband was alive. Otherwise it would be very hard for me to refuse. I have to think of my children. But by refusing to marry I lose any hope of help from him.

If I die, the oldest children will have to take care of the young ones. I cannot trust my husband's brother, and I do not think his first wife would treat them well. My own two sisters cannot take the children because their husbands will not allow this. It is not traditional and they have their own families. The women take care of the children, but it is the husbands who must make the decision about this."

5. Can Women and Men reduce risks and share responsibilities?

The goal of our response to HIV/AIDS and STD is to decrease vulnerability to infection, reduce stigmatization and discrimination and curb the epidemic socio-economic impact. This will be best achieved through gender-based approaches promoting shared responsibility for prevention and care between women and men.

To ensure wider development and implementation of gender-sensitive strategies, collective action is required. Women's organizations and networks can help by reinforcing such strategies, sensitizing and mobilizing women and men, and making linkages to other gender-based initiatives in society. Collaboration and co-ordination between UN system agencies, governments and NGO networks may further serve to reinforce gender-sensitive responses.

Gender-sensitive strategies must address both short and longer-term needs and goals Short-term strategies focus on people immediate needs in specific communities, including obtaining basic information about HIV/AIDS and STD, gaining access to sexual health education, acquiring condoms and obtaining back-up support for home-based care.

Longer-terme strategies are directed at underlying cultural and social structures. They aim to promote mutual respect between men and women and equal access to all types of resources. The goals of longer terms strategies include, but are not limited to:

- changing ideas and social norms that keep women in an inferior social position
- achieving shared decision-making power between women and men at all levels: in relationships, community affairs, political and economic bodies, etc.
- creating structural changes to give women equal access to education, training and income-earning opportunities.
- reallocating work responsibilities so that women and men share them fairly
- encouraging legalization of traditional marriages or

unions where this would strengthen the rights of women to property, inheritance and children.

Governments and NGOs are now beginning to integrate a gender perspective in to their HIV/AIDS/STD programmes. Women living with HIV/AIDS are playing an increasingly important role in this process. Below, examples from programmes around the world show how a gender-based response is being developed. The examples are randomly grouped action areas. Gender-sensitive strategies must be developed simultaneously in all of them:

- creating a supportive and enabling environment
- research
- facilitating access to information and services
- changing the way we think and act
- sensitizing and mobilizing men
- combating discrimination
- developing gender-sensitive care and support
- living positively with HIV/AIDS.

A Supportive and Enabling Environment

The social environment must enable people to achieve effective prevention and care. Policy, legal and human rights, economic, social, cultural and educational structures are needed that benefit women to the same extent as men. If such structures are developed, then women and men will have a much better chance to change the social norms and values oppressing them in their daily lives. Although structural changes take time to achieve, strategies must be developed to address them at the same time as grassroots initiatives improve women's daily life situation.

Structural Measures

Decreasing women's economic dependence is an important step towards enabling them to reduce infection risks for themselves and their families. A credit scheme established by the Grameen Bank and Bangladesh Rural Advancement Committee (BRAC), for example, enables rural women to establish an independent income by offering them loans. The programme has enhanced women's autonomy and self-confidence and led to increased contraceptive use[38].

In addition to income-generating schemes, other structural measures are necessary. These include guaranteeing women:

- better access to schooling, vocational training and higher education

— equal access to employment and equal pay for equal work
— equitable access to social and health services
— legal and human rights protection equal to that of men
— better representation in political and economic bodies
— freedom from restrictive cultural expectations and practices.

Political and Community Support

Broad political and bureaucratic support is necessary if governments are to implement the measures outlined above. This can be facilitated if NAPS are made intersectoral, involving not only the health sector but also ministries and departments such as women's affairs, education, labour, justice, agriculture, defence and social affairs. By creating links among these sectors, the HIV/AIDS epidemic can illustrate why women must gain greater access to education, paid employment and social services. NAPS can further mobilize support for a gender-based response by formulating policies that provide various ministries and NGOs with a framework for action.

INCORPORATING GENDER AND WOMEN'S CONCERNS INTO NATIONAL RESPONSES

The first generation of National AIDS Programmes (NAPS) were gender neutral in their approach. Health education messages ignored gender disparities and roles in sexual and family relations. One and all were simply urged to "stick to one partner", avoid casual sex, reduce the number of sexual partners or use condoms.

As awareness gradually developed, NAPS started to address specific issues confronting women in relation to HIV/ AIDS. The initial approach was to "mobilize women" through women's NGOs as agents of health education and information. When concern arose about women's heightened vulnerability to HIV, interventions were developed to enable women to talk about sexual safety and condom use with their partners. This approach was criticized because it neglected men and the fact that men control the circumstances under which most women are exposed to risk or protected from infection.

Analysis of gender disparities and women's disadvantaged socio-economic status is now being incorporated into national HIV/AIDS policies. The challenge is to integrate gender considerations into all aspects of programme development. Botswana's National Information, Education and

Communication Strategy for HIV/AIDS Prevention places gender prominently among factors related HIV/STD spread. Guidelines for gender interventions for men and women are a key component for district programme planning. By determining how gender disparities affect women throughout their lifetime, interventions can be facilitated at community, school and workplace levels to ensure that girls do not grow into adults with increased vulnerability to HIV/STD infection.

Interventions also need to take account of women's responsibility for providing family and community care. Programmes developed by social welfare agencies, NGOS, employers, etc. should make provision for these responsibilities. Education and communication programmes should encourage sharing of domestic responsibilities and tasks between men and women.

Only when countries address gender disparities squarely in their economic political and social development strategies will incorporation of gender and women's concerns into HIV/AIDS programmes have a sustainable impact.

Tshidi Moeti, former Botswana NAP Manager

"The most critical decision of my life was to reveal to representatives of Caribbean media that I had tested positive for the AIDs virus. Coming face-to-face with a battery of journalists was a nerve-racking experience. I decided to impose this agony on myself in an effort to dispel some of the myths surrounding HIV-positive peoples. During my presentation, information that would usually be regarded by journalists as a 'juicy story' was instead treated as a moving commentary. On the admission of some of the journalists, my presence and commentary were edifying and represented their first opportunity to understand the plight of HIV-infected persons."

A Women living with HIV[39]

CREATING A SUPPORTIVE ENVIRONMENT

When sex workers in Calabar, Nigeria, wanted their customers to use condoms, they failed to get support from the people who influence their working conditions, such as hotel owners, managers and chairladies (head sex workers) . The Cross River State AIDS Programme (CRSAP) therefore approached them on the sex workers' behalf.

A special STD clinic was established to serve the women near their working sites. Collective actions were fostered to protect the sex workers' interests. The hotel managers and chairladies began backing the women's demand for higher fees and their right to refuse clients who wouldn't use condoms. The sex workers also were able to retain fees when clients attempted to renege on condom use. Harassment and extortion by security agents decreased, to.

The women reported more confidence in handling problems with clients, hotel owners and the police. They also organized a self-help group called Nka Iban Uko (Women of Courage), which focuses on skills training and services for their children[40].

Governmental and NGO programmes mobilizing communities to create conditions for effective prevention and care need expansion. Besides serving as a channel for information on HIV/AIDS and STDs, the media can mobilize public support for gender-sensitive programmes by highlighting the effects of the epidemic on women. Media workers may also be enlisted to help create a climate tolerant towards those affected by or responding to HIV/AIDS.

Policy-Making and Agenda-Setting

To ensure broad-based support, all agencies and government ministries must add HIV/AIDS and STDs to their action agendas. In this way, alliances for policy-related advocacy as well as new initiatives will arise at the national and community levels:

— After a national workshop in Malaysia where women were trained to organize HIV/AIDS awareness workshops, such meetings were held even in the most remote parts of the country. By linking women's umbrella organizations, duplication of effort was avoided and time and money saved[41].

— In England, regional seminars were organized on the theme "Women, AIDS and the Future" in collaboration with local women's organizations. Activities carried out by participants afterwards included: reporting on HIV/AIDS to local organizations; planning similar seminars in their area; talking with men, family, friends and colleagues about HIV/AIDS; writing advocacy letters to government ministers; holding study days/meetings with church groups; and writing articles for the press[42].

— The Society for Women and AIDS in Africa (SWAA) raises political awareness concerning gender in relation to HIV/AIDS and STDs and provides a voice for women in many parts of the continent. SWAA has national member organization in more than 20 countries.

Research

Biomedical studies-e.g., on opportunistic infections in women and ways to reduce perinatal transmission (including through breast-feeding)are increasing in scope but need expansion. More support is required for research on female-controlled methods to prevent HIV/STD infection, including the female condom. The current research priority is to develop microbicide, which appear to have great potential for acceptance. Other important topics for a gender-sensitive research agenda include:

- barriers to female control HIV/STD risks and ways to overcome them
- how young women and men define personal risk in relation to different types of relationship
- how men and women currently protect themselves against infection
- barriers to female and male STD treatment and how to improve access
- improving contact tracing for STDs
- the effects of HIV infection during various phases of a woman's life cycle (e.g., in relation to onset of menstruation and menopause)
- the appropriateness of counselling messages and methods in meeting women's and men's specific concerns
- partner notification, confidentiality and information sharing
- the division of labour concerning reproductive and productive tasks at the household and community levels and how these contribute to maintaining women in their current lower status and increase their burdens related to care.

NGOs and research institutes have not waited for international leader ship and donor funding to undertake studies in these areas. Research must be demystified so that more local organizations develop their own research agendas. Some of the most useful findings come from simple small-scale studies, especially when their results are linked directly to the implementing service agencies.

Exciting developments are taking place through participatory action research in which community members explore topics such as differences in knowledge and information sources for boys and girls, traditional communication channels used by women and men and inter generational family communication. The findings indicate how educational programmes can be better structured and channelled.

Dissemination of research results urgently needs expansion. This can be facilitated by linking researchers and NGOs. The International Center for Research on Women (USA) worked with Comprehensive Health for Women (SIPAM) and the Programme in Gender Studies of the National Autonomous University in Mexico to document and analyse their studies and programmes on women and AIDS. A forum held to discuss the results with NGOs, researchers and government institutions resulted in the formation of a permanent researcher NGO network[43].

Establishment of "inter-country" projects is another approach. For example, FEIM in Argentina and the Movimiento Paulina Luisi in Uruguay together planned action research and an intervention to increase gender awareness and prevention possibilities for poor and lower middle-class women[44]. They then compared their findings, identifying concerns that are country-specific and broader in scope.

Donor organizations can contribute to dissemination of research findings by funding the publication of research reports and researchers' participation in national and international meetings. Many UN agencies have distribution channels that might be expanded to include dissemination of studies carried out by governments and NGOS.

Facilitating Access to Information and Services

Information Dissemination

Printed materials can be improved by involving women and men in creating more appropriate messages and materials that address their specific concerns. Funding is also needed for translation of texts into local languages to allow greater access to printed information.

Including HIV/STD information in a variety of health programmes, such as mother and child health and family planning, reaches more people. The Guatemalan Association for the Prevention and Control of AIDS conducted educational sessions and small-group workshops on health and sexuality, self-esteem, partner communication and communication with adolescent children for women waiting at antenatal clinics [45]. Fears that discussions about HIV/STDs would cause the women to worry, increasing their stress levels during pregnancy, appeared unfounded. On the contrary, women reported that they felt relaxed and less apprehensive in talking about condoms, infidelity, STDs and AIDS with their partners. More than half of those interviewed postpartum said they shared written materials with their partners.

Information channels other than health services are also available. Traditional community counsellors, women and men's associations, church-based groups, sports and recreational clubs provide entry points for individual and group educational sessions. Other possibilities include labour and trade unions and groups participating in agricultural and small-enterprise projects. Training peer educators has proved particularly effective among women from various walks of life. NGOs have further explored ways to reach women whose mobility is restricted, e.g., girls living in slums and female prisoners.

REACHING OUT TO WOMEN

Both existing and new communication channels can be used to reach out to women and girls.

Traditional Associations

The Cheikh Anta Diop University in Senegal mobilized members of a well-respected women's association, the Dimba, to help organize community education sessions. Dimba membership is restricted to women who coped well with difficult circumstances, like infertility problems, repeated miscarriages and adopting orphans. They are influential because their members have thorough knowledge of women's and infants' illnesses. The University also worked with women ofthe Laobe ethnic group, who provide advice about reproductive health and sexuality. Laobe women are traders who make and sell products designed to enhance sexual pleasure; they were persuaded to sell condoms as an erotic product [29].

Adolescent Girls

World Vision designed a sex and family education programme for low-income adolescent girls in Bombay, India. The girls had little information about reproduction and almost none about HIV/STDs. They seemed trapped in a "culture of silence" that did not permit them to voice their opinions, feelings or concerns on any issue.

Parental and community support were essential to permit the girls to participate (e.g., providing child care for younger siblings). A community AIDS/STD awareness programme was therefore implemented, including meetings with mothers, teenage boys and young men, and a street play dramatizing women's status at different stages in life. The meetings stressed the value of educational interventions for the girls.

Topics discussed with the girls included: being a woman, female puberty, sexuality, sexual exploitation and harassment, health problems (with specific reference to HIV/STDs) and the development of an action plan to protect oneself against infection. The programme had to encourage the girls to talk. As the sessions progressed, they became more self-confident, freely voicing their opinions, suggestions and criticisms. The feedback was very positive, with the girls asking for more sessions[46].

Women Prisoners

"My partner used a condom because he saw the signs on my arms. That hurt me. Now I know something more about AIDS and I have changed my mind: I think that he did the right thing because both of us ran less risk." This comment came from a participant in the "Women, AIDS, Information" Project at the women's prison Le Nuove in Turin, Italy.

The 3-month project was initiated at the prisoners' request. The project team helped the women discuss HIV-testing, how to reduce infection risks and how to live with seropositive persons without fear or rejection. The women then developed a story that could be used as the basis for a video.

The intervention enabled the women to share their experiences as equals and realize they were capable of carrying out such a project. They began discussing the possibility of having relationships with other groups working on AIDS both inside and outside prison[47].

Reorientation of Services

NAPS, local governments and NGOS are reorienting services to better meet fee needs of women and men. They are providing information and condoms to men and women at sites they regularly visit (e.g., clubs, cafes, hairdressers). Clinics are being located where people live (e.g., STD clinics located in sex worker districts, mobile clinics). This enables people to acquire what they need without much effort.

- A programme in Haiti, which sells condoms in places where women feel comfortable buying them, aims to give women skills in negotiating social and cultural barriers to condom use. Product packaging is discreet, with advertising stressing women's right to control their sexuality [48].
- Government and NGOs in Calcutta, India, have increased female sex workers' access to STD services and health care for their children by opening a general health clinic in a local youth club. The clinic runs during the day and the club at night. Peer educators participate in outreach activities[49].
- The Filipino NGO Kabalikat provides comprehensive

services to female, male and youth sex workers by training peer educators, running a drop-in centre, offering short-term shelter and nutritional support and providing medical and residential care to those who need support[50]. In Colombia, PROFAMILIA runs male family planning clinics, emphasizing that family planning is a right. The men are offered general counselling, STD/HIV diagnosis, vasectomies and a free hotline. The programme has resulted in more early consultations related to STDs and increased condom use[51].

These types of programmes need to be replicated, along with increasing efforts to make the female condom and spermicides more accessible and affordable.

STD diagnosis and treatment are of special importance since STDs increase vulnerability to HIV. Because most STD diagnostic tests are too costly or require equipment unavailable at the primary health care level, WHO recommends syndromic management based on the identification of collections of STD signs and symptoms (syndromes). Any woman presenting with a particular syndrome is treated for all STD infections commonly associated with those symptoms.

To increase the accessibility and acceptability of STD services, stigmatization and the negative attitudes of staff must be reduced. Contact tracing procedures guaranteeing confidentiality also need further development.

Changing the Way we think and Act

Programmes can facilitate community exploration of how gender is related to prevention and care by addressing the following kinds of question: —Beliefs: how can people be assisted to re-examine ideas related to HIV/AIDS/STDs and sexuality which hinder prevention, e.g., men need to release semen to stay healthy, women must receive semen to promote an unborn baby's growth?

— *Relationships*: how are relationships defined, e.g., what kind of contact do the partners have in casual, regular and other types of relationship? What makes a relationship good? Who usually makes decisions in relationships? What circumstances in relationships increase or decrease risks of HIV/STD infection?

— *Sexuality*: why, with whom and in what circumstances do women and men engage in sex? What needs and desires do women and men have regarding sex and what do they understand of each other's needs? What types of sexual practices and needs are or are not considered normal and why? How do various aspects of sexuality affect risks of HIV/STD infection?

— *Power between women and men*: how should power relations between women and men be changed? How can women gain greater control over their lives and situations contributing to their risk of HIV/STD infection, e.g., condom use, types of sexual activity, extra-marital sex?

— *Care and support*: who provides what types of care and support to family members and needy people in the community? Why is caretaking divided between women and men in a particular way? What needs to be done to ensure that women and men both participate actively in providing care and support?

CREATING GENDER AWARENESS AND BUILDING SKILLS TO ACT ON IT

Around the world, communities are becoming more conscious of gender issues and acting to address them:

Women, Children, Citizenship and Health (MCCS), an NGO in Sao Paulo, Brazil, recruits women for sensitization workshops from mothers' clubs, unions, political parties, professional associations, community groups and feminist organizations. MCCS adapted its approach to safer sex when it was recognized that family planning programmes have emphasized use of "long-term" and "inexpensive" methods, such as sterilization and the pill. Barrier methods, such as condoms and spermicides, are frequently identifed as inefficient, inappropriate for lower-income groups and too complex for use by uneducated persons. MCCS encourages women to think about contraception in relation to HIV/STDs in the broader context of their overall health[52].

Julliet Awino, a widowed mother in Uganda, stars in "Strings Attached", a play portraying her personal experience with HIV/AIDS. It emphasizes practices that undermine women's role in society and the home, making them vulnerable to HIV transmission, such as: male pre- and extra-marital sexual activity, hostility from in-laws who blame wives for family problems, abandonment without rights and property if a woman refuses sexual "ritual cleansing" when she becomes a widow. The drama has contributed to an increase in people writing wills to regulate inheritances*[53].

In Kalabo, Zambia, women aware that girls in their area were especially vulnerable to HIV formed a committee to focus on communal attitudes towards sexuality and behaviours affect-

ing women. They organized seminars for more than 600 women, through churches, hospitals and health centres, to stimulate extensive community discussions about female sexuality and gender roles. As a result, the traditional initiation ceremony for girls was revised to include information on reproductive health and HIV/STDs [54].

In Mali, a primary health care project (SSP-Segou) and programme focused on improving women's status (PROFED) generated discussions on gender and sexual health among the general community and young women in particular during a needs assessment study. To break down barriers against discussing sexuality, they developed a drama with the villagers about a woman who has problems giving birth. It was acted out for the entire village, following an introduction by a male village leader concerned about women's situation. The audience became highly involved, worrying about the sick woman and giving advice to the husband. In this climate male and female researchers could address all kinds of topics from the perspective of both sexes. Some previously taboo subjects, like the negative consequences of female circumcision and sexual violence against women as a risk factor for HIV/AIDS, were dealt with publicly for the first time. The group discussions were geared towards analysing the villagers' problems and mobilizing them into action. The first step was to re-establish a village pharmacy [55].

Participatory group methodologies increase awareness and motivate adults and youth to devise solutions to the gender-based problems they identify. Skills building needs to be an important component of such approaches so that women and men learn how to talk about sex and relationships, resist pressure from peers and partners to engage in unwanted practices and stand up for their rights (e.g., resisting service providers' pressure to have an abortion or sterilization). The capacity to practise such skills is based on a sense of self-worth, a perception of one-self as capable and assertive. Examples of approaches that build self-esteem and gender awareness include:

— using drama and visual arts to help women "discover" their abilities and talents.
— role-play (e.g., to develop safer sex negotiation skills)
— vocational training and education (e.g., production skills, relating skills, managing skills)
— peer education programmes.

Ritual cleansing is a custom among some African cultures wherein the spouse of a deceased man or woman has sexual intercourse with a member of the spouse's family in order to allow the dead person's spirit to attain rest; it also ensures that the spirit will not bother the surviving spouse.

Changes in attitudes need to begin in childhood. Although parents are expected to play the primary role, in many societies talking about sexuality and related issues between parents and children is difficult. A study in Zimbabwe, for example, found that parent-child communication is severely limited, especially in the case of fathers, who are often absent, remote and moody.[56] Research in Mexico showed that adolescents want more communication about sex with their parents than they actually have. Obstacles included parental time/work constraints. not being able to reach agreement, lack of trust and knowledge and embarrassment.[57] Such studies indicate that parents want help to improve their ability to communicate, for instance, through NGO and church training activities for couples.

When questioned, many parents indicate they are willing for others to deliver prevention messages to their children as long as they are informed about the content. Media campaigns can help create a supportive environment for this. NGOs and schools can offer courses and activities for schoolchildren and out-of-school youth that explore gender relations, values, sexuality and related issues. Stressing the effects of positive as well as negative peer pressure is an important component of such programmes. As few teachers and youth workers have been trained to deal with such subjects, organizations such as UNICEF, WHO and UNESCO, as well as NGOS, are assisting governments to develop appropriate materials and training programmes for them. Training of youth peer educators has also shown promising results.

HELPING YOUNG PEOPLE

Two programmes in Asia and Africa are teaching young people the skills needed to insist on safer sex. One programme focuses on pre-marital abstinence and fidelity within marriage and the other on condom use.

In Africa, Aid for AIDS fosters the creation of positive self-images among boys and girls, emphasizing respect for girls. "It's great to be a girl" is an attitude crucial for boys and girls to absorb. The programme uses drama, role-play and discussions to teach young people how to resist peers who try to make them do things they don't want to do. The idea of positive peer pressure is promoted through Anti AIDS Clubs, in which friends help one another stand by mutually agreed behaviours, e.g.: 1. We will make friendships with lots of other boys and girls more important than "pairing off'. 2. We will commit ourselves to avoid sex before marriage. 3. We will especially help and care for any of our friends who have HIV infection.

The University of Chiang Mai in **Thailand** *developed special* *materials for young female factory workers. Research had shown that a lack of communication between women and men, reluctance to discuss condom use ("men's business") and misconceptions about moral goodness andAIDS (if someone looks and acts good, they are perceived as HIV-free) were major obstacles to prevention. Two booklets with discussion starters addressing these factors are used by female peer educators trained to facilitate group discussions and lead group activities.*

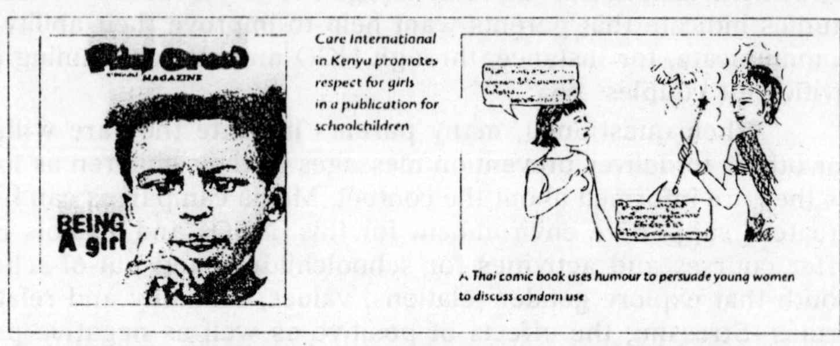

Care International in Kenya promotes respect for girls in a publication for schoolchildren

A Thai comic book uses humour to persuade young women to discuss condom use

A romantic illustrated novel shows the consequences of not discussing sexual behaviour. It tells the story of factory worker Lamyai, who falls in love with Tong Dee. Because he is good, she doesn't ask about his past. Despite warnings from a co-worker, they have unprotected sex. When Tong Dee enters military service to earn money for their marriage, he is tested and found HIV-positive; Lamyai also has the virus and, after working on for a few years, eventually dies.

To demonstrate what girls can say to negotiate condom use, a humorous comic book focuses on a young woman named Jon Di. Before she leaves to work at the factory, Jon Di prays to the Spirit of Good Health: "Please turn something near to me into a living thing —to be my friend—to protect me when I go to Chiang Mai." The Spirit does so, producing Brother Protector Condom, an invisible flying condom. The Spirit promises that if Jon Di and Brother Condom save five young women from AIDS, she will make Brother Condom into a real friend. Jon Di completes the assignment successfully, whereupon the Spirit changes Brother Condom into a young man with a condom head. After protest from Jon Di, the Spirit makes him a completely human companion.

DAVID CUNNINGHAM, Zimbabwe,
KATHLEEN CASH, BUPA ANASUCHATKUL and
WANTANA BUSAYAWONG, Thailand

ENLISTING INFLUENTIAL MEN

The Thai Health Project for Tribal People (HPTP) has trained

influential male community leaders as health educators for isolated hill tribe communities. The headmen, who also act as village counsellors, already have the respect, position and credibility necessary to promote new information. They are also experienced in talking to large groups.

The training seminars include practice teaching sessions. One headman, for example, used a picture of a young girl being sold into sex work to talk about the man who had taken her away and what happened to her once she was in town. HPTP teams visit the headmen several months after the seminars to ask about any problems they have using the materials and what is going well.

Knowledge changes are occurring in villages taught by the headmen. In one tribe, the initial survey showed that 85 per cent of the people had heard of AIDS, but none understood that it could be transmitted from mother to child. After teaching by the headman, 98 per cent of the villagers understood this.

Lori Rowe, Thailand

PARENTS! WHEN YOU CAN'T PROTECT THEM ANYMORE....
...Condoms Can
DO YOU 'VE SPARE CONDOMS MIKA.....?
CONDOMS,!? DO YOU REALLY LOVE YOUR WIFE?
I LOVE MY WIFE THAT'S WHY I ASK FOR CONDOMS...!
!?
© G. Mwampembwa

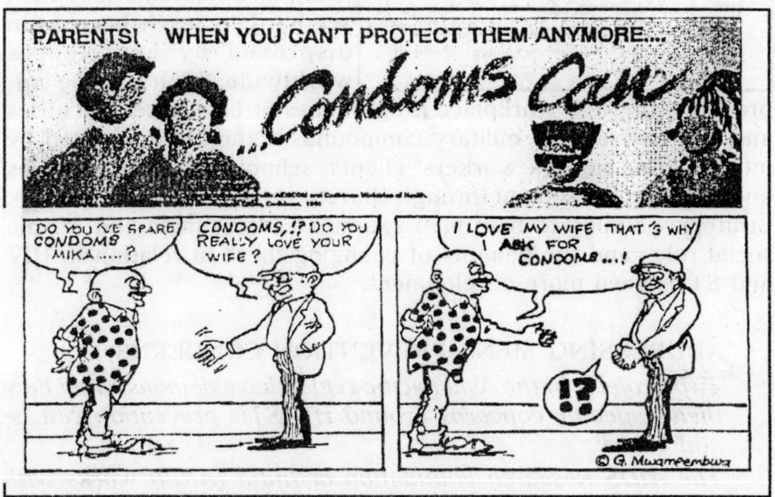

Sensitizing and Mobilizing Men

Men must be sensitized and mobilized to a greater extent for an effective response to HIV/AIDS and STDs. Since men occupy most positions of influence, their participation in advocating gender-sensitive policies and programmes is essential.

Some men are, ofcourse, already aware in this regard. Others, however, have not yet thought about the fact or placing women at a disadvantage. A Filipino NGO, HASIK, has developed a gender training programme for male staff invarious types of organization to address this.[58] Through games, exercises, song, dances and discussions, the men articulate their own ideas about why women are oppressed. Then they address how to change the institutions that determine gender roles, concluding with the formulation of action plans which help the men translate what they have learned into organizational professional goals and schemes.

The collaboration of village headmen, male religious authorities and businessmen in educational interventions and home- and community-based care is most important. They act as role models for the community and can set the example for acceptance of "new" ideas concerning men's and women's responsibilities in preventing HIV transmission and coping with AIDS

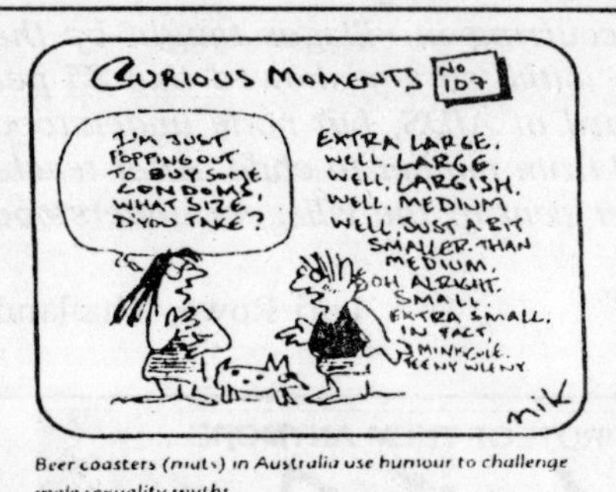

CURIOUS MOMENTS
No 107
I'M JUST POPPING OUT TO BUY SOME CONDOMS, WHAT SIZE D'YOU TAKE?
EXTRA LARGE.
WELL, LARGE.
WELL, LARGISH.
WELL, MEDIUM
WELL, JUST A BIT SMALLER THAN MEDIUM.
OH ALRIGHT. SMALL.
EXTRA SMALL.
IN FACT,
MIK
Beer coasters (mats) in Australia use humour to challenge male sexuality myths

Information and behavioural change programmes specifically targeting men and boys need replication. Objections that men are hard to-reach have been disproved by experiences worldwide. Men can be approached through workplace programmes at businesses, factories and settings such as military compounds. Others are targeted by interventions for sex workers' clients, school-based programmes and activities carried out through churches and recreational groups. Strategies aiming to help men examine current male and female social roles and the benefits of changing these in relation to HIV and STDs need more development.

ADDRESSING MENS PREVENTION CONCERNS

Two projects in the Asia/Pacific region have demonstrated how men's specific concerns around HIV/STD prevention can be addressed:

The AIDS Research Foundation of India (ARFI) works with sex-worker clients in Madras, emphasizing the health benefits of condom use. Truck drivers keep condoms in their trucks to fix radiator hose leaks. ARFI used this practice to start small groups talking about how "leaks during sex" can be fixed. Condoms are provided through transit-stop shops, where they are sold together with items men frequently buy. The truckers also receive key chains containing a compartment for a condom. Since most of the transit-stop teashops play music, a cas-

sette on safety (both on the road and at roadside, "It's all in the rubber", has been distributed with funds from a truck tyre manufacturing company.

Peer opinion leaders tell port/dock workers a story about a man who practices safer sex. To reinforce the message, posters on condom use are displayed in wine shops and barber shops, where the dock workers read the evening newspaper. Some men have been recruited as condom depot holders; a dispensary at the port provides free STD services. Short street plays reinforce the safer sex message. Since the programme started, condom sales have increased at the transitstop and port shops.[59]

The Heterosexual Men's Project in New South Wales, Australia, conducted focus-group discussions with building workers aged between 17-60 years to determine what was important to them in preventing HIV prevention. The groups comprised men from English- and non-English speaking backgrounds and included single, divorced, separated and single men, men in long-term relationships and fathers. Two issues highlighted by the workers were the role of alcohol in promoting unsafe behaviour and difficulties in communicating about sex with women.

Based on the men's suggestions, a campaign was designed using messages on beer coasters and toilet stickers, in pubs and clubs. The beer coasters used "themes" to demystify safe sex and challenge some male sexuality myths. The toilet stickers aimed to facilitate discussion of condom use between men and women by providing humorous ice breakers. Billboard, bus and magazine advertising messages addressed the link between STDs and HIV/AIDS.

HAVING SEX TONIGHT?

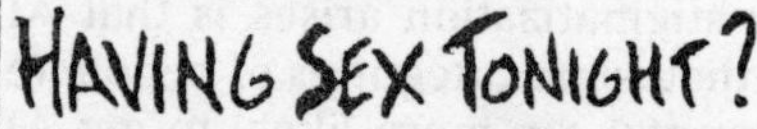

Has your girlfriend read the sticker in the women's toilet?

The one about how hard it is to start talking about safe sex.

This sticker might help break the ice.

..IF HE SEES I'VE GOT CONDOMS HE'LL THINK I'M EASY..
..IF SHE SEES I'VE GOT CONDOMS SHE'LL THINK I'M DESPERATE..
H'MM, THAT REMINDS ME..
Authorised by Family Planning NSW.
Funded by NSW Health Department

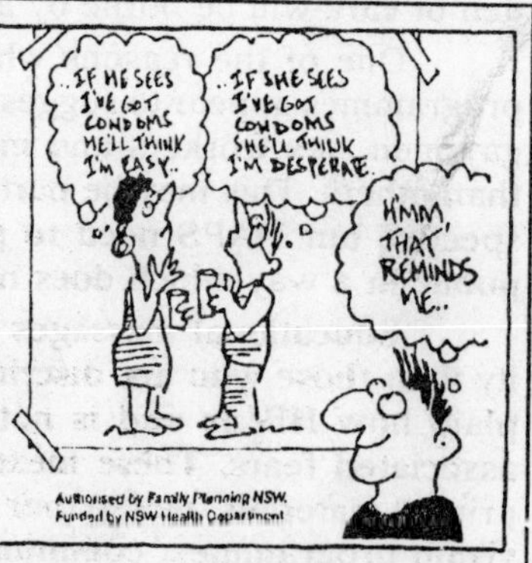

Evaluation showed that 50 per cent of the men familiar with the campaign saw it as personally relevant: 19 per cent of those who had read the beer coasters and stickers said they were

helpful in providing conversation starters on safe sex with their partners: 27 per cent said it led them to discuss this with their colleagues. Generally, the campaign messages were best recalled by men 18 to 24 years old, single men and condom users. Recommendations made for future campaigns included:

- *tailor messages to emphasize that condoms promote health rather than prevent disease*
- *employ humour to challenge aspects of male culture that do not support safer behaviour*
- *develop dynamic and flexible approaches to address men's sexual health needs in the context of changing life roles*
- *use medical centres, youth services and sexual health centres to provide information and resources*
- *use the media, particularly men's magazines, to support sexual health education*
- *locate future campaigns in venues where alcohol is consumed such as clubs and pubs* [60].

Combating Discrimination

Women and men living with HIV/AIDS, their families and people negatively associated with the epidemic (e.g., homosexuals, sex workers, street-children, migrants and foreigners) still face stigmatization and discrimination. Combating this is an important public health strategy. If people are to engage in safer sex, they must feel confident that they will not be abused or abandoned by their partners. If potential careproviders condemn those living with the virus, adequate care and support cannot be given and the burden of care will be borne by a few.

One of the reasons why stigmatization arises is that AIDS programmes appear to suggest that some categories of people (e.g., gay men, sex workers and migrants) are more likely to get AIDS than others. This may be partly true from the epidemiological perspective but NAPS need to present the epidemic to the general public in a way which does not reinforce such perceptions.

Educational messages can emphasize the need for solidarity with those who are discriminated against. A first step is to explain how HIV is and is not transmitted, debunking myths and associated fears. These messages can be communicated through printed materials, newspaper and magazine articles, radio and television programmes, community education sessions, hotlines and word of mouth. Health workers should be taught the principles of universal precautions that should apply to blood and body fluids from all patients, not only those they know or suspect to be HIV-infected.

Personalizing the epidemic also works well: when people tell their stories, they provide concrete examples rather than distant images of "AIDS victims" or "HIV carriers". The first woman to speak out publicly in the Philippines greatly increased the impact of the NAP campaigns, helping raise the general public's awareness in a positive way. Persons living with HIV are often in the forefront of actions to challenge discrimination. A woman working for a care agency in Canada, for example, sued her employer after she was dismissed because her serostatus became known She won her case, simultaneously giving other seropositive women encouragement to stand up for their nights. [61]

NGCs can play a useful "watchdog role" regarding human rights violations. The International Gay and Lesbian Human Rights Commission, for example, publishes an *Act or Alert* bulletin to publicize discrimination and stimulate responses to specific abuses. Amnesty International and many NGOS document discrimination cases so that these can be brought to the attention of the government and press. Lobbying for changes in discriminatory laws and the passage or endorsement of protective ones (e.g., the UN Convention for the Elimination of All Forms of Discrimination against Women) is another important action area. Many NGOs also publish HIV/AIDS rights charters and refer persons suffering discrimination to legal services so that they can pursue their rights.

Further work must be done to change customary and written laws so women have legal recourse in cases of abuse, loss of maintenance and discrimination over inheritance. Many women are unaware of their rights and don't know that they are legally protected against certain abuses. This knowledge gap is slowly being filled by lawyers' groups and NGOs worldwide through "legal literacy" programmes, making the law accessible to women and promoting their capacity to understand and assert their rights.[62]

PROMOTING LEGAL LITERACY

"Ugandan women have almost the same rights as men according to the law books, but in reality tradition rules", says Winnie Sekadde of FIDA, a legal aid organization for women in Uganda. "It means for example that they have no right to property and income."

The HIV/AIDS epidemic has presented FIDA with a growing number of cases regarding property and succession rights, although maintenance money is still the biggest issue. "Women get into trouble when their husbands die because of the gap between traditional customs and official laws. Women in rural areas are not aware of the written laws. Even if they are, the pressure to comply with tradition is enormous."

According to the traditional customs, when a woman marries, her father receives a bride price from her husband. She then belongs to her husband's clan. She must take care of his household and work his land; any earnings go to her husband. "Women are economically and socially completely dependent on their husbands," Sekadde says. "If a man dies, she loses everything to his clan, even the right to custody over her children."

According to written laws in Uganda, women have a right to their own income and a small inheritance. In practice, however, women almost never get this. The amount is divided if a man has more than one wife, which is common in Uganda. Other family members can also claim possessions. In case of doubt, judges may also fall back on customary law, often to the detriment of women. FIDA is therefore lobbying for a women-friendly law, with fewer opportunities for interpretation by judges.

Because not many women know about laws, FIDA educates them through village seminars, radio and television programmes and newspaper articles. FIDA has also formed a team to persuade villagers to write wills.

Cases relating to sexual abuse of children are increasing. Children are regarded as "safe partners" because generally they are notyet infected. Girls have been abused by grandfathers, uncles and teachers. To make pupils aware of these problems, FIDA performs education theatre at schools.[63]

Developing Gender-Sensitive Care and Support

A first step towards making care and support systems more sensitive to the specific needs of women and men is to re-evaluate policies and assess whether they are gender sensitive. Training programmes for care-providers and counsellors need adaptation so that, for example, they respect women's wishes and needs regarding pregnancy, breast-feeding, abortion and sterilization and deal with the potential negative consequences of testing women but not their partners for HIV.

Follow-up counselling and support for women and men living with HIV/AIDS requires expansion. Social and legal assistance must be available even when people cannot pay. Women's lack of money worsens their burden when they care for family members and yet lack care for themselves, especially if the husband dies first. Seropositive women especially need ways to generate an income despite suffering periodic bouts of illness: "When my husband died of AIDS, I found it difficult to make ends meet. I decided to grow tomatoes, but did not have enough money to start the project. When I had almost given up hope, I got into conversation with some women in my village who were in a similar situation as myself. One of them suggested we pool our resources to support one another. The plan worked out quite well. I am now able to take better care of myself and my family. Our group's plan also ended up being an inspiration to other women in the village" (Tanzania).[64]

LIGHTENING THE BURDEN OF CARE

Communities in sub-Saharan Africa recognize that as more households are affected by the epidemic, community life suffers unless affected women and children are supported in coping[65]*:*

In Rakai District, Uganda, men developed an income-generating project to help them support 26 children orphaned due to AIDS. They registered as an association and received training and a loan from the NGO World Vision for a bee-keeping project. In their first season, the association harvested nearly 25 litres of honey to raise funds needed to help them in their role of care-takers.

The University Teaching Hospital in Zambia used to test children suspected of being HIV-positive, then gave the test results only to mothers. Fathers who later learned their children were HIV-positive blamed the mothers and refused to be tested themselves. SWAA helped change this policy. Now, when children show clinical symptoms suggesting HIV infection, the parents are called in together for counselling and both parents and child are tested simultaneously. The test results are given to the parents together during additional counselling. This process has reduced blaming and tension between spouses.

Because much of the care and support for people affected by HIV/AIDS now falls on women's shoulders, a major task is to find ways of lessening women's extra workload. One way is to provide help with home-care nursing. In south Thailand, nurses are assisted by La Trobe University (Australia) in sharing skills with village women so that they can manage those sick with infectious diseases (including HIV/AIDS and STDs) more effectively and efficiently.[66]

Analysis of successful programmes is needed to determine what it is that motivates people (especially men) to volunteer their time, energy and resources to community- and home-based care and support.

In sights then need to be shared widely so that new initiatives can benefit from them and volunteer support can be maintained long term.

Living Positively with HIV/AIDS

Women and men around the world often feel isolated when they learn of their diagnosis. Women especially have difficulties in contacting peers in the same situation. Yet this provides great psychological benefits: "When the woman at the clinic said, 'Would you like to meet another woman with HIV?' and gave me her phone number, I couldn't wait to get home. . . As soon as I met her, it just changed my life. I realized I hadn't done anything wrong, I wasn't a criminal... We've formed a womens group . . . I can talk about problems that have happened. Not just to do with HIV... Just supporting each other, having good fun, having a laugh" (England).[67]

Associations of women living with HIV/AIDS are helping participants find ways to cope. They also give the epidemic a human—and female—face when their members speak out on how HIV/AIDS affects them In 1992, the International Community of Women Living with HIV/AIDS (ICW) was created at the International Conference on AIDS in Amsterdam. Since then, this coordinating body has provided women most directly affected by the epidemic with a voice at global and regional levels. Through a network of worldwide representatives, they provide policy input to UN agencies.

ICW has also inspired the formation of associations of seropositive women in many other countries. At the national and community levels, seropositive women are joining together to make the ideal of living positively with the virus a reality:

- The National Women and HIV Project in Canada created a coalition of Hlv-positive women by supporting regional networks and developing communication tools 168].
- The Argentine Network of Women Living with HIV/AIDS (ANW) gives women information about AIDS, helps access treatments and medications through state and private services and makes referrals to NGOs and governmental social services.[69]
- Many seropositive women who care for their households alone must also plan for their families' future, especially the children. Due to discrimination and frequent illness, their access to the labour market is also restricted. Women Touch in Sao Paulo, Brazil, helps provide them with work, an income and special protection.[70]

Such initiatives demonstrate that women and men living with HIV/AIDS are not the problem but part of the solution. To prove we truly care - not only in the sense of caring for but also caring about people living with HIV/AIDS—we must ensure that our response to the epidemic gives these women and also men a central role in policy and programme formulation, implementation and evaluation.

A PERSONAL TESTIMONY

"I became pregnant with my fourth child in 1988. My health deteriorated and I had persistent vaginal itching and abnormal pains. I complained during antenatal check-ups but didn't get proper treatment for my vaginal infection. They took my blood for an HIV-test without my consent.

After I delivered, they tested my child, too. Then the doctor just told me that they had taken our blood and the results for both of us were positive. When I broke the news to my husband, he left me that very same night, after calling me names and accusing me of being unfaithful and a prostitute. I later learned that he had already been tested and was HIV-positive but didn't have the courage to tell me.

I confided my HIV status to my sister, a nurse. Because of stigmatization and discrimination, she told me not to tell anyone else. I kept quiet but felt as if everybody knew that I was HIV-positive. I was so lonely, isolated and afraid of leaving my children without any information on AIDS. I spent most of my time crying and the loss of my child at five months made my condition worse. Fortunately, I didn't have to give up my job because it was my only source of support.

In 1992, I was invited to attend a conference organized by Dutch seropositive women. I accepted though I was afraid to talk about my status and had never been involved in AIDS activities. I went because I wanted to meet people who were also dying of AIDS. But I was wrong about that. The conference gave me self-confidence and courage to talk about my status to friends and family, including my children and co-workers.

Back home I began giving my personal testimony during workshops, seminars and on national radio. I introduced the idea of forming a support group for women whose husbands had died of AIDS because I saw many widows who were suffering from property-grabbing by the relatives of their deceased husbands. At first we met just to share our personal experiences, give each other moral and psychological support and break our isolation and fear.

Eventually, we established the National Association of People with HIV/AIDS in Malawi (NAPHAM) with the aim to promote health through self-care and support. We care for one another when one falls sick and are now trying to involve our families. Most of the women are poor housewives. NAPHAM therefore promotes self-reliance through income-generating

RESEARCHERS	YES	SOMEWHAT	NO
>Do you explore the implications of gender inequality in relation to HIV/AIDS and STDS?	☐	☐	☐
>Does your research focus on issues of special relevance to women and men:	☐	☐	☐
— Women controlling their risk	☐	☐	☐
— Women's scope for decision-making in different situations	☐	☐	☐
— Women's right to control fertility	☐	☐	☐
— Factors motivating men to share decision-making regarding fertility control	☐	☐	☐
— HIV transmission through breast-feeding	☐	☐	☐
— Female-controlled prevention methods	☐	☐	☐
— Factors motivating women and men to discuss mutual rsponsibility in relation to prevention	☐	☐	☐
— Factors facilitating women's and/or men's ability to undertake prevention			
— Women's and/or men's access to health services that address their specific concerns (including STD treatment)	☐	☐	☐
— Rape and violence	☐	☐	☐
— Sex work	☐	☐	☐
— Sexual practices facilitating HIV transmission	☐	☐	☐
— Female circumcision in relation to HIV/STDs	☐	☐	☐
— Female care roles and their impact on production and education	☐	☐	☐
— Factors motivating men to participate in domestic tasks and care	☐	☐	☐
— Inheritance rights	☐	☐	☐

Question			
>Do you explore which information channels are most appropriate for different age and gender groups?	☐	☐	☐
>Do you use these channels to communicate research findings and other information?	☐	☐	☐
>Have you researched barriers to women's participation in programme activities?	☐	☐	☐

POLICY-MAKERS, PROGRAMME DEVELOPERS AND IMPLEMENTERS

Question			
>Are all programme implementers able to address gender issues?	☐	☐	☐
>Are women's organizations involved in policy and programme development and decision-making processes?	☐	☐	☐
>Do women and men share programme goals?	☐	☐	☐
>Do your interventions combat violence against women and girls (active policy goals, educational programmes, legislation)?	☐	☐	☐
> Do your programmes consider differences in gender roles, access to resources and decision-making that affect women's and men's abilities to protect themselves?	☐	☐	☐
>Do your programmes consider differences in male and female life experiences ?	☐	☐	☐
>Do your programmes differentiate between male and female health needs throughout the life cycle?	☐	☐	☐
>Do your programmes call for gender-based sexual health education in school curricula?	☐	☐	☐
>Do your programmes encourage couples, parents and/or children to discuss sexual health?	☐	☐	☐
>Do your programmes address the need to motivate men to inform their wives if they are HIV-positive?	☐	☐	☐

	Yes	Somewhat	No
>Do your interventions aim to develop and strengthen men's concern and caring for their families?	☐	☐	☐
>Do your education and communication programmes encourage men to share domestic responsibilities and tasks?	☐	☐	☐
>Do your programmes encourage social welfare agencies, NGOs, employers, etc. to provide or make allowances for child and patient care?	☐	☐	☐
PROGRAMME ACTIVITIES			
>Do you organize activities at locations and times convenient to both women and men?	☐	☐	☐
>Do you provide child-care services during activities and meetings?	☐	☐	☐
>Do you create situations in which women and/or men can talk freely about their opinions, feelings and needs?	☐	☐	☐
>Do you try to ensure that men and women hear and respond to one another's concerns and needs in a constructive manner?	☐	☐	☐
PROMOTING SAFER SEX			
Do your programmes:			
>challenge double standards between men and women regarding a) teenage sexuality, b) casual sex, and c) sex outside marriage?	☐	☐	☐
>address difficulties in condom use from women's and men's perspectives?	☐	☐	☐
>teach both women and men how to use condoms?	☐	☐	☐

>promote easy access to condoms for women and men?	☐	☐	☐
>enhance women's and men's skills in negotiating safer sex?	☐	☐	☐
>enhance women's self-confidence?	☐	☐	☐
>address sexual abuse?	☐	☐	☐
>promote attitudes to relationships that meet women's and men's sexual needs?	☐	☐	☐
PROVIDING HEALTH AND CARE SERVICES			
Do your programmes:			
>ensure equal access by men and women, particularly for STD treatment?	☐	☐	☐
>make family planning services attractive and accessible to men?	☐	☐	☐
>encourage men to take on greater care roles in the family?	☐	☐	☐
>address inheritance laws and customs where these put women and children at a disadvantage?	☐	☐	☐
>address the different financial problems affecting women and men?	☐	☐	☐
>ensure that girls' care roles and lack of money do not exclude them from school?	☐	☐	☐
>include men as volunteers in providing community and home care services?	☐	☐	☐

activities. By making soap and raising chickens we are able to pay school fees for some of our members' children.

I know God is keeping me for a purpose which I yet have to fulfil. Today I am in the eighth year from the time I was diagnosed. I'm still living because I have a will to live and want to help those who are suffering as I did."

Winnie Chikafumbwa, Malawi

6. HOW GENDER SENSITIVE IS YOUR WORK?

The enormous cost and suffering caused by the HIV/AIDS epidemic is forcing serious re-evaluation of norms values and conditions related to genden. Such analysis may lead to fundamental improvements that can benefit misions of people—women, men and children—in societies around the world.

The following Checklist is designed to help policy implementers and programme planners assess the gender sensitivity of their HIV/AIDS and STD policies and programmes. First determine which areas pertain to your type of activities. Responses to the questions may then be answrere *"yes"*, *"somewhat"* and *"no"*.

References

1. Reid., E., Gender, knowledge and responsibility. In J. Mann et al., eds., *AIDs in the World*, Cambridge London: Harvard University Press, 1992, p. 657.
2. Heise, L. L. & C. Elias, Transforming AIDs prevention to meet women's needs a focus on developing countries. *Social Science and Medicine*, 1995, 40/7: 931-943.
3. Dabis, F. et al., Estimating the rate of mother to-child transmission of HIV Report of a workshop on methodological issues Ghent (Belgium), 17-20 February 1992 AIDS, 1993, 7:11391148.
4. De Cock, K. M. et al., The public health implications of AIDS research in Africa JAMA, 1994, 272:481.
5. Nyo Nyo, *National Programme for Training Urban and Rural Women on STD/HIV In Myanmar* WHO/GPA Meeting on Effective Approaches for the Prevention of HIV/AIDs in Women, Geneva, February 1995.
6. Reid, E., *Women's dreaming: women, sexuality and development.* Presentation at the Women's Studies Conference, Sydney, Australia, November 1994.
7. Thin, N., Women's status and rights. In: M. de Bruyn, ed., *Advancing women's statues women and men together? Critical reviews and a selected annotated bibliography.* Amsterdam:: KIT Press, 1995.
8. du Guerny, J. & E:. Sjoberg, Inter relationships between gender relations and the HIV/AIDS epidemic: some possible consideration for policies and programmes AIDS, 1993,7/8: 1027 - 1034.

9 Heise, L. L. et al., *Violence against women: the hidden health burden.* World Bank Discussion Paper No. 255. Washington, D.C.: IBRD/World Bank, 1994.

10 Muhindi, B., 'Immoral' female condom. World AIDs, July 1993, p. 3.

11 Marres, D., *AIDS and childbearing: an explorative study among Kenyan women* [Dutch] M.A Thesis. Maastricht: University of Limburg, 1992, p. 27.

12 Marres, p. 33.

13 Flummer, F. A. etal., *The effect of HIV infection on the clinical features and response to treatment of genital ulcer disease (GUD) due to chancroid.* Presentation at the VII International Conference on AIDS, Florence, June 1991

14 Karim, Q.A., personal communication, September 1994.

15 Nataraj, S., No way to treat a woman. *Populi,* November 1994, p. II.

16 PANOS quoted in *Sunday Mail* (Harare), 18 December 1994.

17 Personal communication, November 1994.

18 Karim, Q. A. et al., *Women and AIDS in Natal/KwaZulu, South Africa: determinants of the adoption of HIV protective behaviour.* Washington, D.C.:ICRW, 1994.

19 Soroptomists and SPC co-operate. *Pacific AIDs Alert Bulletin,* 1994, 9:8.

20 Lee, S., ed., *our voices, our lives: life stories of women living with HIV/AIDS in Zimbabwe* Harare: Body Positive, l 994, p 59.

21 Seruunkuma, R., Living with HIV/AIDs :a personal testimony. *AIDs Health Promotion Exchange,* 1994, 3:7

22 Ray, S., personal observation, l 995.

23 Armstrong, S., The last taboo. *World AIDs,* 1993, 29:6-9.

24 Jenkins, C., An epidemic with a future? *World AID,* 1993, 29: 2.

25 Surapaty, R.M. et al., *Knowledge about AIDs and husband-wife communication among married women in. Palembang, Indonesia* Presentation (PD 0132) at the X International Conference on AIDs,Yokohama, Japan, 1994.

26 Personal communication, November 1993.

27 Van den Berg, D. & M. Swenne, Eenzame strijd. *HIV Nieuws,* September-October 1993, pp.13-15.

28 Foppen, R., "Let's form a club of 'sexually-disabled' women". AIDS *Health Promotion Exchange,* 1994, 3: 12-13.

29 Niang, C.I., *Socio -cultural factors favouring HIV infection and the integration of traditional women's associations in AIDS prevention strategies in Kolda, Senegal* Washington, D.C: ICRW, 1994.

30 Apisuk, C. & N. Apisuk, eds., *Living with HIV.* Nontburi: NAAM-CHEWIT Project, 1994, p 6.

31 Berer, M.&S. Ray, *Women & AIDs, an international resource book.* London: Pandora 1993, p. 248.

32 Ngcongco, V.N., *Nursing, home care, and HIV.* X International Conference on AIDS, Yokohama, Japan,1994.

33 Apisuk & Apisuk, pp. 10-11.

34 Topouzis, D., *Uganda: the socio-economic impact of HIV/AIDS on rural families with an emphasis on youth.* TCP/UGA/2256 paper. Rome: FAO, I994, p. 20.

35 Personal communication, London, March, 1994.

36 Sharma, J., Fighting against. *World AIDs,* March, 1994, p.h..

37 Africa's largest population begins AIDS campaign. *Herald* (Zimbabwe), I3 December I99I .

38 Hashemi, S. *Credit programmes, women's empowerment and contraceptive use in rural Bangladesh.* WHO/GPA Meeting on Effective Approaches for the Prevention of HIV/AIDS in Women, Geneva, February I995.

39 Fitzpatrick, L., Reflections from a workshop on the media and AIDS prevention: participation makes a difference. *AIDs Health Promotion Exchange,* 1991, 1: 13-15.

40 Esu-Williams, E.,Country Watch: Nigeria *AIDs Health Promotion Exchange,* I992: 1: 13-14.

41 Shahabudin, S.H., HIV/AIDS awareness workshops for women. *Report of a Consultation on Women and HIV/AIDS,* Geneva: WHO/GPA, December I993.

42 Dibb, L., Country Watch: England.*AIDs Health Promotion Exchange,* I992, 3: 8-9.

43 Weiss, E. & M. Rehra, *Fostering collaboration between researchers and NGOS on women and AIDS,* Washington, D.C., I994.

44 Bianco, M., personal communication, 1995.

45 Bezmalinovic, B. et al., *Guatemala City Women: empowering a vulnerable group to prevent HIV transmission.* Washington, D.C.: ICRW, I994.

46 Bhende, A., *Evolving a model for AIDS prevention education among low-income adolescent girls in urban India.* Washington, D. C., ICRW, 1993.

47 Mazzola, E., Country Watch: Italy. *AIDS Health Promotion Exchange,* I992, 3: 7-8.

48 Surena, Y., *Women's Protection Project: condom social marketing for women in Haiti.* WHO/GPA Meeting on Effective Approaches for the Prevention of HIV/AIDs in Women, Geneva, February I995.

49 Dasgupta, P., personal communication, I995.

50 Urban, M.T., personal communication, I995.

5I Guttierez, A., *Man/Hombre/Homme: meeting male reproductive health care needs in Colombia.* WHO/GPA Meeting on Effective Approaches for the Prevention of HIV/AIDS in Women, Geneva, February I9

52 Kalckmann, S., personal communication, I995.

53 Awino, J., Country Watch: Uganda. *AIDs Health Promotion Exchange.* I992,3:6-7.

54 Blaauw., C., personal communication, I994.

55 Prochaska, R., personal communication, I995.

56 Wilson, D. et al., *Intergenerational communication within the family: implications for developing STD/HIV prevention strategies for adolescents in Zimbabwe.* Washington, D.C.: ICRW, I994.

57 Givaudan, M. et al., *Strengthening intergenerational communication*

within the family: an AIDS prevention strategy for adolescents. Washington, D. C.: ICRW, 1994.

58 Constantino-David, K., A model of gender training for men. In: A. Rao et al., eds., *Reflections and learnings: gender trainers workshop report.* Amsterdam: Royal Tropical Institute, pp. 58-61.

59. Raman, S., Positive reinforcement to promote safer sex among clients *AIDs Health Promotion Exchange,* 1992, I:6-9.

60. Venables, S & J. Tulloch, *Your little head thinking instead of your big head. The Hetero sexual Men's Project.* Australia: Family Planning NSW, 1993.

61. Trudy, personal communication, 1995.

62. Schuler, M. & S. Kadirgamar-Rajasingham, eds., *Legal literacy: a tool for women's empowerment.* New York: PACT Communications, 1992.

63. Ars, B., Alice erfde alleen de ziekte van haar overleden man. *Internationale Samen werking,* February 1995, pp. 2, 3.

64 Msuya,W. et al., *Life first A practical guide for people with HIV/AIDs and their families* Mwanza: AMREF/Kuleana, 1993, p.69.

65 *Action for Children affected by AIDS: Programme Profile and lesson learned* Geneva: WHO/UNICEF, 1994.

66 Parsons, C., personal communication, 1995.

67 Richardson, A. & D. Bolle, *Wise before their time.* London: Fount Paperbacks, HarperCollins Publishers Limited, 1992, pp.77-78.

68 *Canadian women and AIDS projects and committees inventory.* Edmonton: Canadian AIDS Society - National Women and HIV Project, 1995.

69 Perez, P., Country Watch :Argentina. *AIDs Health promotion Exchange.* 1994, 3: 11-12.

70 Eugenia, personal communication, 1995.